Clinical Research Methods
in
Speech-Language Pathology
and Audiology

Fourth Edition

Clinical Research Methods
in
Speech-Language Pathology
and Audiology

Fourth Edition

David L. Irwin, PhD, CCC-SLP, FASHA
Jeremy J. Donai, AuD, PhD, CCC-A

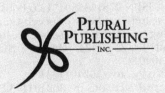

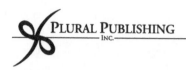

9177 Aero Drive, Suite B
San Diego, CA 92123

email: information@pluralpublishing.com
website: https://www.pluralpublishing.com

Typeset in 10.5/13 Garamond by Flanagan's Publishing Services, Inc.
Printed in the United States of America by Integrated Books International

For permission to use material from this text, contact us by
Telephone: (866) 758-7251
Fax: (888) 758-7255
email: permissions@pluralpublishing.com

*Every attempt has been made to contact the copyright holders for material originally
printed in another source. If any have been inadvertently overlooked, the publisher will
gladly make the necessary arrangements at the first opportunity.*

NOTICE TO THE READER
Care has been taken to confirm the accuracy of the indications, procedures, drug dosages, and
diagnosis and remediation protocols presented in this book and to ensure that they conform
to the practices of the general medical and health services communities. However, the authors,
editors, and publisher are not responsible for errors or omissions or for any consequences
from application of the information in this book and make no warranty, expressed or implied,
with respect to the currency, completeness, or accuracy of the contents of the publication.
The diagnostic and remediation protocols and the medications described do not necessarily
have specific approval by the Food and Drug administration for use in the disorders and/
or diseases and dosages for which they are recommended. Application of this information
in a particular situation remains the professional responsibility of the practitioner. Because
standards of practice and usage change, it is the responsibility of the practitioner to keep
abreast of revised recommendations, dosages and procedures.

Library of Congress Cataloging-in-Publication Data:
Names: Irwin, David (David L.), author. | Donai, Jeremy J. (Jeremy James),
   author.
Title: Clinical research methods in speech-language pathology and audiology
   / David L. Irwin, Jeremy J. Donai.
Description: Fourth edition. | San Diego, CA : Plural Publishing, Inc.,
   [2026] | Includes bibliographical references and index.
Identifiers: LCCN 2024011731 (print) | LCCN 2024011732 (ebook) | ISBN
   9781635507225 (paperback) | ISBN 9781635504712 (ebook)
Subjects: MESH: Biomedical Research--methods | Speech-Language
   Pathology--methods | Audiology--methods | Research Design
Classification: LCC RC423 (print) | LCC RC423 (ebook) | NLM WL 21 | DDC
   616.85/50072--dc23/eng/20240607
LC record available at https://lccn.loc.gov/2024011731
LC ebook record available at https://lccn.loc.gov/2024011732

Contents

List of Tables

**14 Critical Review of Quantitative and Qualitative
Research Articles**

List of Figures

About the Authors

David L. Irwin, PhD, CCC-SLP, FASHA.
Dr. Irwin received his BSE and MS degrees in speech-language pathology from the University of Central Missouri. He earned a PhD degree in communication disorders from the University of Oklahoma Health Sciences Center. He is currently professor of Communication Disorders at the School of Allied Health Professions, Louisiana State University Health at Shreveport, Louisiana. He is a Fellow of the American Speech-Language-Hearing Association and received Honors of the Association from the Louisiana Speech-Language-Hearing Association. His primary areas of research include individuals with autism spectrum disorder, augmentative and alternative communication, professional issues, and ethics. He has been the principal investigator (PI) for approximately $1.8 million in grants from federal, state, and private resources.

Jeremy J. Donai, AuD, PhD, CCC-A.
Dr. Donai is an associate professor and audiology program director at Texas Tech University Health Sciences Center (TTUHSC). Dr. Donai also serves as the director of the Auditory Perception Lab at TTUHSC. Over his career, Dr. Donai has had significant clinical, teaching, and research experience at multiple universities. His research involves the study of high-frequency speech energy. Dr. Donai has taught courses in amplification, psychoacoustics, research, audiology business practice, anatomy and physiology, and counseling. He is the coauthor of *Hearing Science Fundamentals, Second Edition* and *Audiology Review: Preparing for the Praxis and Comprehensive Examinations*, both published by Plural Publishing.

Contributors

Anne Marie Sisk, PhD, CCC-SLP
Speech-Language Pathologist
Monroe City Schools
Monroe, Louisiana
Chapter 4

Tobias A. Kroll, PhD, CCC-SLP
Associate Professor
Speech, Language, and Hearing Sciences
Texas Tech University Health Sciences Center
Lubbock, Texas
Chapter 14

Preface

This book is intended for speech-language pathology and audiology students as well as practicing professionals who wish to learn more about conducting clinical research and its application to the professions. In line with previous editions, more speech-language pathologists and audiologists are being asked to conduct research due to increased interest in evidence-based practice and demands for accountability.

Revisions to the Fourth Edition

As with the third edition, this text begins with a general orientation to research design and statistical analysis, followed by chapters with specific discussion of various types of research methods, and concludes with a chapter focusing on the acquisition of research grants. Furthermore, the utilization of discussion questions at the end of each chapter functions as a guide to focus learning and prompt further inquiry for the reader.

Major changes to the fourth edition include the following: (1) many references to and quotations from the American Speech-Language-Hearing Association (ASHA) and the American Academy of Audiology (AAA) Codes of Ethics (ASHA, 2023 and AAA, 2023); (2) an updated list of databases and sources for research in communication sciences and disorders (CSD); (3) examples to follow regarding integration of citations into a literature review; (4) an updated discussion of types of qualitative research currently being used; (5) additional and updated examples of qualitative research published in speech-language pathology and audiology; (6) a chapter with critical review of both quantitative and qualitative articles; (7) an expanded discussion of types of mixed method designs; (8) additional and updated examples of mixed method designs published in speech-language pathology and audiology; (9) an additional review of textbooks regarding evidence-based practice published in CSD; and (10) online companion materials including student study questions and questions for the instructor to use for examinations.

Preface

Acknowledgments

The authors of this book thank the publishers who granted a waiver or reduction in the fees to publish the materials in this book. The authors also want to acknowledge the wonderful mentoring and motivation for this book from Dr. Mary Pannbacker, CCC-SLP, ASHA Fellow. Dr. Pannbacker gave many people the inspiration to achieve above and beyond for the professions of speech-language pathology and audiology. Many of the chapters continue to include her work and ideas. The authors would also like to thank Dr. Norman Lass, ASHA Fellow, Dr. Mary Ellen Koay, CCC-SLP, and Dr. Jennifer Whited, CCC-SLP for their contributions to previous editions of this text.

David L. Irwin, PhD, CCC-SLP, FASHA
Jeremy J. Donai, AuD, PhD, CCC-A

1

Introduction to Research

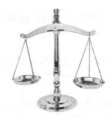

LEARNING OBJECTIVES

Upon completion of this chapter, the reader will be able to:

■ Discuss the importance of research to clinical practice

■ Describe the historical evolution of research in the professions

■ Explain the sources of knowledge used in the professions

■ Describe descriptive research including strengths and weaknesses

■ Discuss exploratory research including strengths and weaknesses

■ Describe experimental research including strengths and weaknesses

■ Discuss survey research including strengths and weaknesses

Introduction

The vitality and endurance of a profession are dependent on the quantity and quality of its ongoing research programs. The curricula of speech-language pathology and audiology programs traditionally have reserved the study of research methods and responsibilities for advanced graduate training. By that time, students may have developed an attitude of apprehension about research. Sometimes, these attitudes develop into sheer terror. Some academic advisors in programs having a thesis option rather than a requirement have difficulty persuading entering graduate students to consider pursuing a thesis project. Sometimes by the time the students become informed and confident about doing research, they are so far along in their graduate programs that doing a thesis would delay graduation.

The purpose of this text is to remove the mystery surrounding research by teaching basic principles and providing practice in gathering and summarizing data. It is hoped that this information will be conveyed to students early in their training in an effort to increase the number of research projects conducted by speech-language pathology and audiology students. Once students have developed research skills under the direction of productive faculty, they are more likely to continue the practice as they move into varied professional settings.

Importance of Research in Communication Disorders

There are a number of reasons for doing research in communication sciences and disorders. Short-term or survival objectives for doing research include doing projects to complete one's education or to improve one's job security in an academic setting where tenure and promotion depend on research productivity.

More important reasons for doing research include contributing to the professional pool of knowledge about treatment of clients presenting a variety of communication disorders and maintaining quality clinical services while realizing a sense of professionalism by active involvement in learning through discovery. For the person who enjoys receiving professional recognition along with the opportunity to be creative, satisfy curiosities, and engage in problem solving with a team of colleagues having similar interests, research provides numerous secondary rewards (Pannbacker & Middleton, 1991–1992).

A profession's image is readily enhanced by the integration of research along with the provision of clinical services. This has become more important with an increased emphasis on the use of evidence-based practice. Such practice increases professionalism, accountability to clients and other professionals, and the social relevance of the health services delivered in an economy with increased costs and decreased resources. Clinical research may readily integrate into the assessment, planning, intervention, and evaluation phases of clinical management (Portney & Watkins, 2009). Findley and DeLisa (1990) stress the importance of integrating clinical and research activities for the following reasons. The best clinicians and strongest researchers are providing clinical services and conducting research. Furthermore, staff training and awareness about new procedures and technology followed by improved client care are direct results. Both lead to the establishment of a rewarding, stimulating professional environment that contributes to improved staff recruitment and retention.

There is also an ethical reason for accepting the challenge of doing research. The speech-language pathologist or audiologist is frequently asked by clients or their relatives, "Does this treatment really work?" or "Is this hearing aid going to make a difference?" These questions are very difficult to answer ethically and truthfully without controlled research to substantiate an affirmative response. Ferketic (1993) stated, "We can't ignore the challenge to promote efficacy research. There are many questions to be answered. We all have something to offer and we need to work together to answer the questions. It's an opportunity to strengthen our professional credibility and viability" (p. 12). Collaboration between researchers and clinicians has been identified as a priority by the American Speech-Language-Hearing Foundation (ASHF; http://www.ashfounda tion.org) and the National Institute on Deafness and Other Communication Disorders (http://www.nidcd.nih.gov). Many members of the American Speech-Language-Hearing Association (ASHA, n.d.) now utilize the Practice Portal to have an evidence-based resource for assessing and treating a variety of communication disorders (http://find .asha.org/asha#q=Practice%20portal &sort=relevancy). Distinguishing two terms at this point is important. In research, efficacy is the benefit of an intervention plan as compared to a control or standard program. This type of research lets us examine theory and draw generalizations to large populations. Effectiveness in research is defined

as the benefits and use of the procedure under "real-world" conditions. Effectiveness involves the expectation that when researchers apply treatments, they do so without being able to control all circumstances (Portney & Watkins, 2000). Understanding the distinction and also the relationship between these two terms helps researchers ask answerable questions that meet the rigor of scientific methods and produce usable results.

Historical Evolution of Research in Communication Disorders

During the academic year of 1968 to 1969, Dr. Elaine Pagel Paden began to write a history of ASHA. In 1970, Paden authored a book that covered the years from 1925 to 1958. This is a summary of the early efforts by the membership to compile completed projects and continue research in speech disorders.

A small group interested in speech disorders met, beginning in 1919, at the annual meeting of the National Association of Teachers of Speech (NATS) and continued meeting until 1925. Lee Edward Travis reported a study in which he described the effects on phonatory pitch of stutterers and nonstutterers following the firing of a blank pistol at close range without warning. The teachers of public address (public speaking) in attendance were outraged at such inhumane treatment of subjects under investigation. Following this incident, it was decided that a separate organization for individuals interested in researching speech disorders should be established.

In December 1925, the American Academy of Speech Correction was organized by 11 individuals, 5 men and 6 women. Conducting research about speech disorders was one of the three minimal requirements for membership. From the very beginning, the group emphasized the importance of a working, productive organization. The projects initially assigned to the membership were all research in nature. They included establishing the classifications and terminology for the field, summarizing thesis projects in progress, developing bibliographies on topics in speech correction, and investigating topics including stuttering, foreign accent problems, and phonetic description of "careless speech." Realizing the need for a vehicle for publishing studies in speech correction, the group initially mimeographed 28 studies and made them available for $3 each. Having made money on the project, the group continued the practice. The *Journal of Speech Disorders* was established in 1935. The University of Illinois library has in its collection the early issues of this journal.

In the first issue of the new journal, published in 1936, three articles appeared covering the topics of foreign dialect, cleft palate, and stuttering. Also, a bibliography covering speech, voice, and hearing disorders was included. Gradually, the journal became less devoted to news items and increasingly dedicated to quality scholarly content. The camaraderie and friendships established among the young energetic contributors with similar professional interests remained. Eventually, the *Journal of Speech Disorders* was renamed the *Journal of Speech and Hearing Disorders*. The majority of articles that appeared in the journal for the first 20 years covered topics on stuttering followed by articles on general topics and therapy and "audiometry."

Also, between 1936 and 1949, the articles were more clinically oriented. In 1950, the journal's focus shifted to articles with a research orientation, until 1957 when the reverse trend began.

With the explosion of submitted research, the *Journal of Speech and Hearing Research* (JSHR) began publication in 1958. This journal adopted a research orientation, whereas the *Journal of Speech and Hearing Disorders* (JSHD) published research with clinical application. Because individuals working in school settings were interested in clinical applications and felt that neither journal served their needs, another ASHA journal, *Language, Speech, and Hearing Services in Schools* (LSHSS), began publication in 1970.

In an effort to increase the relevance of the ASHA journal program to all members, in 1990, the *Journal of Speech and Hearing Disorders* was divided into two separate publications, and its title was discontinued. Two new journals were initiated. The *American Journal of Audiology: A Journal of Clinical Practice* and the *American Journal of Speech-Language Pathology: A Journal of Clinical Practice* were first published in the fall of 1991. With these changes, both audiologists and speech-language pathologists have subject-specific periodicals in which to publish clinical and experimental research. Supporting research by the ASHA will continue to evolve as the needs of the professions change. In 2004, ASHA took action to develop the Advisory Committee on Evidence-Based Practice (ACEBP). This committee has been charged to address several issues relative to evidence-based practice (EBP) in communication disorders. According to Mullen (2005), ASHA has also established the National Center for Evidence-

Based Practice in Communication Disorders (N-CEP). Mullen (2005) stated that ASHA "members will be introduced to the basic principles of EBP and provided with the necessary support tools to assist them with integrating quality evidence into their practice" (p. 1). Duchan (2006) has developed a website that documents the history of speech-language pathology during the 19th and 20th centuries. The historical review contains numerous references and efforts of various fields on the evolution of research in speech-language pathology. These fields include phonetic studies, brain studies, technology, testing, and child study.

The American Academy of Audiology (AAA) was founded in January 1988 when a group of audiology leaders met. The purpose of the study group was to establish an independent freestanding national organization run by and for audiologists. The AAA published the first edition of the *Journal of the American Academy of Audiology* (JAAA) in 1990 (http://www.audiology.org).

Sources of Knowledge

Information used by clinicians and other types of researchers can come from a variety of sources. As consumers of research, we may accept some findings based on tradition, authority, trial and error, and logical reasoning (deductive and inductive). For a summary of these sources, one should consult Portney and Watkins (2009). Each of these sources of knowledge may be limited by a lack of empirical research principles, an unsystematic use of variables, lack of control for critical variables, or stifling of new knowledge and thought.

Research is conducted to answer questions, and it is an increasingly important component in speech-language pathology and audiology, because both basic and clinical questions remain unanswered. In an effort to determine cause-and-effect relationships, researchers conscientiously apply scientific methodology to carefully control variables. Kerlinger (1973) defined the scientific approach as a systematic, empirical, controlled, and critical examination of hypothetical propositions about the association among natural phenomena. Portney and Watkins (2000) assert that the element of control is "the most important characteristic that sets the scientific method apart from the other sources of knowledge" (p. 11). It is important for any researcher to attempt to control factors that are directly related to the variables in question.

Lieske (1986) described the systematic study of a problem or question as a cyclical process beginning with an unanswered question followed by a clear statement of the problem, development of appropriate hypotheses, data collection, and finally interpretation of the information gathered in an effort to accept or reject hypotheses.

Portney and Watkins (2009) caution researchers that the scientific method may have limitations when applied to human behavior. Because humans are unique and capacities vary widely, there will always be some uncertainty regarding the interpretation and generalization of data. It is almost impossible to control for all variables in clinical research. This does not mean that clinicians should allow for less control, but rather that they should recognize that other variables may be happening that could influence results.

Types of Research

Classification of research into specific categories is not easy because there are a number of different research strategies. There is also a lack of agreement about these categories as well as overlap among the various types of research so that specific research projects may fit more than one classification (Ventry & Schiavetti, 1986). Portney and Watkins (2009) view research on a continuum and describe the major categories: descriptive, exploratory, and experimental. Figure 1–1 shows how these types of research may be viewed along a continuum and that some share properties with all three categories (e.g., survey research), whereas others are specific to a particular category (e.g., randomized controlled trials).

Descriptive Research

Descriptive research is designed to systemically describe situations or events as they naturally occur; in other words, the status of phenomena of interest as they currently exist (Polit & Beck, 2010). It is a type of research in which the distributions of selected dependent variables are observed and recorded (Hegde, 2003). Descriptive research is used to study group differences, developmental trends, and relationships among variables (Schiavetti et al., 2011). Sometimes this type of research is called normative or developmental research (Hegde, 2003). Developmental research that focuses on changes over time may be cross-sectional, longitudinal, or semilongitudinal (Maxwell & Satake, 2006; Portney & Watkins, 2009; Schiavetti et al., 2011; Shearer, 1982). Not

all research is developmental in the maturational sense; it may be designed, for example, to study the course of progress for a pathology.

Cross-Sectional Research

Cross-sectional research involves selecting subjects from various age groups and observing differences between the behavior and characteristics of the group. This approach has several advantages: (a) it is less costly and less time consuming than longitudinal research and (b) it is relatively immune to subject attrition. The greatest disadvantage is the possibility that results could be attributable to biased selection of the cross-sectional groups. A variety of terms are used to describe cross-sectional research: disease, frequency, survey, and prevalence study (Rosenfeld, 1991).

Longitudinal Research

Many consider longitudinal research stronger than cross-sectional research because the same group of subjects is followed over time. This approach has the disadvantages of being expensive, time consuming, and vulnerable to subject attrition (subject drop out). Because of these problems, only a small number of subjects can be studied. Synonyms for longitudinal research include cohort study, follow-up study, incidence study, and perspective study (Rosenfeld, 1991).

Semilongitudinal Research

The semilongitudinal approach is a compromise designed to maximize the strengths and minimize the weaknesses of the cross-sectional and longitudinal approaches. This involves dividing the

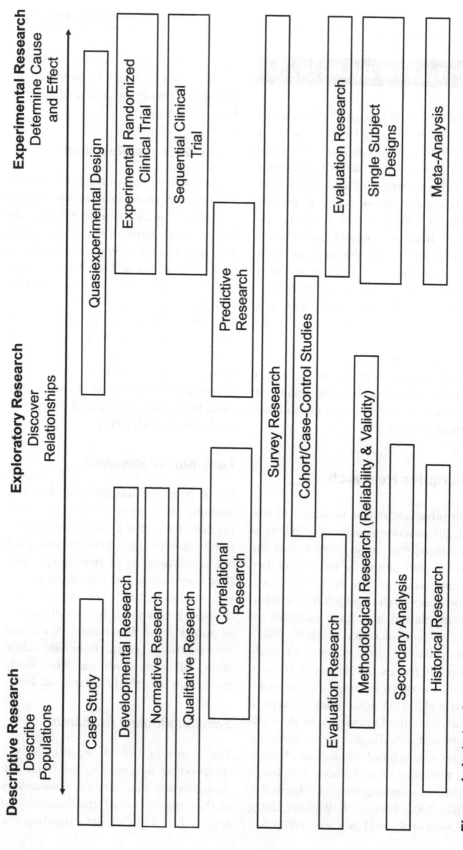

Figure 1–1. A visual representation of the continuum of research.

8

total age span to be studied into several overlapping age spans, selecting subjects whose ages are at the lower edge of each new age span, and following them until they reach the upper age of the span (Schiavetti et al., 2011; Shearer, 1982).

Historical Research

Historical research, sometimes referred to as archival or library research, is a type of research aimed at establishing facts and relationships about past events (Bordens & Abbott, 1988; Portney & Watkins, 2000). It may summarize a specific topic, sometimes in a type of review article entitled "State of the Art" or "Tutorial." Tutorial papers have been published about a variety of topics in communication disorders: facilitated communication (Duchan, 1993) as well as hearing loss, speech, and hearing aids (Van Tassell, 1993). Such papers are often written at the request of a journal editor who wants to present a summary from the viewpoint of a recognized scholar (Shearer, 1982). Shearer (1982) pointed out that "nearly every example of published research contains a miniature library study as part of the introductory section that refers to related research. More extensive reviews of the literature commonly comprise the second chapter of theses and dissertations" (p. 17).

The following characteristics of historical research were identified by Isaac and Michael (1987):

1. Historical research depends on data observed by others rather than the investigator.
2. Historical research must be rigorous, systematic, and exhaustive. Much "research" claiming to be historical is an undisciplined collection of inappropriate, unreliable, or biased information.
3. Historical research depends on two kinds of data: primary sources where the author was a direct observer of the recorded event, and secondary sources where the author reports the observation of others and is one or more times removed from the original event.
4. Two basic forms of criticism weight the value of the data: external criticism, which asks, "Is the document or relic authentic?" and internal criticism, which asks, "If authentic, are the data accurate and relevant?" This critical evaluation of the data is what makes true historical research so vigorous—in many ways more demanding than experimental methods (p. 45).

Case Study Research

Case study research is an intensive study of the background, current status, or environmental interactions of an individual, group, institution, or community (Isaac & Michael, 1987). Most case studies are descriptive studies that examine relationships among different variables or trends over time (Maxwell & Satake, 2006; Polit & Beck, 2010).

The primary strength of case study research is that it may be the only method available for studying some phenomena when few subjects are available or when financial restrictions preclude the use of other types of study (Schiavetti et al., 2002). In some instances, case studies should be considered pilot studies because they need to be combined with appropriate follow-up studies using larger numbers of subjects having the same phenomena and focusing on specific hypotheses (Isaac & Michael, 1987). Table 1–1 presents several case studies that have been done in communication disorders.

Case studies also have weaknesses. Because of their narrow focus on a few subjects, case studies are limited in their generalizability. Also, case studies are vulnerable to subjective bias. This may happen because the subjects were selected because of dramatic or atypical attributes.

Secondary Analysis

Secondary analysis involves research that uses previously gathered data (Polit & Beck, 2010). It may involve examining unanalyzed variables, testing unexplored relationships, focusing on a specific subsample, or changing the unit of analysis. Because secondary analysis uses existing data, it has the advantage of reducing time and cost. It has the disadvantage of little or no control over data collection

Table 1–1. Examples of Case Studies in Communication Disorders

Author(s)	Topic
Adams et al. (2015)	Integrating language, pragmatics, and social intervention for a child with developmental social communication disorder
Budhan et al. (2019)	Use of a novel gaming reinforcement system for oral intake and pediatric feeding therapy
Colemen (2017)	Comprehensive stuttering treatment in adolescents
Dupuis et al. (2018)	Care for older adults with hearing loss in a geriatric audiology clinic
Green & Steele (2019)	Improving morphological skills in a ninth grader with language and reading disabilities
Herbert et al. (2022)	Speech recognition outcomes after cochlear implantation
Jasso & Potratz (2020)	Assessing speech sound disorders in school-age children diverse language backgrounds
Kissel et al. (2023)	Vocal outcomes and voice-related quality of life after bilateral laryngeal reinnervation
Medina et al. (2023)	Mindfulness program for adults who stutter
Salley et al. (2019)	Expertise and collaboration to support students with brain injury
Tyler et al. (2015)	Tinnitus suppression with mixed background stimuli following cochlear implant
Vidal et al. (2020)	Communication profile of a minimally verbal school-age autistic child

(Hearst & Hulley, 1988). There is also the possibility that the data are inaccurate.

Evaluation Research

Evaluation research involves collection and analysis of information related to the effects of a program, policy, or procedure (Hegde, 2003; Polit & Beck, 2010). Four types of evaluation research have been described in the literature: process or implementation evaluation, outcome and impact evaluation, cost-benefit analysis, and comprehensive evaluation. This type of research can be used to ensure compliance with quality assurance policies and third-party payers such as Medicare and Medicaid.

Process or implementation evaluation is designed to answer questions about the function of a program or policy (Polit & Beck, 2010). Typically, this type of research involves intensive examination of a program and often involves collection of both qualitative and quantitative data gathered through interviews with clients and staff, observation of the program in operation, and analysis of records related to the program.

A process or implementation evaluation may focus on improving a new or ongoing program. Such an evaluation is sometimes referred to as a formative evaluation. In other instances, the evaluation may be designed primarily so that the program can be replicated by others (Polit & Hungler, 1999).

Outcome and impact evaluation is concerned with the effectiveness of a program. The purpose is to determine whether a program should be discontinued, replaced, modified, continued, or replicated. The evaluation may be referred to as a summative evaluation. An outcomes evaluation is fairly descriptive but does not utilize a vigorous experimental design (Polit & Beck, 2010). Such an evaluation documents the extent to which the goals of the program are achieved and the extent to which positive outcomes result.

Impact evaluation is designed to identify the impact(s) of an intervention, in other words, the impact(s) that can be attributed to the intervention rather than to other factors. Polit and Hungler (1999) believe that impact evaluation usually involves "an experimental or quasi-experimental design, because the aim of such evaluations is to attribute a casual influence to the specific intervention" (p. 200). Hegde (1994) agrees to an extent because he feels that "in some ways, an impact evaluation resembles experimental research. However, in practice, appropriate experimental methods are not used in impact evaluation" (p. 101).

Evaluations that determine whether the benefits of the program outweigh the cost are referred to as cost-benefit analyses. Such analyses are often done in conjunction with impact evaluations (Polit & Beck 2010).

Evaluation research combines process and outcome-impact evaluations, which were previously described. Hegde (2003) believes that comprehensive evaluation is the only truly useful type of evaluation research, because the usefulness of process or impact evaluation is limited. A comprehensive model of evaluation, which includes multiple types of evaluation, was described by Isaac and Michael (1987) and is presented in Figure 1–2. The greatest problem with evaluation research is that it can be threatening to individuals. Even though the focus of evaluation research is on a program, procedure, or policy, people develop and implement the entity. Some people think

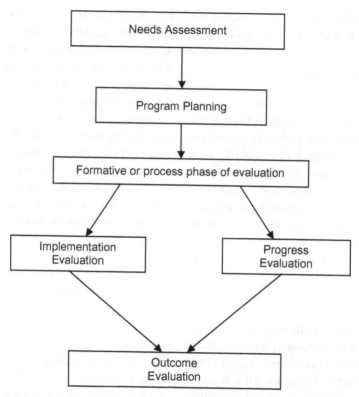

Figure 1–2. Comprehensive model of evaluation from needs assessment to outcome evaluation. From *Handbook in Research and Evaluation* (3rd ed., p. 11), by S. Isaac and W. B. Michael, 1995, San Diego, CA: Edits Publishing. Copyright 1995 Edits Publishers. Reproduced with permission.

they or their work are being evaluated. It can also be difficult to determine goals of the program (Polit & Beck, 2010). Often, the objectives of a program are multiple and diffuse.

Exploratory Research

An exploratory researcher examines how one event or events relate to other factors. Correlational research is used to determine possible relationships among factors (Portney & Watkins, 2009). Examples of correlational research include studying the role of home literacy practices

and children's language and emergent literacy skills (Roberts et al., 2005), frequency processing in listeners with hearing impairment (Healy et al., 2005); and frequency discrimination and literacy skills for children with mild to moderate sensorineural hearing loss (Halliday & Bishop, 2005).

Correlational Research

Portney and Watkins (2000) state that "predictive research studies are designed to predict a behavior or response based on the observed relationship between that behavior and other variables" (p.

278). For example, predictive studies can be used to study the scores achieved on standardized tests (e.g., Graduate Record Examination) and performance in a graduate program. Predictive research is being used more often in outcomes for making clinical decisions. For example, Daniels et al. (1997) studied whether risk factors detected in the clinical examination approximated the videofluoroscopic swallow study in the identification of dysphagia severity. They studied six clinical features: dysphonia, dysarthria, abnormal volitional cough, abnormal gag reflex, and cough after an oropharyngeal evaluation as well as a clinical swallowing examination.

Case-Control Studies

Case-control studies are done when individuals are selected, whether they have a particular disorder or not. Cases have the disorder or disease being studied, and controls are chosen because they do not have the disorder or disease (Portney & Watkins, 2009). The researcher may utilize a variety of techniques—including interviews, questionnaires, or chart review—to determine why an individual may or may not have a disorder/disease based on exposure factors. Tallal et al. (2001) conducted a case-control study in which the current language-related ability of all biological, primary relatives (mother, father, siblings) or probands with specific language impairment was studied and compared to matched controls.

Portney and Watkins (2000) suggest that "one advantage of case-control design is that samples are relatively easy to gather. Therefore, case-control studies are useful for studying disorders that are relatively rare, because they start by

finding cases in a systematic manner" (p. 325). Case-control studies are typically done for diseases or disorders that have a long latency period.

Cohort Studies

A cohort study is where the "researcher selects a group of subjects who do not yet have the outcome of interest and follows them to see if they develop the disorder" (Portney & Watkins, 2000, p. 328). Cohort studies allow the researcher to follow the temporal sequence of factors that may have impacted the development of a disorder. Grievink et al. (1993) examined the relationship between early otitis media with effusion (OME) and later language ability in a group of children systematically documented with bilateral OME. The children in this study received tympanometry every 3 months—between the ages of 2 and 4, and at age 7—three groups participated in language testing.

Cohort studies can be either prospective or retrospective. If a researcher determines that subjects have already been exposed to risk factors, then the study would be retrospective. If the researcher contacts the subjects before they develop the disorder but after exposure to risk factors, then it would be prospective (Portney & Watkins, 2000).

Experimental Research

In experimental research, the independent variable is controlled to measure its effect on the dependent variables (Shearer, 1982). In other words, experimental research is used to examine possible cause-and-effect relationships by exposing one or more experimental groups to one or more conditions and comparing the results to one or more control groups (Isaac & Michael, 1987). This type of research has also been referred to as the cause-and-effect method, the pretest-posttest control group design, and the laboratory method (Leedy, 1989). The distinguishing feature of experimental research is the experiment and control of the main variables; other types of research do not involve an experiment (Hegde, 2003; Shearer, 1982). Experimental research is considered by many to be the best or most powerful research design, but it is not the only acceptable type of research (Hegde, 2003; Ottenbacher, 1990; Portney & Watkins, 2009). Shearer (1982) points out that the most appropriate type "of research is the one that best fits the problem and the situations available" (p. 10).

The three characteristics of experimental research described by Polit and Hungler (1999) were the following: (1) "manipulation—the experimenter does something to at least some of the subjects in the study; (2) control—the experimenter introduces one or more control over the experimental situation, including the use of a control group; and (3) randomization—the experimenter assigns subjects to a control or experimental group on a random basis" (p. 152).

Isaac and Michael (1987) have outlined the steps in experimental research (Table 1–2). This outline is useful in understanding experimental research and knowing the procedures that a researcher might utilize.

Hegde (2003) stated, "The strengths of experimental research are the strengths of science itself" (p. 170). It is the most appropriate method for testing hypotheses of cause-and-effect relationships between variables. Experimental research offers greater corroboration than any other type of research in that if the independent variable is manipulated in a certain way, then certain consequences in the dependent variable may be expected to ensue.

Experimental research has several weaknesses. First, there are many situations in which experimental research cannot be conducted because of ethical or practical considerations (Polit & Beck, 2010; Portney & Watkins, 2009). Another problem with experimental research is the Hawthorne effect. This refers to the effect on the dependent variable caused by changes in subjects' behavior because they know they are participating in a study (Huck et al., 1974; Portney & Watkins, 2000). Despite problems inherent in research, Hegde (2003) believes none of the "weaknesses of experimental research seem to be valid" (p. 169).

Randomized Controlled Trial

The basic structure of an experiment involves the pretest-posttest design (Portney & Watkins, 2009). Some researchers (Portney & Watkins, 2009) regard the "gold standard" for clinical research to include the randomized controlled trial (RCT). This involves the experimental group receiving the variable of interest and the control group not receiving any form of treatment. The differences between the two groups, with all other factors being equal or constant, are due to the impact of the experimental variable. In RCT, the assignment of subjects to groups is randomized. An example for the use of RCT by speech-language pathologists includes Roy et al. (2003), who studied three treatments for teachers with voice disorders. Cohen et al. (2005) used RCT when studying 77 chil-

Table 1–2. Seven Steps in Experimental Research

1. Survey the literature relating to the problem.

2. Identify and define the problem.

3. Formulate a problem hypothesis, deducing the consequences and defining basic terms and variables.

4. Construct an experimental plan.

   a. Identify all nonexperimental variables that might contaminate the experiment, and determine how to control them.

   b. Select a research design.

   c. Select a sample of subjects to represent a given population, assign subjects to groups, and assign experimental treatment to groups.

   d. Select or construct and validate instruments to measure the outcome of the experiment.

   e. Outline procedures for collecting the data, and if possible conduct a pilot or "trial run" test to perfect the instruments or design.

   f. State the statistical or null hypothesis.

5. Conduct the experiments.

6. Reduce the raw data in a manner that will produce the best appraisal of the effect which is presumed to exist.

7. Apply an appropriate test of significance to determine the confidence one can place on the results of the study.

Source: From *Understanding Educational Research* (Rev. ed.), by D. B. Van Dalen and W. J. Meyer, 1966, New York, NY: McGraw-Hill. Copyright 1966 by McGraw-Hill. Reproduced with permission of The McGraw-Hill Companies.

dren between the ages 6 and 10 and the effects of computer-based intervention through acoustically modified speech (i.e., Fast ForWord; Scientific Learning Corporation, 1998). Portney and Watkins (2009) assert that this design is strong in internal validity, and selection bias can be controlled through random assignment of subjects.

Quasi-Experimental

Variations of "true" experimental research are considered quasi-experimental be-cause they have the same degree of experimental control or inferential confidence (Ottenbacher, 1990). This type of research is sometimes referred to as pseudoexperimental or preexperimental (Huck et al., 1974). Quasi-experimental research, like experimental research, involves manipulation of an independent variable but does not have a comparison group or randomization (Polit & Beck, 2010). The two characteristics of quasi-experimental research identified by Isaac and Michael (1987) are "(1) quasi-experi-mental typically involves applied setting where it is not possible to control all the relevant variables but only some of them; and (2) the distinction between true and quasi-experimental research is tenuous, particularly where human subjects are involved" (p. 54).

Sequential Clinical Trials

The use of sequential clinical trials (SCTs) addresses two concerns often seen with experimental designs. First, an SCT does not require a fixed sample size before the study can begin. Subjects can be added to the study as they become available or develop a disease. Second, a SCT allows for the analysis of data to occur when the subject has completed the trial. Other forms of experimental research require the collection of the data from the entire sample before data analysis begins (Portney & Watkins, 2009). The use of SCTs has application to the field of speech-language pathology and audiology because it allows for the comparison of a "new" treatment to an "old" treatment. This may address the ethical concerns of true experimental designs being used in clinical research.

Single-Subject Designs

Single-subject designs focus on the behavior of one or a few subjects. These designs are also referred to as applied behavioral analysis designs or behavioral analysis, idiographic designs, single-subject experimental designs, single-case designs, intrasubject replication designs, small N-approach, and within-subjects designs. It is misleading to consider any design that uses one or a few subjects as a single-subject design. Designs that use single subjects also can be classified as case studies or single-subject designs

(Warren, 1986). Single-subject designs are experimental designs that attempt to establish cause-and-effect relationships (Hegde, 2003).

Meta-Analysis

Meta-analysis is similar to secondary analysis because it also uses previously gathered data. In meta-analysis, statistical techniques are used to compare results across previous studies (Bordens & Abbott, 1988; Cooper, 1993). Meta-analysis by speech-language pathologists and audiologists has included various topics such as clinical outcomes in the treatment of aphasia (Robey, 1998), the efficacy of treatment for children with developmental speech and language delay/disorder (Law et al., 2004), and otitis media and language development (Casby, 2001).

Meta-analysis provides a method for integrating and synthesizing research studies and theory development. It involves (a) identification of relevant variables, (b) location of relevant research to review, and (c) conduction of the meta-analysis (i.e., comparing or combining results across studies; Bordens & Abbott, 1988). Cooper (1993) identified several problems in meta-analysis, including publication bias, missing information, reliability, independent effect sizes, correlated moderators, and interpreting of effect sizes (for details please refer to the original source provided).

Survey Research

Survey research can be used with descriptive, exploratory, and experimental research. Survey research, which is often called sample survey, is designed to provide a detailed inspection of the prevalence of conditions, practices, or attitudes in a given environment by asking people about them rather than observing them directly. Surveys can be classified by the method by which data are obtained: controlled observation, mail questionnaire, panel, personal interview questionnaires, and telephone interviews (Kerlinger, 1973). The most powerful type of survey data is collected through personal interview (Polit & Beck, 2010). This method has the advantage of encouraging subject cooperation, which results in good response rates and a better quality of data (Polit & Beck, 2010). Table 1–3 gives several other advantages. Personal interviews, however, have limitations: they are rather costly and considerable time is required to conduct the interviews. A variety of formats is used for questionnaires: fill in the blank, multiple choice, true/false, and selecting a number to indicate strength of agreement or disagreement with a specific term. There are a variety of methods that can be used to distribute surveys, including the internet (e.g., http://www.surveymonkey.com).

The most important component of any survey, regardless of how it is distributed, is the response rate. High response rates are important for at least three reasons: (a) they increase sample size and statistical power, (b) they tend to produce a more representative sample, and (c) they reduce wasted time and materials (Dodd et al., 1988). A response rate of 50% is considered adequate, a response rate of at least 60% is considered good, and a response rate of 70% or more is very good (Babbie, 1973). Shewan (1986) suggests pretesting questionnaires so that potential problems can be identified prior to disseminating them. Answers to the following questions are requested:

■ How long did it take you to complete the questionnaire?
■ Did you understand the instructions?
■ What, if anything, was unclear?

Table 1–3. Comparison of Personal Interviews and Questionnaires

Advantages of Personal Interviews	Advantages of Questionnaires
Clarity: Clarify questions; avoid problems of illiteracy.	Economy: Self-administration reduces staff time.
Complexity: Obtain more complex answers and observations about respondent's appearance and behavior.	Standardization: Written instruction reduces biases from difference in administration or from interactions with interviewer.
Completeness: Minimize omission and inappropriate responses.	Anonymity: Privacy encourages candid, honest answers to sensitive questions.
Control: Order sequence of questions.	

Sources: From "Planning the Measurements in a Questionnaire," by S. R. Cummings, W. Strull, M. C., Nevitt, and S. B. Hulley. In S. P. Hulley and S. R. Cummings (Eds.), *Designing Clinical Research*, 1988, p. 43, Baltimore, MD: Williams & Wilkins, with permission. Copyright 1988 Williams and Wilkins. Reprinted with permission.

- Did you ever feel forced to make a choice that did not fit your particular situation? If so, on which question(s), and why?
- Were the questions reasonable and appropriate? How, in your judgment, could the questions be improved?

A cover letter should accompany all questionnaires (electronic or paper) briefly explaining the purpose of the survey, conveying researcher's thanks and appreciation for the reply, that the survey has been approved by the appropriate committee or advisor, and offering to provide a summary of the results. Contact information for the researcher should be listed such as telephone number, email, and fax number. A self-addressed envelope should be enclosed for paper questionnaires (to help incentivize participation). There are several resources for conducting surveys (Dillman, 1978; Groves, 1989; Portney & Watkins, 2009). Surveys have been used to study a variety of topics in speech-language pathology and audiology. Garcia et al. (2005) surveyed the practice patterns of speech-language pathologists in their use of thickened liquids. Zipoli and Kennedy (2005) utilized a questionnaire to examine attitudes of 240 speech-language pathologists toward use of research and evidence-based practice. Hoffman et al. (2005) utilized the results from a Medicare Current Beneficiary Survey to determine how many respondents over 65 years of age were categorized by level of communication disability.

The use of surveys makes it possible to obtain a great deal of information from a large population (Kerlinger, 1973). Surveys are also economical because of the amount and quality of information they yield. Surveys, however, have a number of weaknesses. First, survey research tends to be relatively superficial; in other words, it does not usually penetrate much below the surface (Kerlinger, 1973; Portney & Watkins, 2000). Second, survey research does not permit cause-and-effect conclusions because of a lack of experimental manipulations (Hegde, 2003; Portney & Watkins, 2000). A third weakness is that surveys tend to be demanding of time and other resources and tend to focus on "soft" (i.e., opinions) dependent variables (Hegde, 2003).

Summary

This chapter has provided an introduction to the research process, a historical overview of how it evolved during the early years of the professions, a review of various sources of knowledge when making clinical decisions, and an overview of the scientific method and various types of research. It is important for all readers to understand that this chapter is not complete and exhaustive of all aspects related to research. In subsequent chapters, more information is discussed in greater detail. Although many research projects ask very important and viable questions, it is important to remember the following: The best research project is one that is done and properly disseminated. Subsequent chapters are designed to guide students through this process so that they can complete a research project that adheres to standards and answers important questions for the professions of speech-language pathology and audiology.

DISCUSSION QUESTIONS

1. What might be personal, professional, and ethical reasons to conduct research?
2. Differentiate between efficacy and effectiveness. What is used in speech-language pathology and audiology?
3. How did research evolve in the speech-language pathology and audiology professions?
4. What are some sources of knowledge? What might be some problems with these sources?
5. Describe the scientific method. Why is the issue of experimental control difficult for some studies in clinical practice?
6. What are three major types of research? How can these be viewed along a continuum?
7. What is developmental research?
8. Compare cross-sectional, longitudinal, and semilongitudinal research.
9. What are some problems with doing historical research? How might these problems be controlled or resolved?
10. Under what circumstances do researchers tend to use case studies?
11. What are some types of evaluation research? Why might this research be difficult to conduct?
12. Give some examples of exploratory research in speech-language pathology and audiology.
13. What has ASHA done to collect more data using EBP?
14. Compare case-control and cohort studies.
15. What is the distinguishing aspect of experimental research according to Portney and Watkins (2000)?
16. What is considered the "gold standard" for experimental research? Why?
17. Why might sequential clinical trials be valuable to a researcher involved in clinical practice for speech-language pathology or audiology?
18. What are some advantages and weaknesses of meta-analysis?
19. Surveys can be in various formats. Describe the pros and cons of each format.
20. What is considered an "adequate," "good," and "very good" response rate to a survey?
21. Describe why a questionnaire should be tested with some subjects prior to dissemination.
22. What are some weaknesses associated with surveys?

References

Adams, C., Gaile, J., Lockton, E., & Freed, J. (2015). Integrating language, pragmatics, and social intervention in a single-subject case study of a child with a developmental social communication disorder. *Language, Speech, and Hearing Services in the Schools, 46*(4), 294–311.

American Speech-Language-Hearing Association. (n.d.). *Practice portal.* http://find.asha.org/asha#q=Practice%20portal&sort=relevancy

Babbie, E. R. (1973). *Survey research methods.* Wadsworth.

Bordens, K. S., & Abbott, B. B. (1988). *Research designs and methods.* Mayfield.

Budhan, J., Scarborough, D., & Bailey-Van Kuren, M. (2018). The impact of a novel gaming reinforcement on oral intake outcomes in pediatric feeding therapy: A single case study. *American Journal of Speech-Language Pathology, 28*(2), 394–407.

Casby, M. W. (2001). Otitis media and language development: A meta-analysis. *American Journal of Speech-Language Pathology, 10*(1), 65–80.

Cohen, W., Hodson, A., O'Hare, A., Boyle, J., Durant, T., McCartney, E., . . . Naftalin, L. (2005). Effects of computer-based intervention throughout acoustically modified speech (Fast ForWord) in severe mixed receptive expressive language impairment: Outcomes from a randomized controlled trial. *Journal of Speech, Language, and Hearing Research, 48*(3), 715–729.

Coleman, C. E. (2017). Comprehensive stuttering treatment for adolescents: A case study.

Cooper, H. (1993). Children and hospitalization: Putting the new reviews in methodological context. *Developmental and Behavioral Pediatrics, 14*(1), 45–49.

Cummings, S. R., Strull, W., Nevitt, M. C., & Hulley, S. P. (1988). Conceiving the research question and developing the study plan. In S. P. Hulley & S. R. Cummings (Eds.), *Designing clinical research* (p. 43). Williams & Wilkins.

Daniels, S. K., McAdam, C. P., Brailey, K., & Foundas A. L. (1997). Clinical assessment of swallowing and prediction of dysphagia severity. *American Journal of Speech-Language Pathology, 6*(4), 17–24.

Dillman, D. (1978). *Mail and telephone surveys: The total design method.* John Wiley.

Dodd, D. K., Boswell, D. L., & Litwin, W. J. (1988). Survey response rate as a function of number of signatures, signatures ink color, and postscript on covering letter. *Psychological Reports, 63*(2), 538.

Duchan, J. F. (1993). Issues raised by facilitated communication for theorizing research on autism. *Journal of Speech and Hearing Research, 36*(6), 1108–1119.

Duchan, J. F. (2006). *Judith Duchan's short history of speech pathology.* http://www.acsu.buffalo.edu/~duchan/history.html

Dupuis, K., Reed, M., Bachmann, F., Lemke, U., & Pichora-Fuller, M. K. (2018). The circle of care for older adult with hearing loss and comorbidities: A case study of a geriatric audiology clinic. *Journal of Speech, Language and Hearing Research, 62*(4S), 1203–1220.

Ferketic, M. (1993). Professional practices perspective on efficacy. *ASHA, 35*(1), 12.

Findley, T. W., & DeLisa, J. A. (1990). Research in physical medicine and rehabilitation XI: Research training: Setting the stage for lifelong learning. *American Journal of Physical Medicine and Rehabilitation, 68*(5), 240–251.

Garcia, J. M., Chambers, E., IV, & Molander, M. (2005). Thickened liquids: Practice patterns of speech-language pathologists. *American Journal of Speech-Language Pathology, 14*(1), 4–13.

Green, L., & Steele, R. (2019). Improving the derivational morphological skills of a ninth grader with language and reading disabilities: A public-school case study. *Perspectives of the ASHA Special Interest Groups: SIG 1 Language Learning and Education, 4*(5), 759–770.

Grievink, E. H., Peters, S. A., van Bon, W. H., & Schilder, A. G. (1993). The effects of early bilateral otitis media with effusion on language ability: A prospective cohort study. *Journal of Speech and Hearing Research*, *36*(5), 1004–1012.

Groves, R. M. (1989). *Survey errors and survey costs*. John Wiley.

Halliday, L. F., & Bishop, D. V. M. (2005). Frequency discrimination and literacy skills in children with mild to moderate sensorineural hearing loss. *Journal of Speech, Language, and Hearing Research*, *48*(5), 1187–1203.

Healy, E. W., Kannabiran, A., & Bacon, S. P. (2005). An across-frequency processing deficit in listeners with hearing impairment is supported by acoustical correlation. *Journal of Speech, Language, and Hearing Research*, *48*(5), 1236–1242.

Hearst, N., & Hulley, S. B. (1988). Using secondary data. In S. B. Hulley & S. R. Cummings (Eds.), *Designing clinical research* (pp. 53–62). Williams & Wilkins.

Hegde, M. N. (1994). *Clinical research in communicative disorders*. Pro-Ed.

Hegde, M. N. (2003). *Clinical research in communicative disorders* (4th ed.). Pro-Ed.

Herbert, C. J., Pisoni, D. B., Kronenberger, W. G., & Nelson, R. F. (2022). Exceptional speech recognition outcomes after cochlear implantation: Lesson from two case studies. *American Journal of Audiology*, *31*(3), 552–566.

Hoffman, J. M., Yorkston, K. M., Shumway Cook, A., Ciol, M., Dudgeon, B. J., & Chan, X. (2005). Effect of a communication disability on satisfaction with health care: A survey of Medicare beneficiaries. *American Journal of Speech-Language Pathology*, *14*(3), 221–228.

Huck, S. W., Cormier, W. H., & Bounds, W. G. (1974). *Reading statistics and research*. HarperCollins.

Isaac, S., & Michael, W. B. (1987). *Handbook in research and evaluation*. Edits Publishers.

Jasso, J., & Potratz, J. R. (2020). Assessing speech sound disorders in school-age children from diverse backgrounds: A tutorial with three case studies. *Perspectives of the ASHA Special Interest Groups, SIG:14, Cultural and Linguistic Diversity*, *5*(3), 714–725.

Kerlinger, F. N. (1973). *Foundations of behavioral research*. Holt, Rinehart & Winston.

Kissel, I., Van Lierde, K., D'hasseler, A. A., Papeleu, T., Tomassen, P, Marie, J. P., and Meerschmann, I., (2023). Longitudinal vocal outcomes and voice-related quality of life after selective bilateral laryngeal reinnervation: A case study. *Journal of Speech-Language-Hearing Research*, *66*, 1, 1–15.

Law, J., Garrett, Z., & Nye, C. (2004). The efficacy of treatment for children with developmental speech and language delay/disorder: A meta-analysis. *Journal of Speech, Language, and Hearing Research*, *47*, 924–943.

Leedy, P. D. (1989). *Practical research*. Macmillan.

Lieske, A. M. (1986). *Clinical nursing, research: A guide to undertaking and using research in nursing practice*. Aspen.

Maxwell, D. L., & Satake, E. (2006). *Research and statistical methods in communication sciences and disorders*. Thomson-Delmar Learning.

Medina, A. M., Mead, J. S., Comas, K., Perez, G., Prieto, J., & Valencia, I. (2023). Outcomes of a remote mindfulness program for adults who stutter: Five case studies. *Perspectives of the ASHA Special Interest Groups, SIG 4: Fluency and Fluency Disorders*, 1–16.

Mullen, R. (2005). Evidence-based practice planning addresses member's needs, skills. *ASHA Leader*, 1–21.

Ottenbacher, K. J. (1990). Clinically relevant designs for rehabilitation research: The idiographic model. *American Journal of Physical Medicine and Rehabilitation*, *69*(12), 286–292.

Paden, E. (1970). *A history of the American Speech and Hearing Association 1925–1958*. American Speech-Language-Hearing Association.

Pannbacker, M. H., & Middleton, G. F. (1991–1992). Common myths about research. *Journal of the National Student Speech Language-Hearing Association, 19*, 128–137.

Polit, D. F., & Beck, C. T. (2010). *Essentials of nursing research.* Lippincott, Williams, and Wilkins.

Polit, D. F., & Hungler, B. P. (1999). *Nursing research: Principles and methods* (6th ed.). Lippincott.

Portney, L. G., & Watkins, M. P. (2000). *Foundations of clinical research: Applications to clinical practice* (2nd ed.). Prentice-Hall Health.

Portney, L. G., & Watkins, M. P. (2009). *Foundations of clinical research: Applications to clinical practice* (3rd ed.). Pearson.

Roberts, J., Jurgen, J., & Burchinal, M. (2005). The role of home literacy practices in preschool children's language and emergent literacy skills. *Journal of Speech, Language, and Hearing Research, 48*(2), 345–359.

Robey, R. (1998). A meta-analysis of clinical outcomes in the treatment of aphasia. *Journal of Speech, Language, and Hearing Research, 41*(1), 172–187.

Rosenfeld, R. (1991). Clinical research in otolaryngology journals. *Archives of Otolaryngology-Head and Neck Surgery, 117*, 164–170.

Roy, N., Weinrich, B., Gray, S. D., Tanner, K., Stemple, J. C., & Sapienza, C. (2003). Three treatments for teachers with voice disorders: A randomized clinical trial. *Journal of Speech, Language, and Hearing Research, 46*(3), 670–688.

Salley, J., Krusen, S., Lockovich, M., Wilson, B., Eagan-Johnson, B., & Tyler, J. (2019). Maximizing expertise and collaboration to support students with brain injury: A case study in speech-language pathology. *Perspective of the ASHA Special Interest Groups: SIG 2: Neurogenic Communication Disorders, 4*(6), 1267–1282.

Schiavetti, N., Metz, D. E., & Orlikoff, R. R. (2011). *Evaluating research in communicative disorders.* Allyn & Bacon.

Scientific Learning Corporation. (1998). *Fast ForWord—Language* [Computer software].

Shearer, W. S. (1982). *Research procedures in speech, language and hearing.* Williams & Wilkins.

Shewan, C. M. (1986, November). *The survey: An important data collection tool* [Miniseminar]. Annual meeting of the American Speech-Language-Hearing Association, Detroit, MI, United States.

Survey Monkey. (n.d.). http:// www.survey monkey.com/

Tallal, P., Hirsch, L. S., Realpe-Bonilla, T., Miller, S., Brzustowicz, L. M., Bartlett, C., & Flax, J. F. (2001). Familial aggregation in specific language impairment. *Journal of Speech, Language, and Hearing Research, 44*(5), 1172–1182.

Tyler, R. S., Keiner, A. J., Walker, K., Deshpande, A. K., Witt, S., Killian, M., . . . Gantz, B. (2015). A series of case studies of tinnitus suppression with mixed background stimuli in a cochlear implant. *American Journal of Audiology, 24*(3), 398–410.

Van Dalen, D. B., & Meyer, W. J. (1966). *Understanding educational research.* McGraw-Hill.

Van Tassell, D. J. (1993). Hearing loss, speech, and hearing aids. *Journal of Speech and Hearing Research, 36*(2), 228–244.

Ventry, I., & Schiavetti, N. (1986). *Evaluating research in speech pathology and audiology.* Macmillan.

Vidal, V., McAllister, A., & DeThorne, L. (2020). Communication profile of a minimally verbal school-age autistic child: *A case study. Language, Speech, and Hearing Services in Schools, 51*(3), 671–686.

Warren, R. L. (1986). Research design: Considerations for the clinician. In R. Chapey (Ed.), *Language intervention strategies in adult aphasia* (pp. 66–79). Williams & Wilkins.

Zipoli, R. P., & Kennedy, M. (2005). Evidence-based practice among speech-language pathologists: Attitudes, utilization, and barriers. *American Journal of Speech-Language Pathology, 14*(3), 208–220.

2

Ethics of Research in Speech-Language Pathology and Audiology

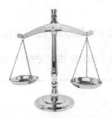

LEARNING OBJECTIVES

Upon completion of this chapter, the reader will be able to:

- Explain the need for ethical research
- Discuss the historical background of ethics in research
- Define responsible conduct of research and research misconduct
- Apply ethical principles to research
- Identify examples of research misconduct
- Compare the AAA and ASHA Codes of Ethics related to research
- Identify content and methods for teaching ethics
- Explain current and future issues related to research ethics

Research requires knowledge about scientific methods as well as the responsible conduct of research. The proliferation of research in speech-language pathology and audiology has increased interest in research ethics. Research requires careful consideration of ethical issues. The American Academy of Audiology (AAA) and American Speech-Language-Hearing Association (ASHA) provide information about the responsible conduct of research. Both the AAA (2023) and ASHA (2023) Codes of Ethics have guidelines, principles, and rules related to research in ethics. The Codes of Ethics for these organizations are found online at https://www.audiology.org/clinical-resources/code-of-ethics/ (AAA) and https://www.asha.org/siteassets/publications/code-of-ethics-2023.pdf (ASHA). It is recommended that students familiarize themselves with each of these documents. This chapter discusses the major ethical issues related to research.

Need for Ethical Guidelines

Research has not always been conducted ethically. Also, there has been inadequate training in the responsible conduct of research. Currently, ethical issues related to research have high visibility because of past ethical transgressions, such as lack of informed consent, unfavorable risk-benefit ratio, and use of vulnerable populations, such as children, students, and prisoners. Furthermore, ethical standards have changed over time. Previously, specific protection of human subjects did not exist, and ethical standards were laxer than today. Last, ethical considerations have not always been given adequate attention. In the follow-

ing section, the historical reasons for the development of ethical guidelines are considered.

Historical Background

There is a long history of research misconduct. Meline (2006) described ethical abuse as early as the first century BC. There has been considerable interest in research ethics since the Nazi medical experiments of the 1930s and 1940s. The Nazi research used prisoners of war and "racial enemies" in studies to test the limits of human endurance and human response to disease and untested drugs. The studies were unethical because "participants" were exposed to permanent physical harm, even death, and not given an opportunity to refuse participation (Polit & Beck, 2010).

There have been numerous reports about unethical research involving humans in the United States. This research has involved surgical experiments; exposure to pathogens, disease, radiation, chemicals, and drugs; and psychological experiments. A historical summary of this research is in Table 2–1. There is limited information about the long-term adverse effects of this research; there is limited information about unethical research in speech-language pathology and audiology except for the Tudor study in 1939. It was not until the 1970s that researchers in the United States considered informed consent and the risks and benefits of research (Horner & Minifie, 2011a). Limited attention has been given to the use of animals in research (Horner & Minifie, 2011a). Relevant issues included the emergence of humane treatment of animals, animal welfare versus

Table 2–1. Chronologic Listing of Unethical Research in the United States 1840–1972

Year(s)	Investigators/Site	Subjects
Surgical Experimentation:		
1840s	Dr. J. Marion Sims	Surgical experiments on enslaved African women without anesthesia; operated on one woman 30 times
1874	Dr. Robert Barthlow Good Samaritan Hospital	Treated Irish woman servant for cancer; cut open head and inserted needle electrodes into exposed brain
1896	Dr. Arthur Wentworth Boston Children's Hospital	Performed spinal taps on 29 children without parental consent
1913–1951	Dr. Leo Stanley San Quentin Prison	Experiments on 100s of prisoners; many involved testicular implants
Pathogens, Disease, and Biological Agents:		
1880s	California physician Hawaii Hospital for Lepers	Injected 12 young girls under 12 with syphilis
1895	Dr. Henry Heiman	Infected two mentally disables boys, 4 and 16, with gonorrhea
1900	U.S. Army doctor Philippines	Infected 5 prisoners with bubonic plague; induced beriberi in 29 prisoners
1906	Professor Richard Strong Harvard University	Infected 24 Filipino prisoners with cholera; all became sick and 13 died
1908	3 Researchers St. Vincent Hospital, Philadelphia	Infected dozens of children with TB causing permanent blindness or painful lesions and inflammation of eyes
1909	C. Knowles	Infected 2 children at orphanage
1911	Dr. Hideyo Noguchi Rockerfeller Institute for Medical Research	Injected 146 patients, some children, with syphilis
1932–1972	U.S. Public Health Service Tuskegee, AL	400 impoverished black males with untreated syphilis

Table 2–1. *continued*

Year(s)	Investigators/Site	Subjects
1941	Dr. Francis and Jonas Salk University of Michigan	Infected patients at several hospitals with influenza virus
1941	Dr. William C. Black	Inoculated 12-month-old with herpes
1943–1970	Statesville Penitentiary Joilet, IL University of Chicago Medical School U.S. Army and State Department	Effects of malaria on 441 prisoners
1944–1946	Dr. Alf Alving University of Chicago Medical School	Infected psychiatric patients with malaria
1946	Guatemala U.S. Public Health Service National Institute of Health Pan American Health Sanitary Bureau	Used prostitutes to infect prisoners, psychiatric patients, and Guatemalans with syphilis and other sexually transmitted diseases
1950	U.S. Navy	Sprayed large quantities of bacteria over San Francisco, CA; numerous pneumonia-like illnesses; killed at least one.
1950	Dr. Joey Stokes University of Pennsylvania	Infected 200 female prisoners with viral hepatitis
1952–1972	Willowbrook State School Staten Island, NY	Mentally disabled children infected with viral hepatitis
1952	Chester M. Southam Sloan-Kettering Institute	Injected live cancer cells into prisoners at the Ohio State Prison, half were black, other half were not
1955	CIA	Released whooping cough bacteria from boats outside Tampa Bay, FL, caused epidemic: killed at least 12
1956–1957	U.S. Army	Released millions of infected mosquitoes on Savannah, GA, and Avon Park, FL; hundreds affected

continues

Table 2–1. *continued*

Year(s)	Investigators/Site	Subjects
1962	Chester M. Southam Jewish Chronic Disease Hospital Brooklyn, NY	22 elderly patients injected with live cancer cells
1966	U.S. Army	Released *Bacillus globigis* into subways of New York and Chicago

Source: From *Children As Research Subjects*, by M. A. Grodin and L. H. Glantz, 1994, New York, NY: Oxford University Press; *Acres of Skin*, by A. M. Hornblum, 1998, New York, NY: Routledge Press; *Sentenced to Science*, by A. M. Hornblum, 2007, University Park, PA: Pennsylvania State University; *Lesser Harms*, by S. A. Halpern, 2004, Chicago, IL: University of Chicago Press; *Medical Apartheid*, by H. A. Washington, 2006, New York, NY: Random House; *Unethical Human Experiments in the United States,* by Wikipedia (n.d.), Retrieved from http://en.wikipedia.org/wiki

animal rights, and evolving regulations and guidelines for animal research. It is noteworthy that the ASHA Code of Ethics did not include the protection of animals until 2003.

There has been little discussion of ethical misconduct in speech-language pathology and audiology except for the Tudor study, which was conducted in 1939 at the University of Iowa. Twenty-two normally fluent children were taught to stutter (Annett, 2001; Dyer, 2001; Yairi & Amrose, 2001). These children were orphans at the Soldiers and Sailors Orphan's Home in Davenport, Iowa. The study was a master's thesis conducted by Mary Tudor, a graduate student, and directed by Wendell Johnson. Ambrose and Yairi (2002) reviewed the Tudor study and concluded that there were "fundamental flaws in its design and execution" (p. 201). They also indicated that their assessment of related ethical issues "should be viewed within the common standards of the period that there is no evidence of intent to harm, and that the

objective in increasing disfluent speech should not be confused with instilling chronic stuttering in normally fluent children" (p. 201). Obviously, such a study would not be permitted under current ethical standards. Ambrose and Yairi (2002) believe that "in spite of the controversy regarding the Tudor thesis, there is no question that Johnson's contribution to the study of stuttering remains very significant in many positive ways" (p. 201). Conversely, Silverman (1988a) reviewed the study and stated: "The implications of the findings seem clear—asking a child to monitor his speech fluency and attempt to be more fluent can lead to increased disfluency and possibly stuttering" (p. 231). Goldfarb (2006) edited a comprehensive review of the Tudor study and current ethical issues in clinical research. Authors of the Tudor study ethics compare favorably not only to the standards of its own time in 1939 but to current standards as well.

It is also important to know about the history of the responsible conduct of research. Horner and Minifie (2011a) provided a detailed chronology of the major documents relevant to the responsible conduct of research pertaining to human and animal experimentation.

Research Misconduct

Research misconduct is rare in speech-language pathology and audiology, although it has increased over the past several years. Horner and Minifie (2011c) noted that "the actual prevalence of misconduct is unknown." Data from the Office of Research Integrity (2018–2023) indicates an increase in research misconduct among public health service researchers. An increase in research misconduct may be related to a number of factors, such as greater attention to responsible conduct of research, awareness and knowledge of research misconduct, and the publish or perish culture. It is possible that junior employees may bear the burden of sanctions for scientific misconduct.

Research misconduct in any form not only threatens to undermine the progress and public support for science, but it also has the potential to cause harm to those who receive the erroneous treatment. Those involved in research must specifically address these issues (Society for Clinical Trials, 2004).

Research misconduct involves fabrication, falsification, or plagiarism in proposing, performing, reviewing, or reporting research. It does not include honest error or differences of opinion. Fabrication is making up data or results and recording or reporting data for experiments that were never conducted. Falsification of data is probably rare (Knapp & Van de Creek, 2006). It involves manipulating research materials, equipment, or processes or altering data or results, such that the research is not accurately represented in the research record. The research record includes, but is not limited to, research proposals, laboratory records, progress reports, abstracts, theses, dissertations, oral presentations, and journals. Plagiarism is the use of another person's ideas, procedures, results, or words without giving appropriate credit. It has been further defined as stealing someone else's work and using it for personal gain. Plagiarism can relate to the theft of ideas as well as text (Association of American Medical Colleges, 1994). In recent years, plagiarism has become more problematic because of the proliferation of documents available on the internet (Knapp & Van de Creek, 2006). Furthermore, some sources offer to sell papers on specific topics or prepare them for a fee. Artificial intelligence software (such as ChatGPT or Google's version known as Bard) also increases the risk of plagiarism.

Self-plagiarism is duplicate submission or publication. Duplicate/previous submission means that the manuscript is simultaneously being considered for publication elsewhere. It is essentially publication of the same content by the same author(s) (Bennett & Taylor, 2003; JAMA, 2006).

Research misconduct is a significant failure to adhere to prevailing, professional standards and is considered a violation of the AAA (2023) and ASHA (2023) Codes of Ethics. The seriousness of research misconduct ranges from obvious to subtle. Several forms of research misconduct have been identified (American Speech-Language-Hearing Association [ASHA], 2008; Bailar, 1995; Sales &

Lavin, 2000). Examples of research misconduct are listed in Table 2–2.

Reporting research misconduct is the responsibility of every speech-language pathologist and audiologist. This is the responsibility of both practicing professionals and students. However, students may be in an especially awkward situation for fulfilling this responsibility. Practicing professionals and students should be aware of AAA (2023) and ASHA guidelines for reporting allegations of research misconduct as well as institutional policies.

Ethical issues and problems related to research were identified and discussed by Hoit (2005). These three issues were self-plagiarism, conflict of interest, and authorship. For each ethical dilemma, a resolution was provided, including issues of the Ethical Principle and Rule. Ethical misconduct in audiology and speech-language pathology has increased. This can be verified by reviewing the *ASHA Leader*, which published sanctions for ethical misconduct of its members. Reynolds (2004) reported that "junior employees may bear the burden of sanction for

Table 2–2. Examples of Research Misconduct

Arbitrary or biased selection of data	Inadequate supervision
Bias in manuscript	Incompetent supervision
Censorship	Lazy writing
Coercion	Misrepresentation
Conflict of interest	Multiple authors
Cyber-cheating	Multiple relationships
Data recycling	Negligent data collection or analysis
Deception	Not fully informing IRB of participant
Duplicate publication	Not maintaining complete records
Dual relationships	Not protecting participants' confidentially
Exploitive supervision	Public bias
Failure to comply with guidelines for handling research misconduct	Role conflicts
	Software piracy
False representation of manuscript	Supervision abandonment
Forging of academic documents	Tardy reviews
Fragmented publication	Unauthorized use of confidential information
Ghost authorship	
Honorary authorship	Undisclosed repetition of study
Improprieties of authorship	Violating research protocol
Inadequate maintenance of records	Wrongful manipulation of data or results

scientific misconduct" (p. 509). The most frequent sanction was the requirement for a plan of supervision. Furthermore, research misconduct frequently involved all members of the research team and not solely those at the doctoral level.

Research misconduct in any form threatens not only to undermine scientific progress and public support for science but also to cause harm to those who use the possible erroneous outcome(s) of this research. Those involved in research must specifically address this issue (Society for Clinical Trials, 2004).

Three types of legal perspectives have influenced selection of sanctions for research misconduct: (a) quasicontractual legal remedy of restitution; (b) philosophy of "just desserts" or retribution based on an intuitive idea that the individual who engages in criminal conduct deserves punishment; and (3) deterrence of misconduct (Dresser, 1993).

Consequences for research misconduct include article retraction, private lawsuits, adverse personal actions, and administrative, civil, and criminal sanctions. The names of individuals guilty of research misconduct are listed in a federal database and published in federal print materials (Horner & Minifie, 2011c).

Issues in Research Ethics

ASHA's 2023 Code of Ethics includes standards for reporting and publishing information. These standards contain sections pertaining to authorship, adherence to basic ethical considerations for protection of human or animals in research, permission about copyrighted materials, dual commitment, and conflicts of interest. The most critical research issues identified by participants in a meeting sponsored by ASHA were authorship, peer review, and handling allegations of research misconduct (Moss, 2006). Other issues include confidentiality, use of controlled groups, institutional review, and documentation. Research requires careful consideration of ethical issues. Recognition and discussion of these issues can reduce the risk of unethical misconduct.

Planning Research

Speech-language pathologists and audiologists design, conduct, and report research in accordance with recognized standards for ethical conduct of research. Research is planned to minimize the possibility that results will be misleading. Planning ethically responsible research involves the application of basic ethical principles (beneficence, respect, and justice) to research activities, which are described in Table 2–3 (Sieber, 1992). In planning research, speech-language pathologists and audiologists consider the AAA (2023) and ASHA Code of Ethics (2023). If an ethical issue is unclear, speech-language pathologists and audiologists seek to resolve the issue through consultation with institutional review boards, the AAA and ASHA Boards of Ethics, or other resources, such as the Publication of the American Psychological Association Manual (APA, 2020). Speech-language pathologists and audiologists take reasonable steps for ethical treatment of all those associated with the research: human and animal subjects, collaborators, assistants, students, and employees.

Ethical issues that may arise during a study should be considered early; that is, these issues should be considered before writing the research proposal (Creswell,

Table 2–3. Scientific Methods Based on Ethical Principles

Valid research design	Only valid research yields correct results: takes account of relevant theory, methods, prior findings (B, R)
Competence of researchers	Investigates capable carrying out procedures validity (B, R)
Identification of consequences	Assessment of risks and benefits; respected privacy, ensure confidentiality, maximize benefit, minimize risk (B, R, J)
Selection of subjects	Subjects must be appropriate to purpose of study, representative of population to benefit from research, appropriate number (B, R, J)
Voluntary informed consent	Obtained in advance
Compensations for injury	Researcher responsible for what happened to subjects. Federal law requires subjects be informed if harm compensated but does not require compensation (B, R, J)

B = beneficence; R = respect; J = justice.

Source: From *Planning Ethically Responsible Research: A Guide for Students and Internal Review Boards*, by J. E. Sieber, 1992, Thousand Oaks, CA: Sage. Copyright 1992 by Sage Publications, Inc. Reprinted by permission of Sage Publications, Inc.

2003). These issues relate to all phases of research and include research sites and potential readers.

Confidentiality

Speech-language pathologists and audiologists have the ethical responsibility to maintain confidentiality in research activities including mentoring, reviewing manuscripts or research grants, consulting, or participating in research (Knapp & Van de Creek, 2006; Lansing, 2002; Lansing & Moss, 2003). Upholding participants' rights to confidentiality and anonymity is a central tenet of research. Speech-language pathologists and audiologists should also be aware of situa-

tions where they have access to confidential ideas, such as hearing ideas during an informal conversation. Maintaining confidentiality in peer review is an ethical responsibility because a manuscript is a privileged communication and represents confidential information (Macrina, 1995c). Reviewers of manuscripts have the ethical responsibility to maintain confidentiality. Speech-language pathologists increasingly are using the internet for online experimentation, chat rooms, and email for collecting research data. This raises new issues of confidentiality and informed consent that will probably require further consideration of existing codes of ethics (Meline, 2006).

Confidentiality is included in the ASHA (2023) Code of Ethics and is mentioned in Principle of Ethics 1, Rule P, which states,

> Individuals shall protect the confidentiality of any professional or personal information about persons served professionally or participants involved in research and scholarly activities and may disclose confidential information only when doing so is necessary to protect the welfare of the person or the community, is legally authorized, or is otherwise required by law. (p. 5)

The AAA (2023) Code of Ethics also addresses confidentiality in Principle 3, "Members shall maintain the confidentiality of the information and records of those receiving services or involved in research" (p. 1).

The Health Insurance Portability and Accountability Act

The Health Insurance Portability and Accountability Act (HIPAA) has had an impact on research practices (Horner & Wheeler, 2005). Research involving the use of protected health information must adhere to both HIPAA's privacy rule and the U.S. Department of Health and Human Services' Common Rule. Information about both of these documents can be found in the U.S. Code of Federal Regulations.

HIPAA protects health coverage for workers and their families and provides standards for transmission of health care records and identification of providers, health care plans, and employers. It also addresses security and privacy (confidentiality of health care data). Although the Act was passed in 1996, the regulations (standards) were not implemented until 1999 (Cornett, 2007). Many aspects of HIPAA are relevant to research. The standards related to research are privacy, security, de-identification, and enforcement.

The Privacy Rule is intended to prevent using or disclosing individually identified health information without consent (Horner & Wheeler, 2005). Ness (2007) believes the intent of the Privacy Rule is "to strike a balance between protecting the privacy of individual's identifiable health information and prescribing the legitimate use and disclosure of this information" (p. 2164).

The Privacy Rule addresses the use and disclosure of all protected health information, including paper and electronic, that is related to the individual's past, present, and future health conditions; treatment for these conditions; and financial history related to health care. A covered entity is a health plan, a health care clearinghouse, or a health care provider that transmits any health care information electronically in connection with a covered transmission (Horner & Wheeler, 2005). HIPAA compliance is required for all covered entities (Romanow, 2011).

Researchers are required to disclose certain information to all research participants. This information includes the following:

- Description of protected health information to be used or disclosed, identifying information in a meaningful, specific way
- Names or other detailed identification of the person(s) authorized to make the requested use of disclosure
- Names or other detailed identification of the person(s) to whom the

covered entity can make a requested use or disclosure
■ Description of every purpose of the requested use or disclosure
■ Authorization expiration date
■ Signature of participants and date (Horner & Wheeler, 2005)

The Security Rule applies only to the protection of electronic health care information. It requires covered entities to meet three standards. The standards for compliance are administration, physical, and technical. Administrative standards are related to policies and procedures designed to describe how the entity complies with HIPAA. Physical refers to controlling physical access to content against inappropriate access to protected health information. Technical standards involve controlling access to computer systems and enabling covered entities to protect communication containing pro-

tected health information transmitted electronically over open networks from being intercepted by anyone other than the intended receiver.

De-identification of health information refers to individually identified information in which all individually identified information is removed. As an alternative to removing all individual identifiers, a researcher may use statistical methods to reduce the possibility that information will identify research participants (Horner & Wheeler, 2005).

The Enforcement Rule became effective in 2006. This rule established penalties for HIPAA violations related to civil violations and compliance. These violations and penalties are shown in Table 2–4.

There are possible changes in HIPAA related to privacy, business associates, and enforcement (Romanow, 2011). The privacy changes are related to the cov-

Table 2–4. HIPAA Violation and Penalties

Violation	Minimum Penalty	Maximum Penalty
Individual unknowingly violated HIPAA	$100 per violation $25,000 annual maximum	$50,000 per violation $1.5 million annual maximum
Reasonable cause, not due to willful neglect	$1,000 per violation Annual maximum $100,000 for repeated violations	$50,000 per violation annual maximum $1.5 million
Willful neglect but violation corrected within required time period	$10,000 per violation $250,000 annual maximum	$50,000 per violation $1.5 annual maximum
Willful neglect not corrected	$50,000 per violation $1.5 million annual maximum	$50,000 per violation $11.5 million annual maximum

Source: From *HIPAA Violations and Enforcement* by American Medical Association. Retrieved from http://www.ama-assn.org/ama/pub/physician-resources/sulutions-managing-our-practice/

ered entity making a reasonable effort to resolve payment issue(s) prior to sending protected health information to the health plan. Business associates would be required to enter into a contract or their agreements with a subcontractor(s) to protect the security of electronic protected health information. The proposed enforcement change addresses civil penalties, complaints, and compliance review. The civil monetary penalty will make a covered entity liable for acts of business associates, which may require covered entities to conduct due diligence. Penalty(s) will also consider previous indications of violations, not just previous violation(s). The secretary of health and human services will attempt to resolve complaints, when possible, but (Romanow, 2011) may directly proceed to formal enforcement without attempting informal resolution.

HIPAA has had considerable impact on research. Several obstacles have been identified in the peer-reviewed literature (Dunlop et al., 2007; Horner & Wheeler, 2005; Ness, 2007; Nosowsky & Giordano, 2006; O'Herrin et al., 2004; WipkeTevis & Pickett, 2008; Wolf & Benett, 2006). These obstacles to research include, but are not limited to, time, delay, cost, subject recruitment and retention, less user friendly, informed consent, and restricted use of databases. Some of the obstacles can be reduced by better education about HIPAA; researchers are working more closely with health care providers and considering the role of researchers in health care (Gunn et al., 2004; Nosowsky & Giordano, 2006). Furthermore, Gunn and associates (2004) provided suggestions for reducing the negative impact of HIPAA on research. These suggestions include using de-identified health information or a limited dataset; requiring the covered entity to develop authorization forms for requesting protected health information; if authorization is impractical, seeking an institutional review board/privacy board waiver; and/or being familiar with burdens the privacy rule imposes on covered entities.

Concern about HIPAA's impact on research is not universal; some believe that HIPAA has not gone far enough to protect privacy and security, especially ensuring patients' rights to control their health information both for research and health care (Nosowsky & Giordano, 2006). Three factors related to HIPAA privacy standards will affect speech-language pathology and audiology research: accessing data from a covered entity; creating data; and disclosing data with a colleague from a different institution (Olsen, 2003).

HIPAA does not define electronic form but does define electronic media relative to storage and transmission. Storage means devices in computers (hard drives) and any removable transportable digital memory medium (magnetic tape or disk, optical disk, digital memory card). Transmission media is used to modify information already in electronic storage and includes the internet, extranet, dial-up lines, leased lines, private networks, and physical movement of removable transportable electronic storage media (Romanow, 2011).

Informed Consent

Most research studies involve informed consent procedures that are designed to provide prospective participants with sufficient information to make a reasonable decision about the potential risks and benefits of participation (Polit &

Beck, 2010). Informed consent should also be sought and documented if a treatment is experimental, that is, if its efficacy has not been established empirically (Silverman, 1998b). According to the ASHA (2005), the key components of informed consent are respect for participants, benefits, and justice.

Informed consent requires that prospective participants sign a consent form. Obtaining informed consent may be complicated for several reasons: the most appropriate method of obtaining informed consent may not be clear, the competency of the patient is in doubt, participants are vulnerable because they are not competent to make an informed decision about participation, and circumstances make participants feel that free choice is constrained or circumstances increase their risk for harm. Children, adults with diminished cognitive ability, and individuals residing in institutions (nursing homes or prisons) are especially vulnerable. A major barrier to informed consent is problems with reading comprehension. Almost half the population of the United States reads at or below the eighth-grade level, and some have little or no reading skills (Meline, 2006). Furthermore, special accommodations are needed for participants from different cultures, ethnic, and socioeconomic groups to avoid misunderstanding. In addition, special accommodations are needed for individuals who are blind, deaf, or hard-of-hearing to ensure comprehension of informed consent.

The AAA (2023) Code of Ethics addressed informed consent in Principle 1, Rule A. The current ASHA (2023) Code of Ethics also contains references to informed consent in Principle of Ethics 1, Rules H and P. Informed consent is usually considered as a means for protecting the rights of research participants (Silverman, 1998b). It also protects the rights of researchers and the institutions where the research is done. Informed consent provides researchers and institutions with some protection from research participants of alleged physical or mental harm.

Deception

One ethical issue that has been debated is the appropriateness of using deception (Mertens, 2005). The justification for deception is that the results of the study would be compromised without it because participants would modify their behavior if they knew what was being studied. Deception is supposed to be reduced by debriefing, misrepresentation, guaranteeing privacy, and obtaining fully informed consent.

Institutional Approval

Speech-language pathologists and audiologists should obtain prior approval for conducting research and provide accurate information about their research proposals (American Psychological Association [APA], 2020). The research should be conducted consistent with the approved research protocol and consultation with the Institutional Review Board (IRB) as needed. Many journals require information about the IRB status of a research report, including the name of the IRB and approval number.

Control Groups

The use of control groups has been a long-standing ethical issue. The most effective design for determining the effect of treatment is to compare subjects who receive treatment with those who receive no treatment or a sham treatment (Portney & Watkins, 2009). It is unethical to withhold treatment, that is, the control group should receive treatment (French et al., 2001). Waiting list control groups are selected from persons on the waiting list for treatment. Furthermore, there is no basis for assuming that no treatment and waiting list control groups are equivalent (Lum, 2002).

Conflict of Interest

ASHA's Board of Ethics (ASHA, 2011a) defines conflict of interest as

> A situation in which personal and/or financial considerations have the potential to influence or comprise judgment in any clinical service, research, consultation, instruction, administration, or any other professional entity (e.g., clinical service, research, consultation, instruction, administration, etc.), or where the situation may appear to provide the potential for professional judgment to be compromised. (p. 1)

Both the AAA (2023) and ASHA (2023) Codes of Ethics address conflicts of interest. The AAA (2023) Code, Rule 4c, indicates that "Individuals shall not participate in activities that constitute a conflict of professional interest" (p. 1). ASHA's Code of Ethics (2023) states that speech-language pathologists and audiologists "shall avoid engaging in conflicts of interest whereby personal, financial, or other considerations have the potential to influence or compromise professional judgment and objectivity" (p. 7). Speech-language pathologists and audiologists should also avoid the appearance of a conflict of interest, although there may not be an ethical violation. Appearance of a conflict of interest can damage the professional reputation of an individual and adversely affect his or her practice and profession (Diefendorf, 2003).

Conflicts of interest involve bias or influencing professional judgment or practice. Some conflicts of interest are obvious, whereas others may be subtle. These conflicts can be intellectual (nonfinancial) or financial and interfere with research conduct or reports. Examples of intellectual conflicts in interest include, but are not limited to, ego, professional advancement, and beliefs (Ludlow, 2001). Financial conflicts include support for research, large honorariums, patents, agreements with industry, and product-oriented research. Scientific conflicts of interest are the use of position to influence publication of manuscripts and review of grant applications (Bradley, 1995).

Conflict of commitment is another aspect of conflict of interest. Also referred to as dual loyalty or dual commitment, it refers to conflicting demands or speech-language pathologists and audiologists who have obligations to their patients and to others, including students and other professionals (Beyrer, 2003). Multiple roles also can contribute to conflicts of interest (Sales & Lavin, 2000). Multiple roles are not unethical if they are not reasonably expected to have adverse effects. Speech-language pathologists and audiologists should be cautious about multiple roles. Guidelines and procedures for addressing personal and professional loyalty, Dual Loyalty, and Human Rights in Health Professional Practice have been developed by the International Dual Loyalty Working Group (2002).

Disclosure is often cited as the key to managing conflicts of interest (Association of American Medical Colleges, 1999; Korn, 2000). ASHA journals require disclosure of any real or potential conflict of interest that could be seen as having an influence on the research, such as financial interests in a test or procedure and funding by an equipment or materials manufacturer for efficiency research. In 2012, submission for the ASHA convention required a disclosure statement.

There are disclosure requirements for presentation of courses offered for ASHA continuing education credits (ASHA, 2012b). These requirements are as follows:

- Presenters must disclose financial or nonfinancial interest
- Focus on one method or device must indicate if information will be given about similar products
- Focus must be on science or contemporary practice, not on sales or promotion
- Should not favor or use, promote, or suggest purchase of a specific product
- Acknowledge if presenting limited or no information about similar products or services
- Disclose relevant financial and nonfinancial relationships or lack of attendees in each session

Accurate outcome research aimed at assessing the efficacy of clinical services is essential to speech-language pathology and audiology. Product-oriented research increases the risk for conflict of interest (Sininger et al., 2004). Responsibility for conducting product efficacy research should be independent of the development and production of these products.

Mentoring

Mentoring is an important part of teaching research. Mentees not only learn scientific expertise from their mentors, but also learn about the reasonable conduct of research, preparing grant applications, interacting with colleagues, and preparing manuscripts for publication (Association of American Medical Colleges, 1994). Unfortunately, sometimes the roles and responsibilities of mentees and mentors are misunderstood. On one hand, the mentee may believe his or her role is passive, not active, and the mentors are responsible for the work. On the other hand, the mentor may view the mentee as inexperienced labor. Therefore, it is important to understand the roles and responsibilities of both mentees and mentors.

Students usually select their mentor based primarily on which faculty member has research interests that most closely align with their interests. Other factors that may be considered in selecting a mentor include the publication record of the faculty member, extramural financial support, national recognition, productivity of the department, atmosphere within the department, current positions of graduates, and opportunities for professional growth (Association of American Medical Colleges, 1994; Macrina, 1995a).

Both mentees and mentors should know what to expect from each other. It is reasonable for mentees to have expectations about the support and advice a mentor can provide. Mentors also have expectations, such as the mentee will work independently and will be enthusiastic about the work.

Supervision is essential to maintaining and facilitating research integrity.

Speech-language pathologists and audiologists often have dual roles as both mentor and supervisor to students whom they also teach in class. It has been suggested that misunderstanding can be avoided by a written agreement outlining the responsibilities of both mentor and mentee. The agreement should also include authorship consideration as well as the amount and type of supervision. It has been suggested that mentors set up periodic and specific meetings to provide mentees feedback and maintain a record of supervision, including meeting times, issues discussed, and duties assigned.

Several problems related to mentoring have been identified by Horner and Minifie (2011b). Among these problems were continued dependency, disparities of power, inadequate accountability, vulnerable subordinates, and failure to give appropriate credit. Recommendations for improving mentoring have been described by Shamoo and Resnick (2003). These recommendations included acknowledging mentors for effective mentoring, developing guidelines for amount and types of responsibilities and intellectual property, ensuring appropriate response to whistleblowing, establishing procedures for evaluating mentees, promoting adverse and nondiscriminatory environment safe from harm, and providing mentors with time for mentoring.

Documentation

Documentation is crucial to research (Macrina, 1995b). Documentation includes IRB approval, informed consent forms on all participants, participant encounters, research protocol, data collection and analysis, and research reports. Confidentiality is a major consideration in creating, storing, accessing, transferring, and disposing of records. According to the AAA (2023) Code of Ethics, "Individuals shall maintain accurate documentation of services rendered, according to acceptable medical, legal, and professional standards and requirements" (p. 2). The ASHA (2023) Code of Ethics also addresses maintenance of records in Principle of Ethics I Rule O.

Referencing Sources

The AAA (2023) Code of Ethics has no specific reference to publication credit or authorship. The 2023 ASHA Code of Ethics states, "Individuals shall reference the source when using other person's ideas, research, presentations, or products in written, oral, or any other media presentations or summary" (p. 8).

Accurate and appropriate referencing of information even in slides and handouts prevents the appearance of plagiarism. Referencing of sources in ASHA journals is based on recommendations and guidelines of the *Publication Manual of the American Psychological Association* (APA, 2020). Speech-language pathologists and audiologists must accept the ethical responsibilities for appropriate referencing of sources.

Stealing ideas, plagiarism, or both is an issue at all levels of education and has increased over the past 10 years (Young, 2003). Plagiarism is not giving credit to someone's ideas, results, or words. Plagiarism can take many forms and ranges from obvious to very subtle. Some plagiarism involves direct verbatim copying of text, or the text can be modified in ways that are not immediately recognizable from the source material (Association of American Medical Colleges, 1994). Other forms of plagiarism include lazy writing and redundant or duplicate publications. Lazy writing or patchwork plagiarism involves overreliance on direct quotations. Duplicate publication or self-plagiarism is repeated publication of previous results (Benninger, 2002). Duplicate publication is also inappropriate because ASHA journals require that submitted manuscripts have neither been previously published nor are currently under review elsewhere. In addition, information about any previous presentation of the data—whether at a professional meeting or in conference proceedings, book chapters, websites, or related media—must be disclosed. Duplicate publications may also contribute to misrepresentation of publication credit, that is, a distorted inaccurate record. Failure to acknowledge the contributions of colleagues, collaborators, or others—whether deliberate or not—can be viewed as a form of plagiarism (Association of American Medical Colleges, 1994). The widespread use of the internet makes using information without acknowledging the source(s) easier. Cyber-cheating or online plagiarism enables cut and paste plagiarism and online paper mills. Plagiarism frequently occurs because of ignorance about appropriate referencing. Ignorance is not an excuse for plagiarism. This can be avoided by learning and using guidelines for referencing sources such as the *Publication Manual of the American Psychological Association* (APA, 2020). Suspected plagiarism can be identified by Google's search engine for scholarship as well as other commercially available software.

Copyright

Copyright is a legal concept protecting exclusive rights, usually for a limited time, of the creator of intellectual work. The American Medical Association (1999) defined copyright as providing "for the protection of rights of parties involved in the creation and dissemination of intellectual property" (p. 115). The Copyright Act of 1976 is a comprehensive law related to permission for quoting, reproducing, or adapting published or unpublished information (APA, 2020). Requirements for obtaining copyright permission vary. It is the author's responsibility to find out if permission is required from the copyright holder.

Exceptions from copyright permission are fair use and public domain (Blessing & Forister, 2012). Fair use provides for limited use of copyrighted materials. According to Horner and Minifie (2011b) fair public domain applies to materials that can be used without permission but must be acknowledged. Additional information about copyright is available in Silverman's (1999) *Professional Issues in Speech-Language Pathology and Audiology.*

Copyright infringement is the use of published or unpublished information without permission. In other words, it is unauthorized use of information, which includes computer software and programs published since 1976 (Blessing & Forister, 2012). Illegal copying of materials is not uncommon in educational and clinical activities. Test forms are often duplicated without authorization.

Authorship

Authorship is the basis by which university faculty are evaluated for employment, promotion, and tenure. Those faculties who do not publish may not be promoted or tenured. Therefore, these faculties may feel pressure to publish. Some faculty, however, believe publishing detracts from teaching and that resources and time are not available for publishing. In addition to promotion and tenure, there are other advantages in publishing research, such as staying current in professionally obtaining funds for research, networking, and collaborating with other professionals.

Authorship credit can be a problem because of the prevalence of honorary and ghost authorship as well as academia's competitive "publish or perish" (Bennett & Taylor, 2003; Macrina, 1995c; Mowatt et al., 2002). The different types of responsibilities are described in Table 2–5.

Several studies have confirmed that a substantial portion of authors listed in multiauthored publications did not meet criteria for authorship (Bennett & Taylor, 2003; Goodman, 1994; Mowatt et al., 2002; Shapiro et al., 1994). Some individuals who do not meet the criteria for authorship may be included, or individuals who should be included as

Table 2–5. Irresponsible Authorship: Types and Definitions

Types	Definitions
Coercion	Use of intimidation or bullying to gain authorship. The white bull effect.
Courtesy	Author who does not meet authorship criteria. Same as Gift, Guest, or Honorary.
Denial	Failure to include or acknowledge individual(s) who should be included as author. Same as Ghost or Silent author.
Duplicated	Publishing the same paper more than once. Sometimes referred to as self-plagiarism.
Gift	Same as Courtesy, Guest, or Honorary
Guest	Same as Courtesy, Gift or Honorary
Honorary	Same as Courtesy, Gift, or Guest.
Mutual support	Agreement by two or more authors to place each other's name on publication to give appearance of higher productivity. May or may not meet authorship criteria. Depending on the later may be a type of Courtesy, Gift, Guest, or Honorary.
White bull	Coercion or intimidation to obtain authorship

Sources: From "Why not just toss a coin?" by K. Strange, 2008, *American Journal of Physiology-Cell Physiology, 295,* pp. 567–575; and "The White Bull Effect: Abusive Co-Authorship and Publication Parasites" by L. S. Kwok, 2005, *Journal of Medical Ethics, 31,* pp. 554–556.

authors are omitted. Honorary or courtesy authorship is naming as an author an individual who does not meet authorship criteria. Ghost authorship is the failure to name an author an individual who has made substantial contribution that merits authorship or an unnamed individual who participated in writing the manuscript. Students are at greater risk for not being given credit for authorship. Furthermore, students should be the principal author on any multiple-authored presentation or publication that is substantially based on the student's thesis or dissertation (Knapp & Van de Creek, 2006). Mere possession of an institutional position, such as department chair, does not justify authorship (APA, 2020). AAA's (2005) guidelines for ethical practice address issues related to authorship in publication and presentation of research, such as disclosure to avoid potential conflicts of interest and determination of authorship. ASHA's (2016) Code of Ethics provides some guidance about authorship: "Individuals shall assign credit only to those who have contributed to a publication, presentation, or product. Credit shall be assigned in proportion to the contribution and only with the contributor's consent" (ASHA, 2016, P-IV, R-J). The ASHA journal requires corresponding authors to affirm that all individuals listed in the byline have made appropriate contributions for authorship, have consented to the byline order, and have agreed to the submission of the manuscript in its current form. These contributions are outlined in Table 2–6.

The American Medical Association (2020) specifies three criteria for authorship: (a) substantial contributions to conception and design or acquisition of data, or analysis, or interpretation of data; (b)

Table 2–6. Author Contributions

Study concept and design
Acquisition data
Analysis and interpretation of data
Drafting of the manuscript
Critical revision of the manuscript for important intellectual content
Obtained funding
Administrative, technical, or material support
Study supervision

drafting or revising the manuscript; and (c) final approval of the version to be published. Other responsibilities of an author include critical review and revision of manuscript; statistical expertise; administrative, technical, or material support; and study supervision (Mowatt et al., 2002; Yedidia et al., 2003).

The order of authorship also warrants consideration because disagreement about authorship can be very bitter and even result in legal action (Gabard & Martin, 2003; Kwok, 2005). The order of authorship should be in descending order based on level of contribution, with the greatest contribution(s) made by the first author. However, the order of authors may be considered relative to an author's university affiliation because some universities only consider first-author publications in determining promotion, tenure, and merit increases.

Journals do not have uniform criteria for designating authorship. For example, ASHA (2011c) requires that a statement about authorship accompany manuscript submission. Specifically, this affirms that all the authors have made contributions appropriate for authorship. Furthermore, the primary author is responsible for assuring that the list of authors includes all and only those persons who have played significant roles in writing the manuscript, designing the study, preparing and executing the plan for data collection, and or interpreting the results in preparation for publication. (p. 4)

Some journals, such as the *Journal of the American Medical Association*, published the author contribution between the last section of a paper or report and the references. More recently, some journals ask the authors to specify individual author contributions (e.g., conceptualization, data collection, data analysis, manuscript writing, etc.) to be published with the article.

Peer Review

Peer review has been a part of the scientific process for over three hundred years, and researchers probably have complained about its shortcomings for nearly as long (Laine & Murlow, 2003). Peer review is the process by which the quality of research is assessed, and it involves multiple activities (Association of American Medical Colleges, 1994). First, there is the peer review of research proposals to assess the scientific merit of grant applications, that is, funding decisions based on peer review. Second, professional journals and other publications use peer review to assess the quality of manuscripts, namely, publication decisions based on peer review. Thus, it is obvious that peer review is an essential component of research. High-quality reviews are those that provide constructive and substantiated comments about

the importance and originality of the research, strengths and weaknesses, and an interpretation of results (Laine & Murlow, 2003).

Issues related to peer review include, but are not limited to, bias on the part of authors, editors, and reviewers; confidentiality; and plagiarism or theft of ideas (Macrina, 1995c; Olson et al., 2002; Scheetz, 2001). Reviewers and editors may be tempted to solicit the opinion of friends and colleagues with expertise in a particular area about a manuscript, which may be a breach of confidentiality. The Scientific Research Society (1986) described several problems related to reviewers and editors. Among the reviewer problems were obtaining a secondary citation for one's own publication in the guise of improving the manuscript; pirating the topic of the manuscript; providing criticism on a subsequent review; excessively delaying review without explanation; and losing manuscripts. Another problem is peer review failure that occurs when a peer-reviewed paper contains several errors. Most journals do not have a policy for peer-review failures other than "Letter to the Editor." Therefore, it becomes the individual reader's responsibility to identify and seek resolution of these failures in the form of a letter to the editor. The author of a quantitative paper usually has the option of publishing a reply to the Letter to the Editor. Peer review is such an important issue that there have been five International Congresses on Peer Review to discuss efforts to systematize reviews and improve reports of research. The first International Congress was in 1989 in Chicago, the second was in 1993 in Chicago, the third in 1999 in Prague, the fourth in 2001 in Spain (Rennie, 2002), and the fifth in 2005 in Chicago. The topics of presentation included authorship, conflicts of interest, journal guidelines and policies, ethical concerns, peer-review process, scientific misconduct, publication bias, and quality of journal articles.

Publication Correction

Research reports may be flawed because of errors in methodology, selective reporting of results, or overuse of or vague citation of references (Altman, 2002). Critical review of published reports and letters to the editor about inaccurate published reports are essential to the integrity of research (Getzsch et al., 2010). Authors are sometimes reluctant to respond to critical reviews of their work. Editors should insist that the authors respond to criticism of their work. Speech-language pathologists and audiologists also have ethical obligations when their research is published. If authors discover or learn of errors in the published data, they are ethically obligated to promptly take reasonable steps to correct the error, retract the error, or use other appropriate publication means (APA, 2020).

Reports also may be retracted or withdrawn because of unsubstantiated or irreproducible data. According to Scheetz (2001), since 1992, findings of scientific misconduct have resulted in 63 revisions to the literature.

Several problems related to mentoring have been identified by Horner and Minifie (2011b). Among these problems were continued dependency, disparities of power, inadequate accountability, vulnerable subordinates, and failing to give credit. Recommendations for improving mentoring have been described by Shamoo and Resnik (2003). These rec-

ommendations include acknowledge mentors for effective mentoring, develop guidelines for amount and type of responsibilities and intellectual property, ensure appropriate response to whistle-blowers, establish procedures for evaluating mentees, promote a diverse and nondiscriminatory environment, secure an environment safe from harm, and provide mentors with time for mentoring.

More subtle issues of research ethics were identified by Rosenthal (1999). These issues were related to inadequacy in research design, hyperclarity, data dropping, outlier rejection, self-censoring, and external censoring. Hyperclarity is suggesting that research is likely to achieve what it is unlikely to achieve. Closely related to hyperclarity, it is the tendency to imply a caused relationship when none has been established. Rosenthal (1999) believes bad science makes for bad ethics.

Reasons for retraction of a report include misconduct or presumed misconduct, significant reporting errors, and inability of author(s) to replicate (Horner & Minifie, 2011c). If there are significant errors or ethical misconduct, published papers should be retracted and citation of retracted papers should not occur.

Evidence-Based Practice

Gupta (2003) believes there has been limited consideration of the ethical issues related to evidence-based practice. Ethical considerations are involved in evidence-based practice as well as in not practicing it. There are several areas for ethical concern. One concern is the potential for patient care to be manipulated by administrators to deprive persons of certain health services. Another area of concern is the effect that evidence-based practice has on the authority and power of health care providers. Evidence-based practice prioritizes certain types of research and, thus, increases the pressure for this research to be funded. There may be publication bias, that is, the publication of positive and statistically significant results. Another area for ethical concern is the uncritical and permissive attitude of evidence-based practice toward private funding of research. Other issues are related to control groups, randomization, need for research or treatment, meaning outcomes, setting (location) of research treatment, strategies for which evidence is not available, and determining risks and benefits. Additional information about evidence-based practice is presented in Chapter 13.

American Academy of Audiology

The AAA (2023) Code of Ethics contains several specific statements related to research. AAA also has guidelines for ethical research: authorship in publication and presentations; adequacy of research design; security of data; and conflicts of interest in product-oriented outcome research.

American Speech-Language-Hearing Association

Standards for the Certificate of Clinical Competence (CCC) in Speech-Language Pathology (ASHA, 2020a) require knowledge of standards of ethical conduct.

Standards for the CCC-Audiology (ASHA, 2020a) also require knowledge about ethical conduct.

The ASHA (2023) Code of Ethics is central to the integrity of research. Twenty-one specific references to research are in the 2023 ASHA Code of Ethics. Ethical responsibilities should be interpreted to include ethical treatment of all collaborators, assistants, and students associated with research (McCartney, 2002). The Issues in Ethics statement about research (ASHA, 2008) discusses and interprets the Code relative to ethics in research. It also provides guidance about teaching ethics to students. Other issues statements related to research are conflict of professional interest (ASHA, 2011a), confidentially (ASHA, 2001), cultural competence (ASHA, 2011b), and protection of human subjects (ASHA, 2005).

Sanctions for Ethical Misconduct

Three types of legal perspectives influence selection of sanctions for ethical misconduct: (a) quasicontractual legal remedy of restitution; (b) philosophy of "just desserts" or retribution based on an intuitive idea that the individual was engaged in criminal activity deserving punishment; and (c) detection of misconduct (Dresser, 1993).

Sanctions for ethical misconduct have been described by both AAA (2023) and ASHA (2023). Part II of the AAA (2023) Code of Ethics includes "procedures for the management of alleged noncompliance" (p. 1). The sanctions are educative letter, reprimand, probation of suspension, suspension of membership, and revocation of membership.

The fundamental purposes of ASHA (2023) include the following: (a) penalize the person in violation; (b) serve as a mechanism to educate and rehabilitate; (c) protect the public; and (d) inform other ASHA members and certificate holders that the Association enforces its ethical standards and alert them that there are penalties for engaging in professional misconduct. Typically, more serious misconduct receives harsher sanctions. The sanctions from least to most severe are reprimand; censure; revocation of membership, certification, or both; suspension of membership, certification, or both; withholding of membership, certification, or both; and cease and desist.

Institutional Review Board

An Institutional Review Board (IRB) is a committee mandated by the National Research Act, Public Law 93-348, to be established within each institution that conducts research involving human and animal subjects and needs federal funding for research (Sieber, 1992). The IRB is a group of individuals who are affiliated with an institution who meet to review research proposals and monitor ongoing research relative to ethical standards. Responsibilities of the IRB include the following:

- Protecting the rights and welfare of subjects
- Ensuring protocols are presented by the sponsor(s)
- Ensuring sponsor(s) of a protocol provide disclosure(s) including areas of concern such as appearance of

a conflict of interest and financial interests
- Reviewing, monitoring, and approving research protocols
- Ensuring that rights including privacy and confidentiality are protected
- Ensuring that all research is conducted within current federal and state guidelines (Pozar, 2012)

The term "research ethics review board," not IRB, has been suggested because the focus is on ethics rather than the institution. HIPAA has had a significant impact on IRB (see the HIPAA discussion earlier in this chapter).

IRBs are often viewed negatively by researchers because of delays and requirements that provide limited protection of subjects (Azar, 2002). However, delays and revisions can be reduced by using understandable language in the consent form, explicitly describing the research protocol submitted to the IRB, and submitting all required documents (Sharp, 2001). Furthermore, many of the ethical problems related to research are resolved during the IRB review, that is, appropriate risk-to-benefit rating, details about informed consent, and appropriateness of compensation (Jonsen et al., 2006).

The IRB is responsible for making decisions about research plans at convened meetings. In making decisions, the following are considered: scientific merit, competence of the investigator(s), risk to subjects, feasibility based on identified reasons, procedures for selecting subjects, voluntary informed consent based on complete understandable descriptions, and confidentiality. The required elements of informed consent are listed in Table 2–7. In addition, the informed consent must be written in lay language; that is, the language must be clear and basic so that it can be understood by the average participant (Portney & Watkins, 2009). Many believe that informed consent makes research ethical; however, informed consent is neither necessary nor sufficient for ethical research.

IRB members must be able to adequately review research proposals. The IRB must be composed of at least five members and may not consist entirely of males, females, or members of one profession. At least one IRB member must be primarily concerned with nonscientific areas; many are lawyers, clergy, or ethicists. One member may not be affiliated with the institution where the research is to be conducted or be a member of the immediate family of a person who is affiliated with the institution (Polit & Beck, 2010; Sales & Folkman, 2000).

Many research plans require a full review by the IRB. For a full review, the IRB must meet with a majority of the members present. In order for the research plan to be approved, it must receive approval of the majority of IRB members present at the meeting.

Table 2–7. Elements of Informed Consent

Purpose	Clear explanation of research and its importance reason for selecting individual
Procedures	Clear explanation of what will be done to or by individual
Risks and discomforts	Truthful and inclusive statements
Benefits	Description of potential benefits to individual, general knowledge, or future of health care
Alternative to participation	Description of reasonable alternative procedures that might be used in treatment with treatment is being started
Confidentiality	Statement of procedures used to ensure anonymity for collecting, storing, and reporting information and who (persons or agencies) will have access to information
Request for more information	Statement that individuals may ask questions about or discuss study participation at any time, naming an individual to contact
Refusal or withdrawal	Statement that individual may refuse to participate or discontinue participation at any time without prejudice
Injury statement	Description of measures to be taken if injury occurs as direct result of research activity
Consent statement	Confirmation that individual consents to participation
Signatures	Participants; patient or guardian, assent of minor over age 7; witness

IRBs are often viewed negatively by researchers and administrators. The major reasons for these negative views are increased delays, added costs, and limited protection of subjects. There have also been complaints about differences between federal regulations and IRBs (Azar, 2002). Several strategies have been suggested for improving IRBs. One strategy is modifying the local independent IRB system and replacing it with a central IRB plus a local option. Education and dissemination of guidelines about IRBs have also been suggested (Green et al., 2006). Delays and revisions of research protocol can be reduced by using understandable language in the consent form, providing specific descriptions of the research methodology, and submitting all associated documents (Sharp, 2001). Last, many problems are resolved during the IRB review. These problems include risk to benefit, details about informed consent, and suitability of compensation (Jonsen et al., 2006).

Some research plans qualify for expedited review or exempted status. For certain types of research involving no more than minimal risk, the research plan may be expedited. An expedited review is conducted by the IRB chair or another IRB member designated by the chair. The advantage of an expedited review is that it usually is completed in less time than a full review.

Research plans may be exempted from full review if there is no apparent risk. Surveys, interviews or studies of existing records may be exempt from full review if data are collected so that subjects cannot be identified and the study does not involve sensitive issues such as criminal activity, drug abuse, or sexual behavior (Portney & Watkins, 2009).

Before implementing a study, the researcher must submit a research proposal to the IRB. An IRB can approve the proposed research plan, require restriction(s), or disapprove the plan. The main requirements governing IRB decisions are summarized in Table 2–8.

Recent issues about IRB include the cost of operation, local versus central IRB, and characteristics of IRB members. It was reported that high-volume IRBs were more expensive than low-volume IRBs but more economically efficient. The potential savings of large IRBs may encourage small IRBs to merge, which could reduce local review, control, and oversight. Christian and associates (2002) advocate both central and local IRBs. Central IRBs review large, national, multicenter clinical studies, whereas local

Table 2–8. Major Requirements Governing IRB Decisions

Risks to participants minimized
Risks to participants reasonable in relation to anticipated benefits, if any, and importance of knowledge that may reasonable be expected to result
Equitable selection of participants
Informed consent appropriately documented
Adequate provisions for monitoring research to ensure safety of participants
Appropriate provisions to protect privacy or participants and confidentiality of data
When vulnerable subjects involved, appropriate additional safeguards to protect their rights and welfare

IRBs continue to be a key component of the review system. This approach preserves local autonomy and responsibility for local matters, reduces the workload of local IRBs, and eliminates duplication of effort. McWilliams and associates (2003) believe that there are serious differences in the review process between local and central IRBs for multicenter studies. Conversely, Rose (2003) opposed central IRBs and suggested that reviews by local IRBs could be improved by education, consultation, and funding. Campbell and associates (2003) studied the characteristics of medical school faculty members serving on IRBs. Faculty members serving on IRBs have research experience and knowledge, but almost half of all faculty IRB members were consultants to industry, which raises the possibility of the potential for conflict of interest.

Teaching Research Ethics

Professional ethics begin on the college campus (DeRussy, 2003). Therefore, higher education has a critical role in teaching ethics. Furthermore, ASHA's certification standards for speech-language pathology and audiology require training in research and ethics. This involves integrating ethical principles into research. This requires that students in speech-language pathology and audiology be able to understand and integrate ethical principles into research. Educational training programs must have curricula and experiences in the ethical conduct of research. This section addressed topics related to teaching research ethics. First, content is considered and then methods for teaching about ethics in research are considered. Goals for teaching ethics are listed in Table 2–9. Their goals should also be reviewed periodically by practicing speech-language pathologists and audiologists.

The goal of teaching research ethics is to apply ethical principles in making decisions about research.

Emanuel et al. 2000) identified seven requirements for evaluating the ethics of research studies: (a) value—enhancement of health or knowledge must be derived from the research; (b) validity—methodological rigor; (c) fair subject selection—scientific objectives, not privilege or vulnerability, and potential

Table 2–9. Goals for Teaching Research

Examine and make distinctions between ethical concepts such as beneficence, nonmalfiecence, justice, fidelity, respect. Patient rights, confidentiality
Know that ethical certainty is often impossible but ethical reasoning about choice can be precise.
Serious consideration of personal and professional ethics
Identify ethical dilemmas and seek resolution of these dilemmas

for and distribution of risks and benefits should determine selection; (d) risk-benefit ratio within context of standard clinical practice and the research plan, risks must be minimized, potential benefits enhanced, and potential benefits to individual and knowledge gained for society must outweigh the risks; (e) independent review—unaffiliated individuals must review the research and approve, amend, or terminate it; (f) informed consent—individuals should be informed about the risks and provide voluntary consent; and (g) respect for enrolled subjects—subjects should have confidentiality protected, opportunity to withdraw, and their well-being monitored.

Content

The teaching of ethics cannot be separated from the Codes of Ethics of AAA (2023) and ASHA (2023), which contain several references to ethics in research. There is a wide range of information about the responsible conduct of research, such as the following: (a) topic related to conduct and reporting of research; (b) ethical dilemmas presented by certain types of research; and (c) responses to research misconduct. Ingham and Horner (2004) identified eleven core areas for teaching the responsible conduct of research, which include the following: ethics and morality; research misconduct; protection of human subjects; publication practices and responsible authorship; peer review; mentor/trainee relationships; conflict of interest and commitment; data acquisition, management, share, and ownership; collaborative research; animal subjects protection; and guidelines and regulation.

In addition to the AAA (2023) and ASHA (2023) Codes of Ethics, it is helpful to be aware of the ethical issues that may arise during a research study. These issues are usually related to specifying the research problem; identifying a purpose statement and research questions; and collecting, analyzing, and writing up the results of the study (Creswell, 2003). By anticipating these issues in advance, ethical problems may be prevented or reduced. There is also a need for information about research ethics in dissertations. Krellstrom et al. (2011) reported that ethical concerns about dissertations are often related to inadequate supervision. It was suggested that ethical issues be emphasized in graduate and postgraduate studies.

Topics about conducting and reporting research are presented in Table 2–10. The second classification is related to ethical dilemmas associated with certain types of research that could become the focus of public debate.

These topics included the use of humans and animals in research. The third area addressed is recognizing and responding to research misconduct, such as plagiarism and fabricating or falsifying research data. This involves institutional policies and guidelines for the responsible conduct of research and guidance from the AAA (2023) and ASHA (2023) Codes of Ethics. The American Medical Association (Iverson et al., 1998) has guidelines for ethical and legal considerations in publishing papers. These topics and subtopics are listed in Table 2–11.

There is a need for information about ethical issues related to specific populations and work settings. Moss (2011) and Jakubowitz (2011) described ethical research practices in pediatric popula-

Table 2–10. Topics Related to Conducting and Reporting Research

Reasonable performance of research	Research design avoids subjectivity and minimizes bias
	Unbiased data selection and analysis
	Data management, storage, retrieval, ownership
	Sharing research methods, information
	Adherence to rules about safety, animal use, etc.
Responsible reporting of research	Authorship criteria
	Recognizing contributions of others
	Crediting previous work
	Duplicate and fragmented publication
	Avoidance of premature reporting or publishing
	Reporting in the public media
Ethical training practices	Fair performance evaluations, compensation, and benefit
	Responsibility to teach
	Responsibility to mentor
	Responsibility to give credit
	Avoidance of exploitation
Maintaining confidentiality	In reviewing submissions for publication
	In reviewing grant proposals
	In privileged personal communication

Source: Adapted from *Teaching the Responsible Conduct of Research Through a Case Study Approach*, by Association of American Medical Colleges, 1994, Washington, DC: Author.

tions. Work settings such as the schools (Watson et al., 2011) and health care settings (Kummer & Turner, 2011; Larsen & McMillin, 2011) are considered ethical research in multidisciplinary clinics. A comprehensive survey of students and faculty in communication sciences and disorders by Minifie and associates (2011) found that students were not receiving adequate information about mentoring, research collaboration, conflicts of interest, and humane treatment of animals in research. These findings provide a basis for including and expanding this information.

There is also a need for continuing education about research ethics. Speech-language pathologists and audiologists need to periodically review and monitor information about professional ethics. The quality of instruction in ethics should be considered.

Ethical consultations are being used more frequently to resolve ethical dilemmas (Schneiderman et al., 2003). Lo (2003) suggests that ethics consultation fosters more effective education because it may identify areas needing improvement such as misunderstandings about ethics or limitations in communicating

Table 2–11. Ethical and Legal Considerations in Publishing

Authorship Responsibility	Authorship criteria
	Guest and ghost authors
	Unsigned editorials
	Number of authors
	Order of authorship
	Group/collaborative authorship
Acknowledgments	Permission to name individuals
Duplicate Publications	Secondary publication
	Editorial policy or preventions/handling allegations of duplicate publication
Scientific Misconduct	Misrepresentation
	Misappropriation
	Editorial policy for scientific misconduct
Conflict of Interest	Author's disclosure
	Peer reviewer's disclosure
	Editor's disclosure
	Editorial policy for failure to disclose financial interest
Copyright	Ownership and control of data
	Copyright
	Types of works; copyright duration
	Copyright assignment or licensure
	Copyright notice/resignation
	Copying, reproducing, adapting
	Publishing discussions from symposia, conferences
Reprint permissions, Intellectual Property	Standards for reprints
	Standards for licensed international editors
Ownership rights, Management	International copyright
	Moral rights
	Patent
	Trademark
	Peer review
	Allegation of scientific misconduct
Confidentiality	Selecting editors, editorial board members
	Legal petitions, claims privileged information

Table 2–11. *continued*

Protecting Individual's Rights in Publication	Informed consent
	Patient's rights
	Rights to publish reports
Defamation Libel	Living persons, existing entities
	Public, private figures
	Statements of opinion
	Editorials, letters, reviews
	Works of fiction
	Republication, news reporting
	Defense against libel
	Other liability concerns
Editorial Freedom and Integrity	Policy on editorial freedom
Editorial Responsibilities, Procedures, Policies	Editor's responsibilities
	Rejection
	Acknowledging manuscript receipt
	Revisions
	Manuscript assessment
	Peer review
	Acceptance
	Correspondence column, corrections
	Disclosure of practices
	Audits, reviews
	Quality reviews
Advertisements, Suppliers Sponsored Supplements	Advertisements
	Criteria of advertisement
	Advertorials
	Sponsored suppliers
	Advertising, sponsorship
	Release of information to public
	Embargo
	Dealing with news media
	News release

Source: From *American Medical Association Manual of Style*, by C. Iverson, 1998, Philadelphia, PA: Lippincott Williams & Wilkins.

with patients and families. Kenny et al. (2010) found that experienced speech-language pathologists more frequently used informal support networks to resolve ethical dilemmas than consulting work-based committees or their professional associates.

Methods

There is literature available about a variety of methods for teaching ethics. These methods include role-playing, discussion groups, mentoring, case studies, self-directed learning, and computerized reference searches (ASHA, 2002; Association of American Medical Colleges, 1994; Bulger, 2001; Bulger et al., 2002; Canter et al., 1999; Davies, 1999; Hamilton, 2002; Huffman, 2003; Jefferies & Bauer, 2003; Macrina, 1995a; Moss, 2010). The National Institutes of Health have online training for the protection of human subjects at no cost (http://cme.cancer .gov/clinicaltrials/learning/humanpar ticipants/protection.csp). Analysis and discussion about cases and situations are essential to teaching the responsible conduct of research (Heitman, 2002). Ethics courses and programs in many professions, including speech-language pathology and audiology, use the case study method to illustrate ethical issues in the field and to teach a system for ethical decision-making in professional practice.

Another approach to teaching research ethics is on-site observation of ethical misconduct. This can be modified and based on role-playing or case-based observations (Oberman et al., 2011).

Other resources for teaching research ethics are online print syllabi. McCarthy et al. (2007) developed a model for teaching professional issues in university audi-

ology and speech-language pathology training programs. The issues included ethical conduct and dilemmas and professional writing. Activities for these issues were based on Bloom's taxonomy ranging from one (knowledge) to seven (evaluation). A syllabus for research ethics committee training was developed by Cairoli and associates (2011). Training needs and competencies were identified. Funding for this training was reported to be a major problem. The University of Pittsburgh designed, implemented, and evaluated an institution with web-based training for the responsible conduct of research (Barnes et al., 2006).

Current and Future Issues

There are several unresolved issues related to the responsible conduct of research. These issues should be recognized and appropriate strategies for resolution be developed. Two surveys have identified relevant issues (Ingham et al., 2011; Minifie et al., 2011). Ingham and associates (2011) completed a two-part survey of ASHA members about research principles of publishing research. Several of the topics considered important were included in ASHA policy documents, although some topics were not adequately addressed; recommendations were to have ASHA create a single comprehensive publication policy document, implement and enforce the policy, develop formal procedures for processing alleged ethical misconduct, and foster collaboration of communication sciences and disorders programs to design and implement long-term educational programs about research ethics. Minifie and associates (2011) used a web-based survey to assess the perceptions of students and faculty about the responsible conduct of research in communication science and disorders. Coverage of eight topics related to the responsible conduct of research was rated as adequate: fabrication, falsification, reporting research misconduct, interpreting and reporting findings, confidentiality, protecting vulnerable subjects, alternative treatments, and data accuracy. Two topics did not receive adequate coverage: protection of electronic research information as well as recognizing and disclosing conflicts of interest. This information should be useful for improving instruction about the responsible conduct of research.

In a comprehensive review about research ethics, Minifie and associates (2011) identified "a host" of ethical issues. These issues were balance between risk and benefit, vulnerability and protection of subjects, conducting research with deceased subjects, protection of children, adequacy of federal regulations, appropriate limits of consent by parents and other legally authorized representatives, waive consent in intensive care, appropriate limitation of coercion and deception, representation of minorities, ethical and legal responsibilities of researchers, nature of research setting, social behavioral protection of subjects, harmful effect of randomization, and access to experimental pharmaceutical devices or alternative treatments when studies show no benefits.

There is a need for professional universities and professional organizations to develop a consensus on the best ethical practices (Steneck & Bulger, 2007). There is also a need to assess the quality of ethical instruction and the effect of training. Ethical training of students and professionals may be a way to decrease the need for regulation (Body

& McAllister, 2009). Therefore, there should be increased self-assessment and monitoring.

Case studies should be detailed enough to provide meaningful ethical decisions but general enough for students to analyze from their own knowledge and experience. The goal of case studies is to determine an ethical resolution to the problem(s) pertinent to the case and to define appropriate action for resolving the problem(s). The basic steps of case study and analysis are outlined in Table 2–12. Yin (2003a, 2003b) provided extensive guidelines about designing case studies. Case studies in research

Table 2–12. Steps for Case Study

1. Recognize and identify issues and specific ethical problems in the case.

2. Identify key facts, establish important definitions, and obtain other necessary information.

3. Identify professional ethical principles, standards or practice, and law relevant to ethical issues of the case.

4. Identify possible alternative courses and action, ethical arguments for and against implementation, and the likely outcome.

5. Choose the course of action best supported by the preceding analysis.

6. Evaluate the actions taken and the subsequent outcome.

Source: From *The Ethical Dimensions of the Biology and Health Science* (pp. 349–364), by E. Heitman, In R. E. Bulger, E. Heitman, & S. J. Reiser (Eds.), 2002, Cambridge, UK: Cambridge University Press.

ethics are available in the Association of American Medical Colleges (1994), Hamilton (2002), Heitman (2002), Jonsen et al. (2006), and Macrina (1995a).

Summary

Speech-language pathologists and audiologists face multiple ethical issues in planning, designing, and implementing research. There is a need for ethical guidelines because research has not always been conducted ethically. There are three major types of research misconduct: (a) fabrication, (b) falsification, and (c) plagiarism. The Codes of Ethics of AAA (2023) and ASHA (2023) have several standards related to responsible conduct of research and scholarly activities. The role and scope of the Institutional Review Board (IRB) and HIPAA are considered.

This chapter also included discussions of ethical issues related to research: (a) planning research, (b) confidentiality, (c) informed consent, (d) deception, (e) control group, (f) institutional approval, (g) conflicts of interest, (h) mentoring, (i) referencing of sources, (j) authorship, (k) copyright infringement and plagiarism, (l) peer review, (m) publication correction, and (n) evidence-based practice. Last, content and methods for teaching the responsible conduct of research and current and future issues are considered.

❓ DISCUSSION QUESTIONS

1. Define the responsible conduct of research.
2. Explain the need for ethical guidelines.
3. Trace the historical background of research conduct.
4. What is the impact of research misconduct?
5. How does research misconduct affect professional status?
6. Describe the major types of research misconduct.
7. Define fabrication, falsification, and plagiarism.
8. Explain ASHA's (2002) ethical standards for reporting and publishing research.
9. Describe the ethical bases for the responsible conduct of research.
10. Why is confidentiality related to research?
11. Why does peer review fail?
12. How can confidentiality be maintained in research?
13. Why can obtaining informed consent be difficult?
14. How do professional codes of ethics address informed consent?
15. Define conflict of interest.
16. How can conflict of interest affect research?
17. What can be done to minimize conflicts of interest?

18. What factors should be considered in selecting a mentor?
19. Why should research records be maintained? For how long should they be maintained?
20. How can and why should plagiarism be avoided?
21. Why can authorship be a problem?
22. What is irresponsible authorship?
23. Describe the types of irresponsible authorship.
24. What is peer review?
25. What issues are related to peer review?
26. What should be done if authors discover or learn of errors in their published reports?
27. What guidelines for research are in the AAA (2023) Code of Ethics?
28. What guidelines for research are in the ASHA (2023) Code of Ethics?
29. What is IRB?
30. What are the major responsibilities of an IRB?
31. What are the essential elements of informed consent?
32. What requirements affect IRB decisions?
33. What are the types of IRB reviews?
34. Discuss recent issues related to IRB.
35. How could these issues be resolved?
36. How can the ethics of research studies be evaluated?
37. What issues affect the content of teaching ethics?
38. Discuss the major topics related to conducting and reporting research.
39. Describe methods for teaching ethics.
40. How can case study and analysis be used to teach ethics?
41. What is the procedure for case study and analysis?
42. How can peer review fail?
43. What can be done to eliminate or resolve failed peer reviews?
44. What is copyright? Copyright infringement?
45. Why should and how can copyright infringement be avoided?
46. What is HIPAA?
47. How are HIPAA regulations enforced?
48. What are the penalties for violating HIPAA regulation?
49. List and briefly describe the three major HIPAA rules.
50. What is protected health information?
51. How has HIPAA affected research?
52. What are the reasons for "Letter to the Editors"?
53. What are the current issues relative to the responsible research?
54. How can these issues be resolved?

References

Altman, D. G. (2002). Poor quality medical research. *Journal of the American Medical Association, 287*, 2765–2767.

Ambrose, N. G., & Yairi, E. (2002). The Tudor study: Data and ethics. *American Journal of Speech Language Pathology, 11*, 190–203.

American Academy of Audiology. (2005). *FAQs for publishing.* http://www.audiology.org

American Academy of Audiology. (2023). *Code of ethics.* AAA-Code-of-Ethics-and-Non-Compliance-Procedures-2023-04-1.pdf

American Medical Association. (2020). *Manual of style.*

American Medical Association. (2011). *HIPAA violations and enforcement.* http://www.ama-assn.org/ama/pub/physician-resources/solutions-managing your practice

American Psychological Association. (2020). *Publication manual of the American Psychological Association* (7th ed.).

American Speech-Language-Hearing Association. (2001). *Conflict of interest.* http://www.asha.org

American Speech-Language-Hearing Association. (2002). Ethics in research and professional practice. *ASHA Supplement, 1*(7), 63–65.

American Speech-Language-Hearing Association. (2005). *Protection of human subjects.* http://www.asha.org

American Speech-Language-Hearing Association. (2008). *Ethics in research and professional practice.* http://www.asha.org

American Speech-Language-Hearing Association. (2011a). *Conflicts of professional interest.* http://www.asha.org

American Speech-Language-Hearing Association. (2011b). *Cultural competence.* http://www.asha.org

American Speech-Language-Hearing Association. (2011c). *Instruction for authors.* http://www.asha.org

American Speech-Language-Hearing Association. (2011d). *Texas state characteristics of licensure law.* http://www.tdlr.texas.gov/slpa/slparules.htm

American Speech-Language-Hearing Association. (2012a). *How ASHA's board of ethics sanctions individuals found in violation of the Code of Ethics.* http://www.asha.org

American Speech-Language-Hearing Association. (2012b, July 31). Presenter disclosure debut at convention. *ASHA Leader, 19.*

American Speech-Language-Hearing Association. (2016). *Code of ethics.* http://www.asha.org

American Speech-Language-Hearing Association. (2020a). *Standards and implementation for the Certificate of Clinical Competence in audiology.*

American Speech-Language-Hearing Association. (2020b). *Standards and implementation for the Certificate of Clinical Competence in speech-language pathology.*

American Speech-Language-Hearing Association. (2023). *Code of ethics.* https://www.asha.org/policy/et2016-00342/

Annett, M. M. (2001). Article alleges 1939 study taught children to stutter. *ASHA Leader, 6*(13), 1, 17.

Association of American Medical Colleges. (1994). *Teaching the responsible conduct of research through a case study approach.*

Azar, B. (2002). Ethics at the cost of research? *Monitor on Psychology, 33*(2). http://www.apa.org/monitor/feb02/ethicscost.aspx

Bailar, J. C. (1995). The real threats to the integrity of science. *Chronicle of Higher Education*, B1–B2.

Barnes, B. E., Fredkaj, C. P., Rosenberg, J. L., Russell, J., Beedle, A., & Levine, A. S. (2006). Creating an infrastructure for training in the responsible conduct of research. *Academic Medicine, 81*, 119–127.

Bennett, D. M., & Taylor, D. M. (2003). Unethical practices in authorship of science papers. *Emergency Medicine, 15*(3), 563–570.

Benninger, M. S. (2002). Duplicate publications in peer-reviewed journals. *Otolaryngology Head and Neck Surgery, 126*(2), 209–210.

Beyrer, C. (2003). Dual loyalty and human rights in health professional practice: Proposed guidelines and institutional mechanisms. *Journal of the American Medical Association, 290*(5), 671–672.

Blessing, J. D., & Forister, J. G. (2012). *Introduction to research and medical literature.* Barlett and Jones.

Body, R., & McAllister, L. (2009). *Ethics in speech and language therapy.* Wiley & Blackwell.

Bradley, S. G. (1995). Conflict of interest. In F. L. Macrina (Ed.), *Scientific integrity* (pp. 166–188). American Society for Microbiology.

Bulger, R. E. (2001). The ethics of teaching and learning. In American Speech-Language-Hearing Association (Ed.), *Promoting research integrity in communication sciences and disorders and related difficulties* (pp. 37–54). American Speech-Language-Hearing Association.

Bulger, R. E., Heitman, E., & Reiser, S. J. (2002). *The ethical dimensions of the biological and health sciences.* Cambridge University Press.

Cairoli E., Davies, H. T., Helm, J., Hooke, G., Knupfer, P., & Wells, F. (2011). A syllabus for research ethics committees: Training needs and resources in different European countries. *Journal of Medical Ethics, 10,* 136–138.

Campbell, E. G., Weissmen, J. S., Clarridge, B., Yucel, R. M., Causino, N., & Blumenthal, D. (2003). Characteristics of medical school faculty members serving on Institutional Review Boards: Results of a national survey. *Academic Medicine, 878,* 831–836.

Canter, M. B., Bennett, B. E., Jones, S. E., & Nagy, T. F. (1999). *Ethics for psychologists.* American Psychological Association.

Christian, M. C., Goldberg, J. L., Killen, J., Abrams, J. S., McCabe, M. S., Mauer, J. K., & Wittes, R. E. (2002). A central institutional review board for multi-institutional trials. *New England Journal of Medicine, 346*(18), 1405–1408.

Cornett, B. S. (2007). Service delivery in health care settings. In R. Lubinski, L. A.

Golpher, & C. M. Frattali (Eds.), *Professional issues in speech-language pathology and audiology* (pp. 279–328). Plural Publishing.

Creswell, J. W. (2003*). Research design.* Sage.

Davies, P. (1999). Teaching evidence-based health care. In M. Daws, P. Davies, Gray, J. Mart, K. Seers, & R. Snowball (Eds.), *Evidence-based practice* (pp. 223–242). Churchill Livingstone.

DeRussy, C. (2003). Professional ethics begin on the college campus. *Chronicle of Higher Education,* B20.

Diefendorf, A. O. (2003). Ethics: Professionalism and conflicts of interest. *ASHA Leader, 25.* http://www.asha.org

Dresser, R. (1993). Sanctions for research misconduct: A legal perspective. *Academic Medicine, 68,* S39–S43.

Dunlop, A., Graham, T., Leroy, Z., Glanz, D., & Dunlop, B. (2007). The impact of HIPAA authorization on willing to participate in clinical research. *Annals of Epidemiology, 17,* 899–905.

Dyer, J. (2001, June 10). Ethics and orphans: The "monster study." *San Jose Mercury News.* http://www.umn.edu

Emanuel, E. J., Wendler, D., & Grady, C. (2000). What makes clinical research ethical? *Journal of the American Medical Association, 283,* 2701–2711.

Fifth International Congress on Peer Review. (2005). http://www.ama assn.org/public/peer/peerhome.htm

French, S., Reynolds, F., & Swain, J. (2001). *Practical research.* Butterworth.

Gabard, D. L., & Martin, M. W. (2003). *Physical therapy ethics.* F. A. Davis.

Getzsch, P. O., Delamothe, T., & Goodlec, T. (2010). Adequacy of authors replies to critical or unfriendly electronic letters to the editor. *British Medical Journal, 5, 3.*

Goldfarb, R. (2006). *Research ethics: A case study for fluency.* Plural Publishing.

Goodman, N. W. (1994). Survey of fulfillment of criteria for authorship in published medical research. *British Medical Journal, 309,* 1482.

Green, A., Lowery, J. C., Kowalski, C. P., & Wyszewianski, L. (2006). Importance of institutional review board practice variation on observational health services research. *Health Science Research, 41,* 214–230.

Grodin, M. A., & Glantz, L. H. (1994). *Children as research subjects.* Oxford University Press.

Gunn, P. P., Fremont, A. M., Bottrell, M., Shuga, L. R., Galegher, L., & Biks, T. (2004). The Health Insurance Portability and Accountability Act privacy rule. *Medical Care, 42,* 321–327.

Gupta, M. (2003). A critical appraisal of evidence-based medicine: Some ethical considerations. *Journal of Evaluation of Clinical Practice, 9,* 111–121.

Halpern, S. A. (2004). *Lesser harm.* University of Chicago Press.

Hamilton, N. W. (2002). *Academic ethics.* American Council on Education.

Heitman, E. (2002). Cases for discussion. In R. E. Bulger, E. Heitman, & S. J. Reiser (Eds.), *The ethical dimensions of the biological and health sciences* (pp. 349–364). Cambridge University Press.

Hoit, J. D. (2005). Write right. *American Journal of Speech-Language Pathology, 14,* 171.

Hornblum, A. M. (1998). *Acres of skin.* Routledge Press.

Hornblum, A. M. (2007). *Sentenced to science.* Pennsylvania State University.

Horner, J., & Minifie, F. D. (2011a). Research ethics I: Responsible conduct of research (RCR)—History and contemporary issues pertaining to human and animal experimentation. *Journal of Speech, Language, and Hearing Research, 54,* S303–S329.

Horner, J., & Minifie, F. D. (2011b). Research ethics II: Mentoring, collaboration, peer review and data management and ownership. *Journal of Speech, Language, and Hearing Research, 54,* S330–S345.

Horner, J., & Minifie, F. D. (2011c). Research ethics III: Publication practice and authorship, conflict of interest, and research misconduct. *Journal of Speech, Language, and Hearing Research, 54,* S346–S362.

Horner, J., & Wheeler, M. (2005). HIPAA: Impact on research practices. *ASHA Leader,* 8–9, 26–27.

Huffman, N. P. (2003). Ethics: Employers, employees, and ethics. *ASHA Leader,* 23. http://www.asha.org

Ingham, J, C., & Horner, J. (2004). Ethics and research. *ASHA Leader, 9,* 10–25.

Ingham, J. C., Minifie, F. D., Horner, J. C., Robey, R. R., Lansing, C., McCartney, J. C. . . . Moss, S. E., (2011). Ethical principles as associated with the publication of research in ASHA's scholarly journals: Importance and accuracy of coverage. *Journal of Speech, Language, and Hearing Research, 54,* S394–S416.

Institute of Society, Ethics, and the Life Sciences. (1980). Applied ethics: A strategy for fostering professional responsibility. *Carnegie Quarterly, 28,* 1–7.

International Dual Loyalty Working Group. (2002). *Dual loyalty and human rights in health professional practice: Proposed guidelines and institutional mechanisms.* University of Cape Town Health Sciences Faculty.

Iverson, C., Flanagin, A., Fontanarosa, P. B., Glass, R. M., Glitman, P., Lantz, J. C., . . . Young, R. K. (1998). *American Medical Association manual of style.* Lippincott, Williams, & Wilkins.

Jakubowitz, M. (2011). Ethical issues in pediatric practice. *Seminars in Speech and Language, 32,* 347–356.

Jefferies, M., & Bauer, J. J. (2003, November). *Research ethics in graduate education* [Seminar presentation]. Annual meeting of the American Speech-Language-Hearing Association, Chicago, IL, United States.

Jonsen, A. R., Siegler, M., & Winslade, W. (2006). *Clinical ethics.* McGraw Hill.

Journal of the American Medical Association. (2006). Instructions for authors. *Journal of the American Medical Association, 295*(1), 103–116.

Kenny, B., Lincoln, M., & Balandin, S. (2010). Experiencing speech-language pathologist response to ethical dilemmas. An integrated approach to ethical reasoning.

American Journal of Speech-Language Pathology, 19, 121–134.

Knapp, S. J., & Van de Creek, L. D. (2006). *Practical ethics for psychologists.* American Psychological Association.

Korn, D. (2000). Conflicts of interest in biomedical research. *Journal of the American Medical Association, 284*(17), 2234–2237.

Krellstrom, S., Ross, S. N., & Fridland, R. (2011). Research ethics in dissertations: Ethical issues complexity of reasoning. *Journal of Medical Ethics, 36*, 425–430.

Kummer, A. W., & Turner, J. (2011). Ethics in the practice of speech-language pathology in health care settings. *Seminars in Speech and Language, 32*, 330–337.

Kwok, L. S. (2005). The white bull effect: Abusive co-authorship and publication parasitism. *Journal of Medical Ethics, 31*, 554–556.

Laine, C., & Mulrow, C. (2003). Peer review: Integral to science and indispensable to annals. *Annals of Internal Medicine, 139*(12), 1038–1040.

Lansing, C. R. (2002). Ethics: Loose lips: Confidentiality in relationships with colleagues. *ASHA Leader.* http://www.asha.org

Lansing, C. R., & Moss, S. (2003). Survey to determine knowledge of research ethics. *ASHA Leader, 8.* http://www.asha.org

Larsen, J., & McMillin, A. (2011). Ethical issues in the conduct of research at a multidisciplinary clinic. *Seminars in Speech and Language, 32*, 338–346.

Lo, B. (2003). Answers and questions about ethics consultation. *Journal of the American Medical Association, 290*(9), 1208–1210.

Ludlow, C. L. (2001). Responsible conduct of clinical research. In American Speech-Language-Hearing Association (Ed.), *Promoting research integrity in communication sciences and disorders and related disciplines* (pp. 29–45). ASHA.

Lum, C. (2002). *Scientific thinking in speech and language therapy.* Lawrence Erlbaum.

Macrina, F. L. (1995a). Mentoring. In F. L. Macrina (Ed.), *Scientific integrity* (pp. 15–40). American Society for Microbiology.

Macrina, F. L. (1995b). Scientific record keeping. In F. L. Macrina (Ed.), *Scientific integrity* (pp. 41–68). American Society for Microbiology.

Macrina, F. L. (1995c). Authorship and peer review. In F. L. Macrina (Ed.), *Scientific integrity* (pp. 69–96). American Society for Microbiology.

Mattick, K., & Blight, J. (2011) Teaching and assessing medical ethics: Where are we now? *Journal of Medical Ethics, 36*, 181–185.

McCarthy, M. P., Poole, K. L., & Solomon, B. (2007). Ethics: A model curriculum for teaching professional issues in university speech-language pathology and audiology programs. *Perspective on Administration and Supervision, 20*, 20–34.

McCartney, J. (2002). ASHA Code of Ethics and research. *ASHA Leader, 12.* http://www.asha.org

McWilliams, R., Hoover-Fong, J., Hamosh, A., Becik, S., Beaty, T., & Cuting, G. R. (2003). Local vs. central Institutional Review Boards for multicenter studies—Reply. *Journal of the American Medical Association, 290*(16), 2126–2127.

Meline, T. (2006). *Research in communication sciences and disorders.* Pearson.

Mertens, D. M. (2005). *Research and evaluation in education and psychology.* Sage.

Minifie, F. D., Robey, R. R., Horner, J., Ingham, J. C., Lansing, C., McCarthy, J. H., . . . Moss, S. E. (2011). Responsible conduct of research in communication sciences and disorders: Faculty, student perceptions. *Journal of Speech, Language, and Hearing Research, 54*, S363–S393.

Moss, S. (2006). Researchers discuss integrity in publications practices. *ASHA Leader, 26*, 34.

Moss, S. (2011). Promoting ethical research practices: Perspectives from pediatric populations. *Seminars in Speech and Language, 32*, 207–289.

Moss, S. E. (2010). Research integrity in communication sciences and disorders. *Journal of Speech, Language, and Hearing Research, 54*, S300–S302.

Mowatt, G., Shirran, L., Grimshaw, J. M., Rennie, D., Flanagin, A., Yank, V., . . . Bero, L. A. (2002). Prevalence of honorary and ghost authorship in Cochrane reviews. *Journal of the American Medical Association, 287*(21), 2769–2771.

Ness, R. B. (2007). Influence of the HIPAA privacy rule on health research. *Journal of the American Medical Association, 298*, 2164–2170.

Nosowsky, R., & Giordano, T. (2006). The Health Information Portability and Accountability Act of 1996 (HIPAA) privacy rule: Implication for clinical research. *Annual Reviews of Medicine, 57*, 575–590.

Oberman, A. S., Bosh-Missimov, T., & Ash, N. (2011). Medicine and the Holocaust: A visit to the Nazi death camps as a means of teaching ethics in the Israel Defense Forces' medical camps. *Journal of Medical Ethics, 36*, 826.

O'Herrin, J. K., Fost, N., & Kudson, K. A. (2004). The Health Insurance Portability and Accountability Act (HIPAA) regulations: Effect on medical record research. *Annals of Surgery, 239*, 772–778.

Olsen, D. P. (2003). HIPAA privacy regulations and nursing research. *Nursing Research, 52*, 344–348.

Olson, C. M., Rennie, D., Cook, D., Dickerson, K., Flanagin, A. &, Magen, J. W., . . . Pace, B. (2002). Publications bias in editorial decision making. *Journal of the American Medical Association, 287*(21), 2825–2828.

Polit, D. F., & Beck, C. T. (2010). *Nursing research: Principles and methods.* Lippincott.

Portney, L. G., & Watkins, M. P. (2009). *Foundations of clinical research.* Prentice-Hall Health.

Pozar, G. D. (2012). *Ethical and legal issues for health professionals.* Jones and Barlett.

Rennie, D. (2002). Fourth International Congress on peer review in biomedical publication. *Journal of the American Medical Association, 287*(21), 2759–2760. http://www.audiology.org

Reynolds, S. M. (2004). ORI findings of scientific misconduct in clinical trials and public funded research 1992–2001. *Clinical Trials*, 509–516.

Romanow, K. (2011). Bottom line: Possible HIPAA changes ahead. *ASHA Leader.*

Rose, C. D. (2003). Local vs. central Institutional Review Boards for multicenter studies. *Journal of the American Medical Association, 290*(16), 2126.

Rosenthal, R. (1999). Science and ethics in conducting, analyzing, and reporting psychological research. In D. N. Bergoff (Ed.), *Ethical conflicts in psychological* (pp. 127–133). American Psychological Association.

Sales, B. D., & Lavin, M. (2000). Identifying conflicts of interest and resolving ethical dilemmas. In B. D. Sales & S. Folkman (Eds.), *Ethics in research with human participants* (pp. 109–128). American Psychological Association.

Scheetz, M. D. (2001). Research integrity issues in the publication of research. In American Speech-Language-Hearing Association (Ed.), *Promoting research integrity in communication sciences and disorders and related disciplines* (pp. 46–54). ASHA.

Schneiderman, L. J., Glimer, T., Teetzel, H. D., Dugan, D. O., Blusten, J., Cranford, R., . . . Young, E. W. (2003). Effects of ethics consultations on nonverified life-sustaining treatments in the intensive care setting. *Journal of the American Medical Association, 290*(9), 1166–1172.

Scientific Research Society. (1986). *Honor in science.* Author.

Shamoo, A. E., & Resnik, D. B. (2003). *Responsible conduct of research.* Oxford University Press.

Shapiro, D. W., Wenger, N. S., & Shapiro, M. F. (1994). The contributions of authors to multiauthor biomedical research papers. *Journal of the American Medical Association, 271*(6), 438–442.

Sharp, H. (2001). Issues in ethics: Institutional Review Boards. *Cleft Palate Newsletter, 274*(4), 8.

Sieber, J. E. (1992). *Planning ethically responsible research.* Sage.

Silverman, F. H. (1998a). The "monster" study. *Journal of Fluency Disorders, 13*, 225–231.

Silverman, F. H. (1998b). *Research design and evaluation in speech-language pathology and audiology.* Allyn & Bacon.

Silverman, F. H. (1999). *Professional issues in speech-language pathology and audiology.* Allyn & Bacon.

Sininger, Y., March, R., Walden, B., & Wilber, L. A. (2004). Guidelines for ethical practice in research for audiologists. *Audiology Today, 15*(6), 14–17.

Society for Clinical Trials. (2004). Lying, cheating and stealing in clinical research. *Clinical Trials, 1*, 475–476. https://doi.org/10.1191/ 1740774504cn056ed

Steneck, N. H., & Bulger, R. E. (2007). The history, purpose, and future of instructions in the responsible conduct of research. *Academic Medicine, 82*, 829–834.

Strange, K. (2008). Authorship: Why not just toss a coin? *American Journal of Physiology–Cell Physiology, 295*, 567–575.

Washington, H. A. (2006). *Medical apartheid.* Random House.

Watson, J. B., Byrd, C. Y., & Moore, B. J. (2011). Ethics in stuttering treatment in schools. *Issues and Instruction Seminars in Speech and Language, 32*, 319–329.

Wikipedia. (n.d.). *Unethical human experiments in the United States.* http://en.wikipedia.org/

Wipke-Tevis, D. D., & Pickett, M. A. (2008) Impact of HIPAA on subject recruitment on retention. *Western Journal of Nursing Research, 30*, 39–53.

Wolf, M. S., & Benett, C. L. (2006). Local perspective of the impact of the HIPAA privacy rule on research. *Cancer, 106*, 474–479.

Yairi, E., & Ambrose, N. (2001). Longitudinal studies of childhood stuttering: Evaluation of critiques. *Journal of Speech Language and Hearing Research, 44*(4), 867–867. doi:10.1044/1092-4388(2001/069)

Yedidia, M. J., Gillespie, C. C., Kechur, E., Schwarz, M. D., Oakene, J., & Chepaitis, A. E., . . . Lipkin, M., Jr. (2003). Effects of communications training on medical student performance. *Journal of the American Medical Association, 290*(9), 1157–1165.

Yin, R. K. (2003a). *Application of case study research.* Sage.

Yin, R. K. (2003b). *Case study research: Design and methods.* Sage.

Young, J. R. (2003). The cat and mouse game of plagiarism detection. *Chronicle of Higher Education, 47*(43), A26.

3

Research Problems

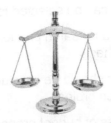

LEARNING OBJECTIVES

Upon completion of this chapter, the reader will be able to:

- Define and provide examples of independent and dependent variables
- Describe how variables and confounding factors may be controlled in a research project
- Describe how a topic can be selected for a research problem
- Discuss how to state a research problem, null hypothesis, and alternative hypothesis
- Describe what factors should be considered regarding the feasibility of a research project
- Discuss the six phases of budget preparation for a research project

Basic Concepts and Terms

Science is the search for knowledge. Orlikoff et al. (2022) described the scientific method as a method of efficiently or methodically generating knowledge by recognizing a problem capable of objective study, collecting data by observation or experimentation, and drawing conclusions based on analysis of the data. Silverman (1998) further described the scientific method as a set of rules used for describing, explaining, and predicting "events" that are observable and occur over time.

The scientific method is an effective tool for answering the types of questions that it was designed to answer. However, as Siegel (1987) points out, some questions in communication disorders (e.g., those involving social or personal values and attitudes) cannot be answered using pure methods of science.

Theoretically, studies can be classified as basic or applied experimental research. **Basic research** focuses on answering important questions or deciphering the laws of nature (Hegde, 2003; Shearer, 1982). **Applied research** employs the answers to basic questions of future research to practical problems, such as questions involving clinical practice.

Questions involving clinical management are answered using clinical or applied research models. Furthermore, clinical research may be experimental or descriptive. **Experimental studies** involve the use of rigorous design in which variables are carefully controlled. Experimental research in speech-language pathology and audiology is often weakened somewhat statistically because some variables cannot be controlled (Shearer, 1982).

Variables are capable of change or modification and may vary in quality or quantity. Examples of qualitative variables might include the gender of an individual, the disorder of speech or language with which an individual has been diagnosed, or the type of clinical management selected for patients. Quantitative variables such as intelligence can be measured quantitatively or numerically. **Discrete quantitative variables** are not expressed in decimals or fractions. Examples include the number of subjects in a study, scores on some tests, or the number of times a treatment is administered. **Continuous quantitative variables** can be expressed in any numerical value, including fractions. Examples include the age of subjects (i.e., 1.5 or 1½ years), scores on some tests that allow results to be expressed in whole numbers or in fractions, or subjects' height and weight data. Variables describe the population investigated by a study. Variables that do not change from individual to individual (such as a diagnosis of stuttering) are called **constant variables**.

Research in speech-language pathology and audiology is designed to investigate the cause(s) of specific communication disorders and the effect(s) of various phenomena on behaviors associated with communication disorders. *Dependent variables*, sometimes called outcome variables, are the effect of unknown etiology(ies). An example of a dependent variable is a hyperfunctional voice disorder characterized by a rough voice quality and accompanied by frequent upper respiratory infections, coughing, allergies, and laryngitis. The dependent variable must be described in operational terms so that it is clear how the variable will be identified and measured for a particular study (Hegde, 2003). An operational definition should have sufficient detail so that other researcher(s) can replicate the procedure or condition (Portney & Watkins, 2009). *Independent variables* explain the dependent variables. For example, an individual's vocal habits (talking frequently, loudly, and with excessive laryngeal tension) along with behaviors associated with a medical condition (laryngitis) might constitute identified independent variables explaining the dependent variable (a voice disorder defined according to description and accompanying medical condition). By manipulating independent variables, an investigator may change dependent variables involving disorders of communication. For example, reducing abusive vocal habits and medically testing the laryngitis may successfully affect a change in voice characteristics to a smooth, more relaxed, and pleasant voice production. Another example would be studying speech recognition scores at various signal-to-noise ratios (level of signal relative to the noise). In this example, speech recognition is dependent upon the signal-to-noise ratio used.

Hegde (2003) described three types of independent variables in communication disorders research, those that

1. explain the cause of normal parameters of communication;
2. explain the development of abnormal communication; or
3. identify treatment techniques that create optimal changes in communication.

The independent variables that can be manipulated (e.g., vocal habits and medical condition of the larynx and surrounding tissues) are active variables (Hegde, 2003). Some independent variables may be impossible to change (e.g.,

a predisposition for laryngeal vulnerability to abusive vocal habits)—these are called assigned variables (Hegde, 2003). They may play a role in determining outcome but cannot be controlled by the researcher. The experimental researcher attempts to rule out assigned variables. For example, if patients identified as having a predisposition or vulnerability to some voice problems and patients identified as having no predisposition or vulnerability to some voice problems and both improve by changing vocal habits and receiving medical intervention, the vulnerability variable may be ruled out, as the assumption that it causes hyperfunctional phonation is reduced.

Control of Variables

According to Portney and Watkins (2009), "an extraneous variable is any factor that is not directly related to the purpose of the study, but may affect the dependent variable" (p. 153). When extraneous variables are not controlled, they can have a confounding influence on the independent variable. For example, if a patient has a history of sinus congestion and drainage, then this extraneous variable could influence vocal quality.

Complete control of all confounding variables is usually not possible, which may lead to results that are inconclusive and difficult to interpret. Portney and Watkins (2009) suggest several methods that may help control for extraneous or confounding variables, such as random assignment of subjects, use of a control group, a well-defined research protocol, and blinding.

Random assignment of subjects means that each subject has an equal chance of being assigned to any group and ensures that assignments will be independent of personal judgment or bias. However, clinical research in speech-language pathology and audiology often involves using small numbers of subjects, and randomization can result in groups with disparate differences on critical variables. Researchers may use statistical means of comparing groups on initial values regarding the dependent variable to determine if the influence of any extraneous variable did balance out (Portney & Watkins, 2009). Control groups are frequently used by researchers to rule out the influence of extraneous variables. In a classic experimental design, subjects in a control group receive no form of treatment. This contrasts with the experimental group, which is targeted to receive the "new" treatment. This type of design strategy would lead the researcher to safely assume that if the treatment group is significantly different from the control group, then that is probably attributable to the influence of the "new" treatment. Portney and Watkins (2000) state that "the use of a control group is often unfeasible in clinical situations, for practical or ethical reasons" (p. 157). Because of such reasons, clinical researchers have a control group receive a "standard" form of treatment with the experimental group receiving a "new" form of treatment. Without comparison of these two groups, it is difficult to conclude that any form of treatment is responsible for an observed change.

A well-defined research protocol usually ensures that many extraneous variables have been considered and controlled. The protocol should have each procedure explained and detailed for another researcher to critically analyze what was done, for an Institutional Review Board (IRB) to make decisions, and to improve reliability. Research protocols should also include a description of all limitations in the study. Limitations would not prevent a study from being conducted but may help to recognize that other variables may not have been controlled, which may have influenced the obtained results.

It is preferable that blinding be used in studies whenever possible to avoid the possibility of consciously or subconsciously influencing the performance of a subject or the recording of data by a researcher. According to Portney and Watkins (2000), double-blind studies are "where neither the subjects nor the investigators are aware of the identity of the treatment groups until after the data are collected" (p. 159). In some cases, single-blind studies can be conducted where only the investigator or research team is blinded. A further discussion about how these aspects of research control might influence the validity and reliability of studies occurs later in this chapter.

Figure 3–1 demonstrates a model of the research process. Phases need to be completed in a sequential manner. This model is referenced in other parts of this text.

Selecting a Topic

Selecting a topic for a research project is influenced by many factors. First, it may be that a researcher or group of researchers share(s) a curiosity about a given topic. Second, it may be that a student must choose one topic to complete an academic requirement for a course or a degree. Third, a topic may be selected because clinical experiences have led a clinician to ask questions about the

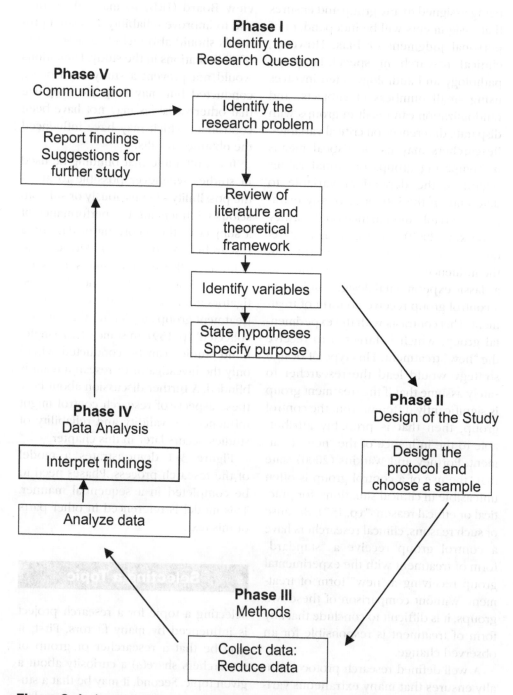

Phase I
Identify the
Research Question

Phase V
Communication

Identify the
research problem

Report findings
Suggestions for
further study

Review of
literature and
theoretical
framework

Identify variables

State hypotheses
Specify purpose

Phase IV
Data Analysis

Phase II
Design of the Study

Interpret findings

Design the
protocol and
choose a sample

Analyze data

Phase III
Methods

Collect data:
Reduce data

Figure 3–1. A model of the research process. From *Foundations of Clinical Research: Application to Practice* (2nd ed., p. 16), by I. G. Portney and M. P. Watkins, 2000, Pearson. Copyright 2000 Pearson Education, Inc. Adapted with permission.

impact of various treatment protocols. Whatever the reason for selecting a topic, it is important that it be something the researcher(s) is/are very interested in doing. Intrinsic motivation and the willingness to know why or how something occurs will drive other decisions in the problem-solving process. There are numerous topics that may be selected, and it may be challenging to determine which problem needs to be addressed first. Discussion with other researchers, faculty, and students should provide productive decision-making.

Selecting a Research Problem

Topics provide a general foundation to determine which *area* may be researched, but this then must be narrowed into a research *question*. A research question is usually answered in a single study (Portney & Watkins, 2000). It may start out very broad, but it does require refinement so that specific variables may be defined. The process of narrowing the research question can be facilitated by a review of the literature or "landmark" studies. Frequently, a review of studies relevant to the topic can provide good examples of the questions that have previously been asked and investigated.

The role of clinical experience may influence the type of research question that is asked (Maxwell & Satake, 2006). Clinicians often encounter situations with patients that are not easily explained. The clinician may believe that it is important to explain unexpected results to the patient and/or family. Research questions have been generated based on everyday clinical experiences.

Research questions may also result from working with different patient populations. For example, a clinician may find that a particular treatment protocol is very effective with one group of patients but does not have a similar impact on another group of patients. These situations can lead a clinician to question which variables differentiate the patients and necessitate the need to modify procedures.

Research is conducted to answer questions and is an increasingly important component of the field of communication sciences and disorders. To determine cause-and-effect relationships, researchers conscientiously apply scientific methodology to carefully control variables. Because of federal laws governing the education of individuals with disabilities and the importance of documenting outcome measures for treatment, it is imperative that the scientific method be implemented in basic and applied research projects.

Johnson (2006) proposed that, when posing an answerable question, a key starting point for evidence-based practice (EBP), the method known as PICO should be used: P = patient/population, I = intervention/ treatment/exposure, C = comparison, and O = outcome. Johnson (2006) stated that "The following is a PICO question of possible relevance to childhood speech-language disorders: 'Does group, as compared with individual, language intervention result in greater expressive language growth for preschool children with delays in language production'?" (p. 23). For this example, Johnson identified the following: "P = preschool children with delays in language production, I = group language intervention, C = individual language intervention, and O = expressive language growth" (p. 23).

Clinical theory is often used as a resource for developing research questions. Theories will guide and sometimes explain relationships between variables. In addition, they also may enhance the prediction of outcomes based on certain information (Portney & Watkins, 2009). However, it should be noted that research will not "prove" that a theory is or is not correct. Research either will or will not support the theoretical principles. Therefore, it is important that researchers carefully word the findings of a study in order to have any consumer of the research understand that nothing has been "proven" but can only support or refute a clinical theory.

Hypotheses and Theories

Hypotheses are often formulated for the purpose of testing theories that explain a phenomenon, event, or condition. Questions may be stated in the form of a formal or working hypothesis. The formal or **null hypothesis** to be accepted or rejected by a study is stated in negative terms. A null hypothesis states that there is "no statistically significant difference" or "no statistically significant relationship" between groups or variables. For example, to test the theory that phonological errors may be caused by the presence of a hearing loss, a null hypothesis attempts to eliminate bias from the hypothesis by declaring that no relationship exists between the variables (Hegde, 2003). Thus, the researcher attempts to reject the null hypothesis that there is no relationship between phonological

development and the presence of a hearing loss. Hegde (2003) cautions, however, that the null hypothesis does not eliminate or control for examiner bias. Objective interpretation of the results of a study requires objective, ethical research practices by a researcher with research education and experience, preferably initially in collaboration with experienced, objective researchers.

A working hypothesis, sometimes known as a **research hypothesis**, may simply ask a question, "Is there a difference?" or "Is there a relationship?" between groups or variables? When a researcher states in a hypothesis that there will be a change or describes a relationship in a certain direction, this is known as a **directional hypothesis**. For example, if the hypothesis states that "there is a high relationship" or "there is a low relationship," this would indicate that the researcher would believe the results of the study will not only be statistically significantly different, but also in a certain direction.

Research hypotheses should include the description of the **independent** and **dependent variables** (Portney & Watkins, 2000). A simple hypothesis includes one independent variable and one dependent variable, while a complex hypothesis contains more than one independent and dependent variables.

The acceptance or rejection of hypotheses (**null, nondirectional, directional, simple,** or **complex**) based on the results of one study are always interpreted as tentative. The findings of current studies may be replaced or expanded by future findings based on new theories, different clinical practice procedures, or changes in research methods. Like the records set by athletes, research findings often do not withstand expansion and changes in the knowledge bases. As Silverman (1998) stated,

> The final aspect of the scientific approach is being aware of the tentative nature of answers and hypotheses because it indicates that no answer to a question or test of a hypothesis is final. Thus, the language used to convey the conclusions reached by a researcher conducting any study revolves around the words "suggest," "support," or "refute" rather than "prove." (p. 33)

Feasibility of a Research Project

The feasibility of a research study needs to be considered very early in the research process (Portney & Watkins, 2000). Any research project that is worthy of investigating and investing of time and resources must undergo a "feasibility" test. The researcher may need to consider several factors when determining feasibility (Johnson, 2004):

- What previous experience does the researcher have with this topic?
- What are the risks/benefits for the subjects?
- What is the duration of the project?
- Does a "pilot study" need to be conducted? If so, will subjects require screening?
- Will an Institutional Review Board (IRB) approve the protocol?
- Will the consent form need to be translated for non-English speakers?

What about consent for subjects with mental disabilities or learning disabilities?
- Can the research protocol be adequately integrated with routine standards of care?
- Is specialized equipment required? If so, how will it be calibrated and maintained?
- Are outside personnel required to conduct special procedures or efficacy measures?
- What are the frequency and severity of an adverse event (AE)?
- Are the inclusion/exclusion criteria reasonable to meet anticipated subject enrollment?
- Will the following factors impede subject enrollment: age, duration of participation, frequency of visits, and procedural discomfort?
- Will extended hours be required? If so, is current staffing adequate to conduct the protocol?
- Will personnel requirements compete with other research projects?
- How much funds will be necessary to conduct the project? Who will pay for them? What about personnel time? What if there is a long-time lag between receiving budgetary funds and initiating the study? Will subjects need to be paid for their time?

Feasibility of a research study needs to be carefully discussed with all involved parties during the planning phase. After several discussions with key personnel, a "go/no go" decision is made by all parties. The next phase involves the development of a budget, which encompasses several phases.

Budgetary Considerations and Preparation

Rowell (2004) suggests that there are six phases when developing a research budget (Figure 3–2). Phase one is the preparation phase. During this time, the researcher(s) should have a good idea of what they can and cannot do, know the costs of services that will be necessary to complete the project, and develop a "charge master." It is important to determine start-up costs by considering the following: IRB fees, IRB preparation, protocol review time, copies, equipment (and any upgrades), chart reviews, database reviews, prestudy visits, any pharmacy and lab setups, administrative oversight, and regulatory requirements.

When considering the per-patient cost, it important to determine direct cost (what will be involved with direct subject contact), variable costs (charges that depend on items that the subject may or may not require), and time for the researcher to conduct the experiment. Rowell (2004) states that time is the most underestimated value when considering per-patient costs. This may not only include researcher salary, but fringe benefits that must be paid for a researcher. In addition, close-out costs need to be considered and include administrative costs, closing out records, and long-term storage of records.

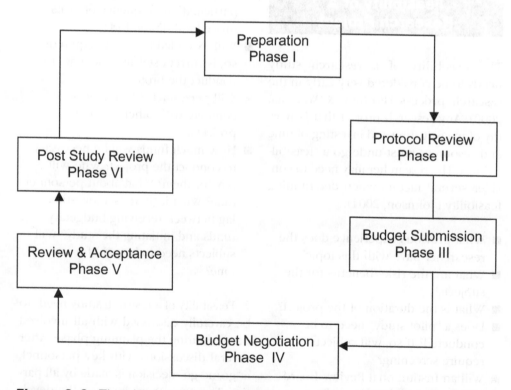

Figure 3–2. The six phases of a research site budget. From *Clinical Research Workshop,* by J. Rowell, 2004, LSU School of Medicine, Division of Research and Department of Pediatric/Section on Clinical Pharmacology. Copyright 2004 LSUHSC-Shreveport. Adapted with permission.

Phase two involves the protocol review phase. It is important that the principal investigator (PI) choose realistic timelines for completion of the study. Time is one variable that can be easily under- or overestimated. During this phase, it is important to consider the amount of time for the following:

- **Consent process**—may take approximately 45 min to 1 hr, including a discussion about the Health Insurance Portability and Accountability Act (HIPAA)
- Screening failure compensation—if a subject does not meet the criteria for inclusion in the study, how is the subject compensated?
- Payments for unscheduled procedures such as adverse events, tests, and failures
- Advertising for subjects, including print and electronic media
- Costs that may be necessary if the study runs longer than expected
- Time for the "coordinator" or someone who has administrative oversight of the project, which includes protocol revisions, meetings, consent or reconsent forms, audits, training, travel, faxing, and preparing source documents

Phase three includes the budget submission to the funding source. There are various ways this may be done, including flat rate (nonnegotiable), small up-front payments, competitive bidding, high performance, and speedy enrollment performances. Rowell (2004) suggests requesting more funding than may be expected is possible. However, any sponsor or supporter of the research may require a single cost figure per patient and justification for each cost.

Phase four includes budget negotiation. In some instances, a sponsor or funding source may allow for some negotiation before support will be provided. It is important that, during negotiation, the sponsor understand the commitment of the researcher toward the project. Enthusiasm and dedication can lead a sponsor or funding agency to support the project at the level required to be successful. If adjustments are necessary by the researcher, it is important that they be carefully considered so as not to jeopardize the completion of the protocol or violate IRB rules and regulations.

Phase five of the process includes the review and acceptance of the budget. During this time, be sure to use your Charge Master (spreadsheet) to determine that all charges are accurate. Carefully review the contract and seek legal counsel when necessary. Does the contract state a startup date? How will the contract be paid? What are the milestones for payment? Payment method can vary, but it may include one-fourth of the budget to cover start-up and screening costs or payment when one-half of the enrollment target is completed.

Phase six is also called the "poststudy" phase of the budget. This phase takes place when all obligations have been met and all payments have been received. At this time, the researcher(s) should review the Charge Master to see if it was indeed accurate, asking, for example, the following questions: Did the budget reflect the work performed? Have all fees been paid? Were there extra procedures that were not requested in the original budget?

Budgetary issues should not be an afterthought. Careful planning of time commitment, supplies, administrative costs, and site preparation need to be included early when discussing the feasibility of a study. Failure to carefully consider these issues could result in some projects being initiated but not completed, thus resulting in a waste of time and resources. Furthermore, all subjects should clearly understand any type of compensation that is due and what is not to be paid. Further examples and information regarding the use of a Charge Master can be found at https://www.researchgo.ucla.edu/research-billing-and-coding (UCLA CTSI ResearchGO, 2022).

Summary

By the time a research project is published, it has been organized and presented in an established, straightforward format. However, the actual process of conducting research is not as organized as one might think after reading numerous published articles that have been repeatedly edited. Hegde (2003) described a formative view of research as an evolving process. After much discussion and pondering, numerous false starts, and repeated attempts, a project may emerge and develop. However, many worthy projects are abandoned in the process. Braddom (1990) provides an in-depth outline or guide to assist in the identification of specific omissions or errors in the major sections of a completed research project.

Some significant findings in science over the years have been based on accidental discoveries. Hegde (2003) refers to serendipity in research as evidence that worthwhile projects are not always carefully planned. Accidental discoveries may be the reward for flexibility and a creative sense of inquiry on the part of observers when conducting a research project.

(?)

DISCUSSION QUESTIONS

1. What is an independent variable? Provide an example of it in research.
2. What is a dependent variable? Provide an example of it in research.
3. What is meant by experimental control? What are some examples of things that can be controlled in a research project?
4. What is the purpose of a control group? Why might it be difficult to have a control group involved in clinical research?

5. How might a researcher decide on a general topic for inquiry? How might the researcher decide on a specific problem to study?
6. What is the difference between a null hypothesis and a research hypothesis? Provide an example of each.
7. Why would a conclusion that forms a hypothesis only "suggest" rather than "prove" something?
8. What are some variables to consider when determining the

feasibility of a study? When is feasibility determined? Who makes the decision for "go/no go"?

9. What are the six phases of planning a budget?
10. What is a Charge Master? What variables might be included in it?

References

Braddom, C. (1990). A framework for writing and/or evaluating research papers. *American Journal of Physical Medicine, 69,* 333–335.

Hegde, M. N. (2003). *Clinical research in communicative disorders* (3rd ed.). Pro-Ed.

Johnson, C. J. (2006). Getting started in evidence-based practice for childhood speech-language disorders. *American Journal of Speech-Language Pathology, 15,* 20–35.

Johnson, V. A. (2004, March). *Feasibility and risk management in clinical trials* [Paper presentation]. Clinical Research Workshop, Louisiana State University Health Sciences Center, Shreveport, LA, United States.

Maxwell, D. L., & Satake, E. (2006). *Research and statistical methods in communication sciences and disorders.* Thomson Delmar.

Orlikoff, R. F., Schiavetti, N., & Metz, D. A. (2022) *Evaluating research in communication disorders.* Pearson Education.

Portney, L. G., & Watkins, M. P. (2000). *Foundation of clinical research: Applications to practice* (2nd ed.). Prentice-Hall Health.

Portney, L. G., & Watkins, M. P. (2009). *Foundation of clinical research: Applications to practice* (3rd ed.). Prentice-Hall Health.

Rowell, J. P. (2004, March). *The six phases of a successful research budget* [Paper presentation]. Clinical Research Workshop, Louisiana State University Health Sciences Center, Shreveport, LA, United States.

Shearer, W. S. (1982). *Research procedures in speech, language, and hearing.* Williams & Wilkins.

Siegel, G. M. (1987). The limits of science in communication disorders. *Journal of Speech and Hearing Disorders, 52*(3), 306–312.

Silverman, F. H. (1998). *Research design and evaluation in speech-language pathology and audiology* (4th ed.). Allyn & Bacon.

UCLA CTSI ResearchGO. (2022). *Research billing and coding.* https://www.researchgo.ucla.edu/research-billing-and-coding

4

Locating, Accessing, and Assessing Information

Anne Marie Sisk and David Irwin

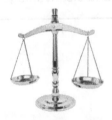

LEARNING OBJECTIVES

Upon completion of this chapter, the reader will be able to:

- Discuss the methods involved in a successful literature search
- Describe speech-language pathology and audiology journals that allow online access
- List some commonly used databases
- List some commonly used tools of critical appraisal
- Describe the content of critical appraisal of topic (CAT)
- List the advantages and disadvantages of using a CAT

Introduction

Locating information for a research project can be done efficiently and effectively if the speech-language pathologist or audiologist applies some basic principles regarding literature searches. Furthermore, after the literature is obtained, it is important that assessment of the research reports involves a systematic approach to summarizing and organizing the evidence. There are many tools available to critically appraise evidence-based information for clinical practice. This chapter provides information about locating, accessing, rating, classifying, and reporting levels of evidence that can be used for clinical practice. It also provides an example of a critical appraisal of a study.

Locating Information

Speech-language pathologists and audiologists should utilize a variety of methods when locating information for research and consumer health materials. As computers and various databases are now available for professionals to utilize, it is not possible to know all information that has been published. For example, the Cumulative Index to Nursing and Allied Health Literature (CINAHL) has a Subject Heading List of over 16,000 headings, nearly half of which cover unique nursing and allied health topics (https://www.ebsco.com/products/research-databases/cinahl-database). According to Portney and Watkins (2009), there are numerous sources such as indexes and abstracts that provide bibliographic listing of several thousand articles and conference proceedings.

Clinicians and students conducting research are busy and need strategies to locate and access critical information. Furthermore, more researchers are expecting full-text online articles after completing the bibliographic search. It is important that a researcher utilize all sources of information when locating sources. A reference librarian at a university library is a valuable resource in learning to conduct effective and informative literature searches. The reference librarian will help guide literature searches and provide instruction about using the various databases that include research in health sciences. It is important that any researcher have a topic and utilize the strategies presented in Chapter 3 to determine a topic of interest. Specificity about a topic facilitates any literature search and provides the reference librarian with key word information.

In Figure 4–1, CINAHL (2001) provides a strategy for a successful literature search that should be used when locating resources. Figure 4–1 emphasizes the importance of using a logical sequence when conducting literature searches. Subject headings need to be carefully worded utilizing key words that will allow the search process to specifically pull articles, abstracts, or books relevant to the topic. If a literature search utilizing an online system is not successful in retrieving information, then it may require rephrasing the heading or reconsidering the topic (CINAHL, 2001).

Databases

Numerous databases can assist the researcher when locating information. These databases may include literature

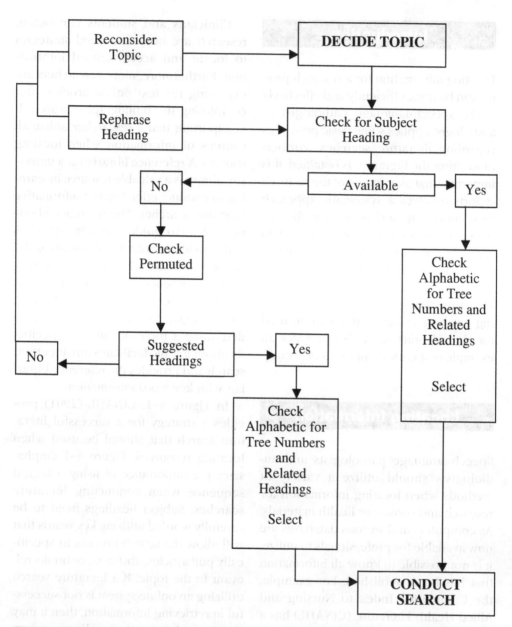

Figure 4–1. Strategies for a successful literature search. From "Strategies for a Successful Literature Search," by CINAHL Information Systems, 2001 (https://health .ebsco.com/products/the-cinahl-database). Flow Chart Copyright © 2001 Cinahl Information Systems. Reprinted with permission.

from around the globe, and some allow for online access. Johnson (2006) also provides a list of databases that may be utilized regarding children with speech and language disorders. Table 4–1 lists some commonly used indexes and databases for references and abstracts in science and related areas.

Table 4–1. Commonly Used Indexes and Databases for References and Abstracts in Science and Related Areas

Database	Description
Academic Search Premier	A multidisciplinary database that covers scholarly journals in biomedical fields, social sciences, humanities, education, physical sciences, and engineering.
ASHAWire	A collection of research, publications, and other publications from the American Speech- Language-Hearing Association at https://pubs.asha.org/index.aspx
CINAHL: Cumulative Index to Nursing & Allied Health Literature	Available from several vendors, CINAHL indexes journals in nursing and allied health. Some versions provide full text of many articles.
Clinical Research Education (CREd) Library	The newest addition to ASHA Wire, the CREd Library hosts a dynamic collection of resources on topics critical to the conduct and advancement of high-quality clinical practice research in the communication sciences and disorders (CSD) domain.
Cochrane Library	The Cochrane Library is a collection of databases created to supply evaluated, high- quality information in support of evidence- based medicine. Although its focus is necessarily broader, it does contain material relevant to communication disorders.
Dissertation Abstracts	A bibliographic database that indexes doctoral dissertations and master's theses from about 1,000 graduate schools and universities. About 47,000 new dissertations and 12,000 new theses are added annually.
EBSCO Information Services	EBSCO offers library resources to customers in academic, medical, K–12, public library, law, corporate, and government markets. Its products include EBSCONET, a complete e-resource management system, and EBSCOhost, which supplies a fee-based online research service with 375 full-text databases, a collection of 600,000-plus e-books, subject indexes, point-of-care medical references, and an array of historical digital archives. In 2010, EBSCO introduced its EBSCO Discovery Service (EDS) to institutions, which allows searches of a portfolio of journals and magazines.
ERIC (Educational Resources Information Center)	ERIC indexes information from education journals, including articles on communication disorders in an educational context.

continues

Table 4–1. *continued*

Database	Description
JSTOR	A series of full-text archives covering scholarly journals. Subscriptions are available for discipline-specific or multidisciplinary subsets of the archive, some of which contain journals relevant in communication disorders.
Linguistics & Language Behavior Abstracts	This database indexes and provides summaries of journal articles in the language sciences, including communication disorders as well as broader subjects such as linguistics.
PsycINFO	PsycINFO contains over two million citations and abstracts of journal articles, book chapters, books, and dissertations. More than 65,000 new records are added each year.
PubMed	PubMed, produced by the National Library of Medicine and available to the public without charge, indexes about 4,000 journals covering all aspects of the health sciences. Much of this content is also licensed to commercial vendors for use on their database platforms for a fee.
Web of Science	A bibliographic database that covers many scholarly journals in the sciences.

Data Mining

Data mining, generally, is the process of analyzing data from different perspectives and discovering new patterns from large datasets involving the intersection of several areas of science procedures and related databases (Wikipedia, 2012). This term is also called *data fishing* and *data snooping*.

Technically, data mining can be used to find correlations or patterns in field in large relational databases. Data mining can be conducted in a variety of different ways with the use of more advanced software and machine learning. In general, the relationships are sought among the following areas: (1) Classes: stored data in predetermined groups. For example, a researcher may be concerned with the variables of individuals with stuttering and perceptions that potential employers have toward such individuals. (2) Clusters: data items are grouped according to logical relationships and determine potential markets. For example, an audiologist may be interested in determining which groups are best for dispensing hearing aids. (3) Associations: data can be used to identify associations such as the relationship between hearing loss and the development of phonological development in children. (4) Sequential patterns: data are used to anticipate behavior patterns and trends. For example, a researcher may study the identification of hearing loss and how many batteries are purchased in a month by various clients (Frand, 2012).

The use of data mining methods in communication sciences and disorders is an emerging field of interest. A study by Danubianu et al. (2010) utilized the association portion of data mining with a case study. The authors used associative data mining with a method of speech-language treatment. They used the database developed from a single-subject case study to answer the following questions: What is the predicted final state for a child or what will his or her state be at the end of various stages of therapy? Which are the best exercises for each case? Which factors might be associated with certain family characteristics and the success of therapy? In general, the authors determined that associative data mining can be used in communication sciences and disorders. However, more research is needed to explore the use of data mining in the use of finding effective assessment and treatment procedures. Similarly, Danubianu et al. (2018) found that data mining could be used to create personalized therapy programs adapted to specific patient characteristics.

The application of data mining has occurred frequently in business, with Walmart pioneering massive amounts of datasets to transform its supplier relationships. Data mining is also being used in sports, gaming, and health care. The more data being processed and the more complex the queries to do data mining are require a more powerful system (Frand, 2012).

Online Journals

Online journals may or may not be free. The American Speech-Language-Hearing Association (ASHA) offers online access to its membership (http://www.asha.org). Access to online journals is sponsored by ASHA, and some date back from 1980 to the present. These include *American Journal of Audiology* (AJA); *American Journal of Speech-Language Pathology* (AJSLP); *Journal of Speech, Language, and Hearing Research* (JSLHR); *Language, Speech, and Hearing Services in the Schools* (LSHSS); and ASHA Leader Online (more information can be found at https://pubs.asha.org/). "CiteTrack" provides email alerts when new content is published that matches specific selected parameters, quick and advanced searches from http://www.highwire.org, improved "Googling," and personal folders (ASHA, 2006). The American Academy of Audiology (AAA) allows access to the *Journal of the American Academy of Audiology* online at http:// www.audiology.org, and it does not require membership in AAA.

Many journals are subject to a publication embargo. This means that access to the full text becomes available only after a specified period—generally 6 to 12 months, but up to 2 years for a few journals. Most databases that contain free journal access online are identified by the "free" icon. Open access journals are free to the public and rapidly increasing in popularity. In 2012, there were 327,766 articles available on this platform, and by 2017, there were 563,146 available (Crawford, 2018). Today, there are over 9 million articles available by simply accessing the *Directory of Open Access Journals & Articles* (https://doaj.org/).

Use of the World Wide Web (Internet)

The World Wide Web (WWW) is frequently one of the first sources that researchers and/or consumers of health information utilize when locating information. Although, the internet provides an excellent source of information, it "must be recognized that this resource cannot replace the quality materials accessible from professional organizations, peer-reviewed health-care journals, the Cochrane Library, etc." (Levy, 2002, p. 1).

O'Brien (2001) made the point that

> information on the WWW needs to be evaluated because, while some of it is accurate, some of it can be potentially dangerous as there can be a lack of peer review or regulation and because the information can be inaccurate and misleading. (p. 42)

Levy (2002) provides a credibility checklist that can be utilized when evaluating research on the internet.

The checklist includes the following:

- Look at the URL. These include .gov for government sites, .edu for educational sites, or .org for not-for-profit organizations (O'Brien, 2001).
- Look for information from trained and licensed health professionals. Cooke (1999) suggests that affiliations be noted.
- The mission and objectives of any organization should be given at the website so conflicts of interest and advertising can be considered (Cooke, 1999; O'Brien, 2001).
- Statements about any website limitations, scope, or purpose should be carefully considered (Cline & Haynes, 2001).
- Be certain that the information has been peer reviewed. Review the credentials of the reviewers and determine if conflicts of interest might be present (Levy, 2002).

- Although the website may look professional, be sure that references and sources are clearly listed. Also, check when the site was last updated.

It is important for researchers and consumers of health-care research to understand that the acceptance rate on the internet for information is probably 110%. Therefore, all information should be carefully scrutinized when reviewing information from any website. The use of the internet may be one of the first resources used, but it certainly should not be the only one.

Interlibrary Loan

Interlibrary loan is one method of obtaining information that may not be available in electronic format or books that may have limited editions. A reference librarian can help when making requests for an interlibrary loan. Charges for the interlibrary loan may or may not exist depending on the agreement the libraries have with each other. Many libraries allow for online requests for interlibrary loan through the ILLiad system. Many loans can be delivered to the user's desktop, depending on the delivery method used by the library that filled the request.

Manual Searches

Manual searches involve going to the periodical sections of a library and reviewing articles that are bound into annual issues. This method may seem somewhat antiquated compared to the use of computerized databases, but it still provides an excellent method to review literature. Probably the most useful aspect of a manual search includes the review of more "classic" studies and other types of research that have not been transferred to electronic formats. Furthermore, photographs and other types of visual information that may not be available in online searches can be reviewed during a manual search. It is important that any researcher not be limited to publications that are available only in electronic format. According to Galvan (2006), landmark studies and theorists with historical importance in developing an understanding of a topic or problem can be achieved by utilizing a manual search.

Social Media

The use of social media—such as email, message boards, Skype, Instagram, X, and Facebook—is one method for expanding research. The use of these methods for communication has increased dramatically within the last few years. Quinnell (2011) discussed that using social media for research and researcher development allows for collection of data from a wide range of stakeholders. The author conducted interviews using asynchronous message boards, Skype, and email conversations. In addition, this author was able to network with other policymakers and organizations on a variety of topics and related issues. There are ethical and logistical issues associated with the use of these types of social media that must be considered. However, as these methods become more widely used, more platforms become available that are reliable and secure.

Evaluating Research

Evaluating research evidence is important for several reasons. First, sources of evidence are heterogeneous; in other words, not all sources of evidence are equal. Second, the quality of clinical services is related to evidence and the manner in which it was obtained and presented. Third, application of research to clinical practice is related to the level of evidence (Finn et al., 2005). Last, the use of high-level evidence in making clinical decisions is an ethical responsibility; that is, evidence-based practice is fundamental to ethical practice.

There is a need for speech-language pathologists and audiologists to utilize evidence-based results to make clinical decisions. Unfortunately, this is not always the case. Zipoli and Kennedy (2005) found that speech-language pathologists used clinical experiences and opinions of colleagues more frequently than research studies or clinical practice guidelines to make clinical decisions. Utilization of research reports can be facilitated by a step-by-step process. These steps include (a) asking a question, (b) finding the highest level of evidence, (c) critically appraising the evidence, (d) integrating the evidence with clinical experience and client values, and (e) evaluating the decision-making process (Boswell, 2005; Johnson, 2006; Kully & Langeven, 2005). Evaluating research reports requires critical analyses. Methods of evaluating research reports can be classified as traditional, evidence based (levels of evidence), and criterion based in distinguishing between science and pseudoscience. Clinical Appraisals of Treatment Evidence (CATEs) are a format for evaluating a treatment study for evidence-based information.

Several systems have been developed for classifying levels of evidence (Agency for Healthcare Research and Quality, 1999; ASHA, 2004; Hadorn et al., 1996; Ottenbacher, 2002; Queensland Center, 2000). The systems are generally based on levels of evidence according to quality and credibility from highest/most credible to lowest/least credible.

Rating the Evidence

Rating the level of evidence is challenging (Yorkston et al., 2001). Hadorn and associates (1996) believe that it is not clear as to what counts as evidence, and evenless clear what weight to assign to different types of evidence. Four questions are usually considered in evaluating the literature for strength of evidence. These questions and more description of the criteria are in Table 4–2 (Yorkston et al., 2001). Chambless and Hollon

(1998) rated the level of evidence based on guidelines of the American Psychological Association. Three questions were considered: (a) Has the treatment been shown to be beneficial in controlled research?; (b) Is the treatment useful in applied clinical settings, and if so, with what patients and under what circumstances?; and (c) Is the treatment efficient in the sense of being cost-effective relative to other alternative treatments? Dawes et al. (1999) also described questions that are important when reviewing a paper on treatment. These questions are listed in Table 4–3.

Levels of Evidence

It is important to recognize the level of evidence in evaluating research. Typically, research evidence is classified according to levels based on the type and quality of research (ASHA, 2004).

Table 4–2. Four Questions Used in Evaluating Literature for Strength of Evidence

How well were the subjects described?

How well was the treatment described?
- Rationale for treatment
- Replication of treatment

What measures of control were used in the study?
- Reliability and stability of outcome measures (inter- or intrarater reliability, dispersion of scores)
- Support for internal validity (outcome measures obtained with or without treatment; improved performance with treatment in progressive disorders)
- Presence of comparison or control group

Are the consequences of the treatment well described?
- Outcome measures at levels of impairment, activity limiting, restriction in participation
- Risks and complication of treatment

Table 4–3. Important Questions When Reviewing a Paper on Treatment

Did the authors answer the question(s)?

Were groups of patients randomized?

Are the comparison groups similar?

Were patients "blinded"?

Was it placebo-controlled?

Was evaluation of efficacy "blinded"?

Was the length of study appropriate?

What was the follow-up rate?

Are there clear measures of outcomes?

The earliest evidence scale was published in 1994 by the American Academy of Neurology. This evidence scale has a hierarchy of three levels of evidence. These levels of evidence are on a continuum of hierarchy, based on study design; that is, evidence based on opinion of respected authorities, evidence from case-controlled studies, and evidence from randomized controlled clinical trials. Class III, the lowest level of evidence, is evidence provided by expert opinion, case studies, case reports, and studies with historical controls. Class II evidence is that provided by at least one or better designed, observational, clinical studies with concurrent controls, that is, single case-control or cohort-control studies. Class I, the highest level of evidence, is provided by at least one well-designed, randomized controlled clinical trial (ASHA 2005; Wertz, 2002).

Hadorn and associates (1996) described a hierarchy of seven levels of evidence based on study design (Table 4–4). The seven levels of evidence were collapsed into three levels: A, B, and C. "A"-level evidence consisted of levels one through three, "B"-level evidence consisted of levels four through six, and "C"-level evidence was seven or expert opinion. "A" is most rigorous, and "C" is least rigorous. Four levels (A–D) of evidence for intervention were described by Ottenbacher (2002). Minor and major flaws were identified for eight aspects of study methodology: selection of patients, allocation of patients to treatment group, treatment regimen, study administration, withdrawal from the study, patient blinding (randomized clinical trials only), outcome measurement, and statistical analysis. Minor flaws include deviations from good practice that do not create a potential for bias large enough to cast doubt on the validity of a study. Major flaws create a potential for bias large enough to question a study's results.

Critical Appraisal

Unfortunately, published papers can have flaws that may occur anywhere along the publication process (Dawes et al., 1999). Critical appraisal is important in examining the rigors with which a study was conducted, and thus the amount of confidence placed in the findings. Speech-language pathologists and audiologists should read and critique the literature to stay current on prevailing clinical research findings and apply what is known to clinical practice (Frattali & Worrall, 2001). Critical appraisal involves the application of knowledge about research design to the literature (Gallagher, 2001).

There are several tools available for the critical appraisal of published papers.

Table 4–4. Hierarchy of Seven Levels of Evidence Based on Study Design

---

1. Supportive evidence from well-conducted randomized controlled trials that included over 100 patients or more.

   a. Evidence from a well-conducted multicenter trial

   b. Evidence from a meta-analysis that incorporated quality ratings in the analysis and included a total of 100 patients in its estimates of effect size and confidence intervals.

2. Supportive evidence from well-conducted randomized controlled trials that included fewer than 100 patients.

   a. Evidence from a well-conducted trials at one or more institutions

   b. Evidence from a meta-analysis that incorporated quality ratings in the analysis and included fewer than 100 patients in its estimate of effect size and confidence intervals

3. Supportive evidence from well-conducted cohort studies

   a. Evidence from a well-conducted prospective cohort study or registry

   b. Evidence from a well-conducted retrospective cohort study

   c. Evidence from a well-conducted meta-analysis of cohort studies

4. Supportive evidence from a well-conducted case-control study

5. Supportive evidence from poorly controlled or uncontrolled studies

   a. Evidence from randomized clinical trials with one or more major or three or more minor methodological flaws that could invalidate the results

   b. Evidence from observational studies with high potential for bias (such as case studies with comparison to historical controls)

   c. Evidence from case studies or case reports

6. Conflicting evidence with the weight of evidence supporting the recommendation

7. Expert opinion

Sources: From "Rating the Quality of Evidence for Clinical Practice Guidelines," by J. S. Hodges and N. Hicks, 1996, *Journal of Clinical Epidemiology, 49*(7), pp. 749–754; and "Identification and Nursing Management of Dysphagia in Adults with Neurological Impairment," by the Queensland Center of the Joanna Briggs Institute, 2000, *Best Practice Information Sheets for Health Professions, 4*(2). Retrieved October 10, 2002, from http://www.joannabriggs.edu/BPFSdysl.html

ASHA (https://www.asha.org/research/ebp/bias-appraisal-tools-and-levels-of-evidence/) links to several user-friendly tools on their website, including Appraisal of Guidelines Research and Evaluation (AGREE II), CATmaker, and Duke Critical Appraisal Worksheets. All of these tools provide a set of critical appraisal tools with specific questions that walk the user through the analysis.

CATmaker uses a well-established format known as a Critically Appraised Topic (CAT). A CAT is a summary of a critical review of the best evidence on a specific topic (Worrall & Bennett, 2001). It is a written outcome of the evidence-based practice (EBP) process. A CAT begins with a declarative title and then indicates a "clinical bottom line," which describes the clinical action that results from the report (Sackett et al., 2000). There are five major types of CATs: (a) diagnosis/screening, (b) progress, (c) evaluating risk and harm in case-controlled studies, (d) evaluating risk and harm in a control study, and (e) intervention (treatment, prevention, and screening; Law, 2002). An example of a CAT on treatment of voice problems of teachers is shown in Table 4–5. Another example of a critical review-based format is presented in Table 4–6. Johnson (2006) suggests the development of collaborative working groups to develop a system for developing a large database of CATs (Johnson, 2006).

Critical appraisals are not without critics. Several problems have been identified that warrant discussion (Woolf, 2000; Yorkston et al., 2001). First, there

is frequent reliance on a single indicator of study quality, that is, marked emphasis on one type of research—randomized controlled trials. Second, individuals are strikingly heterogeneous despite common diagnostic categories. Third, there is an incomplete base of evidence; that is, the research literature is not sufficiently current and complete to answer all clinical questions; there are important gaps in evidence. Fourth, not all sources of information are readily available through electronic searches. Excessive and inadequate critical appraisal can lead to premature adoption or abandonment of treatment and result in overlooking potential harms of more effective treatment alternatives. In addition, critical appraisal can do harm if valid evidence is rejected. Last, critical appraisal lacks systematic application. Criteria to determine which studies are rated "bad" or "good" should be specific and consistent.

Another criticism is the amount of time to write and apply CATs. Worrall and Bennett (2001) suggested that CATs

Table 4–5. Example of a Critically Appraised Topic (CAT) on Treatment of Teachers with Voice Problems

Clinical Bottom Line:	Amplification for teachers with voice problems yields better outcome than vocal hygiene instruction for six weeks.
Citation:	Roy, N., Weinrich, B. Gray, S. P., Tanner, K., Toledo, S. W., Dove, H., Corbin-Lewis, K., & Stemple, J. C. (2002). Voice amplification versus vocal hygiene instruction for teachers with voice disorders: A treatment outcomes study. *Journal of Speech-Language-Hearing Research, 45,* 625–638.
Clinical Question:	Which is more effective for treatment of teachers with voice problems, voice amplification (VA) or vocal hygiene (VH) instruction?
Search Terms:	Voice disorders, treatment, teachers, voice amplification, vocal hygiene.
Design:	Prospective, randomized control group.

Table 4–6. Example of a Critical Review-Based Format

Study	Class I
Study Title:	Voice amplification versus vocal hygiene instruction for teachers with voice disorders: A treatment outcomes study.
Authors:	Roy, N., Weinrich, B., Gray, S. D., Tanner, K., Toledo, S.W., Dove, H., Corbin-Lewis, K., & Stemple, J. C.
Year of Publication:	2002
Source:	*Journal of Speech-Language-Hearing Research, 45*, 625–638.
Design:	Prospective, randomized clinical trial
Subjects:	44 voice disordered teachers randomly assigned to one of three groups: voice amplification (VA, *n* = 15); vocal hygiene (VH, *n* = 15), nontreatment control group (*n* = 14).
Treatment:	VA consisted of using Chatter Box portable amplifier. VH program was adapted from Morrison et al.'s (1994) program
Duration and Intensity of Treatment:	6 weeks
Outcome Measures:	Voice Handicap Index; voice severity self-rating scale; audio recording for later acoustic analysis
Analysis:	Descriptive statistics
Results:	Clearly support clinical validity of amplification as alternative for treatment of voice disorders in teachers

can be undertaken by groups of speech-language pathologists and audiologists. Students and practicing professionals are involved with interest groups and journal clubs. Resources and expertise can be shared in developing CATs. CATs can be the product of one individual or a small group of individuals, and may be subject to error, bias, and other limitations inherent in non-peer-reviewed materials (Law, 2002). CATs can also be flawed because of the speed in which they are created.

Summary

Locating, accessing, and assessing the evidence is an essential part of evidence-based practice. Appropriate clinical decisions require systematic evaluation and integration of evidence from published research studies, reports, and other sources. It is important to summarize the results of critical appraisal and share this information with practicing speech-language pathologists and audiologists.

DISCUSSION QUESTIONS

1. Describe the strategy for a successful search.
2. Discuss how databases are utilized for literature searches.
3. What are some of the types of data mining being used for research? How might these be used for communication sciences and disorders?
4. Discuss some uses of social media that can be used for research and researcher development.
5. What are some journals that are available online? Are these always free?
6. Who is the person in a library who will probably help the most when doing a literature search?
7. Why is rating the level of evidence from a body of literature difficult?
8. What are some key questions to ask when rating the strength of evidence?
9. How can evidence be classified?
10. What is a critical appraisal?
11. What are the key components of a critically appraised topic or paper?
12. Discuss the relative advantages and disadvantages of using CATs.

References

Agency for Healthcare Research and Quality. (1999). *Diagnosis and treatment of swallowing disorders (dysphagia) in acute care stroke.* http://ahrq .gov/clinic/spcsums/dysphsum.htm

American Speech-Language-Hearing Association. (2004). *Evidence-based practice in communication disorders: An introduction* [Technical report]. https://www.asha .org/topicindex/

American Speech-Language-Hearing Association. (2005). *Evidence-based practice in communication disorders* [Position statement]. http://www.asha.org/members/deskrefjournals/deskref/ default

American Speech-Language-Hearing Association. (2006). Online access expands for journals. *ASHA Leader.* http://www.asha.org/about/publications/leader-on-line/archives/2006/060411b.htm

Boswell, S. (2005). Finding the evidence for school-based clinical decision making. *ASHA Leader*, 26–27, 39.

Chambless, D. L., & Hollon, S. D. (1998). Defining empirically supported therapies. *Journal of Consulting and Clinical Psychology, 66*(1), 7–18.

Cline, R. J. W., & Haynes, K. M. (2001). Consumer health information seeking the Internet: The state of the art. *Health Education Research, 16*(6), 671–692.

Cooke, A. (1999). Quality of health and medical information on the Internet. *British Journal of Clinical Governance, 4*(4), 155–160.

Crawford, W. (2018). *Gold open access journals 2012–2017.* Cites & Insights Books. https://waltcrawford.name/goaj3.pdf

Cumulative Index in Allied Health Literature Information Systems. (2001). *Strategies for a successful literature search*. CINAHL Information Systems.

Danubianu, M., Pentiuc, S. G., Tobolcea, I., & Schipor, O. A. (2010). Advanced information technology-support of improved personalized therapy of speech disorders. *International Journal of Computers Communications and Control, 5*, 684–692.

Danubianu, M., Pentiuc, S. G., Tobolcea, I., & Soraciu, T. (2018). Model of a data mining system for personalized therapy of speech disorders.

Dawes, M., Davies, P., Gray, A., Mant, J., Seers, K., & Snowball, R. (1999). *Evidence-based practice*. Churchill Livingstone.

Finn, P., Bothe, A. K., & Bramlett, R. E. (2005) Science and pseudoscience in communication disorders. *American Journal of Speech-Language Pathology, 14*, 172–186.

Frand, J. (2012). *Data mining: What is data mining?* http://www.anderson.ucla.edu/faculty/Jason.frand/teacher/technologies/palace/datamining

Fratalli, C., & Worrall, L. E. (2001). Evidence based practice: Applying science to the art of clinical care. *Journal of Medical Speech Language Pathology, 9*(1), ix–xi.

Gallagher, T. M. (2001). Implementation of evidence-based practice communication disorders course work and practicum. In P. Hargrove, R. McGuire, C. O'Rourke, & W. Swisher (Eds.), *Proceedings of the Council of Academic Program in Communication Sciences and Disorders* (pp. 29–45). Council of Academic Programs in Communication Sciences and Disorders.

Galvan, J. L. (2006). *Writing literature reviews* (3rd ed.). Pyrczak.

Hadorn, D. C., Baker, D., Hodges, J. S., & Hicks, N. (1996). Rating the quality of evidence for clinical practice guidelines. *Journal of Clinical Epidemiology, 49*(7), 749–754.

Johnson, C. J. (2006). Getting started in evidence-based practice for childhood speech-language disorders. *American Journal of Speech-Language Pathology, 15*, 20–35.

Kully, D., & Langeven, M. (2005). Evidence-based practice in fluency disorders. *ASHA Leader*, 10–11, 23.

Law, M. L. (2002). *Evidence-based rehabilitation*. Slack.

Levy, J. R. (2002). Searching the CINAHL database Part 4: Accessing consumer health information and patient education materials. *CINAHLnews, 21*(4), 1–3.

Mason, P. (2011). *How to grow social media leads: New research*. https://pdfs.semanticscholar.org/45c7/bc8513109888ce36e6d3085ff52c439c8c7f.pdf

O'Brien, K. (2001). The World Wide Web and consumer health information. *Collegian, 8*(4), 42.

Ottenbacher, K. J. (2002, June). *Critical appraisal of evidence-based intervention* [Paper presentation]. Boston University Faculty Summer Institute, Boston, MA, United States.

Portney, L. G., & Watkins, M. P. (2009). *Foundations of clinical research: Applications to clinical practice* (2nd ed.). Prentice-Hall Health.

Queensland Center for the Joanna Briggs Institute. (2000). *Identification and nursing management of dysphagia in adults with neurological impairment. Evidence-based Practice Information Sheets for Health Professions*. http://joannabriggs.org/contact.html

Quinnell, S. L. (2011). *Using social media for research and researcher development*. https://onlinelibrary.wiley.com/doi/abs/10.1002/meet.2011.14504801283

Sackett, D. L., Strauss, S. E., Richardson, W. S., Rosenberg, W., & Haynes, R. B. (2000). *Evidence-based medicine*. Churchill Livingstone.

Wertz, R. T. (2002). Evidence-based practice guidelines: Not all evidence is created equal. *Journal of Medical Speech-Language Pathology, 10*(3), xi–xv.

Wikipedia. (2012). *Data mining*. http://en.wikipedia.org/wiki/Data_ mining

Woolf, S. H. (2000). Taking critical appraisal to extremes. *Journal of Family Practice, 49*(12), 1081–1085.

Worrall, L. E., & Bennett, S. (2001). Evidence-based practice: Barriers for speech-language pathologists. *Journal of Medical Speech Language Pathology, 9*(2), xi–xvi.

Yorkston, K. M., Spencer, K., Duffy, J., Beukelman, D., Golper, L. A., Miller, R., & Sullivan, M. (2001). Evidence based medicine and practice guidelines: Application to the field of speech-language pathology. *Journal of Medical Speech-Language Pathology, 9*(4), 243–256.

Zipoli, R. P., & Kennedy, M. (2005). Evidence-based practice among speech language pathologists: Attitudes, utilization, and barriers. *American Journal of Speech-Language Pathology, 14*(3), 208–220.

5

Literature Review

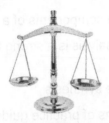

LEARNING OBJECTIVES

Upon completion of this chapter the reader will be able to:

- Prepare and organize various types of literature reviews
- Explain the limitations of narrative reviews
- Describe the difference between narrative and systematic reviews
- List and describe the components of a systematic review
- Explain why meta-analysis is a strong technique for making clinical decisions
- Define best evidence synthesis
- Discuss the limitations of practice guidelines
- Select best available practice guidelines

Literature reviews are at the core of any research. There are two broad types of literature reviews. First, they can be completed to guide primary, original research (Mertens, 2005). This category of literature reviews can be completed to ensure a research project is focused and relevant. This first type of research is typically referred to as a "review of the literature" and is integrated with the introduction of most research articles. A literature review of this nature might also be referred to as a background literature review. The second broad type of literature reviews are those that can be research in and of themselves. These include narrative or traditional; systematic; meta-analysis, best evidence synthesis; and practice guidelines. All have potential limitations, many of which can be overcome by using an evidence-based approach. The more rigorous the method of reviewing the literature and the quality of the primary research that is reviewed, the more evidence-based the review will be (Cook et al., 1997).

Reviewing the literature involves consideration of potential biases related to publication practices, variable quality of the studies involved in the review, and inclusion-exclusion criteria (Mertens, 2014). For example, there is a tendency for research with statistically significant results to be published (referred to as publication bias). Conversely, research studies that show no difference are published less frequently because they either are not submitted or are rejected more often. Literature reviews can be biased by data exclusion that is methodologically questioned or subjective selection of studies for inclusion in the review. Watching for these biases is a necessary part of reviewing literature for any reason.

In this chapter, we will first discuss general principles that apply to organizing literature reviews, then discuss how to conduct a review of the literature or background literature review, and finish with a description of literature reviews that are research in and of themselves: narrative review, systematic review meta-analysis, best-evidence synthesis review, and clinical practice guidelines.

Organizing Literature Reviews

A number of steps are involved in preparing and organizing a literature review as summarized in Figure 5–1. As the figure shows, after identifying potential sources, references need to be located and screened for relevancy to the topic being reviewed. References that seem appropriate are read, notes are taken, and inappropriate references are discarded.

As mentioned in the previous chapter, one reference may provide citations to several other relevant references. After all relevant references have been reviewed they are organized, analyzed, and synthesized. Organization facilitates analysis of the topic or evidence and synthesizes the literature. Information can be organized into four categories based on relevance: A-pile: highly relevant; B-pile: somewhat relevant; C-pile: might be relevant; and X-pile: not relevant (DePoy & Gitlin, 2011). Also, there are several ways literature can be organized to provide a visual summary of research and it is typically represented as a table or figure (Creswell, 2003).

One approach to organizing and integrating the literature is a chart summarizing each study (DePoy & Gitlin, 2011).

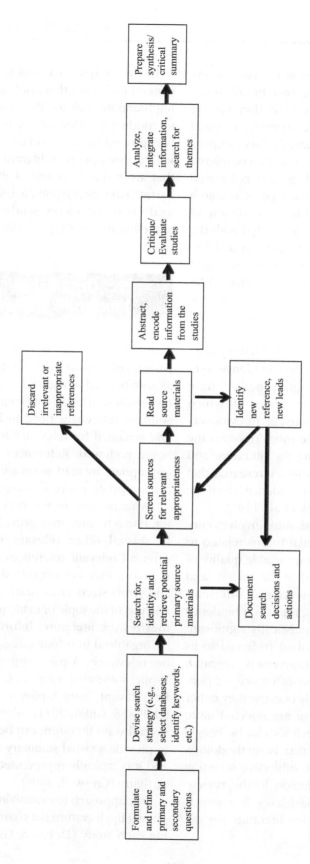

Figure 5–1. Steps in preparing a literature review. From *Nursing Research: Principles and Methods* (p. 105), by D. F. Polit and C. T. Beck, 2004, Lippincott Williams & Wilkins. Reprinted with permission from Lippincott Williams & Wilkins.

The figure shows the following boxes and flow:

- Formulate and refine primary and secondary questions
- Devise search strategy (e.g., select databases, identify keywords, etc.)
- Search for, identify, and retrieve potential primary source materials
- Document search decisions and actions
- Screen sources for relevant appropriateness
- Discard irrelevant or inappropriate references
- Read source materials
- Identify new reference, new leads
- Abstract, encode information from the studies
- Critique/Evaluate studies
- Analyze, integrate information, search for themes
- Prepare synthesis/critical summary

These charts are sometimes referred to as evidence tables (Golper et al., 2001). A chart is used in considering the literature as a whole as well as critically evaluating and identifying research gaps. An example of a literature review table is presented in Table 5–1.

Another approach to organizing the literature is a concept/construct matrix in which information is organized by key concept (*x*-axis) and source (*y*-axis). A matrix helps in identifying specific concepts that need to be discussed in the written report (DePoy & Gitlin, 2011). This approach can be a preliminary step in developing a concept map, which is described in Chapter 11.

Background Literature Reviews

Literature reviews that serve as a background for research papers are an important part of any research project. Background literature reviews are also referred to as "reviews of the literature" in speech-language pathology and audiology. They are typically part of the introductory section of any research article, and they serve three main purposes. The first purpose is that they report on research that has been previously done on a topic to ensure a specific project focuses on the best aspect of a particular issue. The second purpose is to describe the theoretical and conceptual background of the research project. The third reason for a review of the literature is to demonstrate the purpose and significance of the research project.

Prior to beginning a search for literature to serve as background for a research project, it is recommended to establish a topic area by creating a working title to the research project (Creswell, 2014). When creating a title, it is helpful if a researcher can finish the following statement: "my study is about . . ." (Creswell, 2014). For example, if a researcher wanted to study early childhood literacy issues, an initial statement could be, "my study is about early childhood literacy." After more information is gathered from a search based on these terms, a statement such as this could then lead to the development of a working research project title that includes more specific information such as, "An ethnography: Preschool education teachers' early childhood literacy knowledge."

Individuals writing a literature review as part of reporting the results of a research project should review and include all relevant research on a topic

Table 5–1. Literature Review Table

Type of Study	Primary Focus	Number of Subjects	Measures	Conclusions
Randomized Clinical Trials	Voice amplification resonance therapy	6+	Voice Handicapped Index Voice Severity Self-Rating	Voice resonance therapy group improved

area as well as cite sources that help explain to the reader the reasons for the study. It should be noted that once an article related to the overall topic is found, the references cited in that article can serve as a starting point to collect other relevant information to include in the research project literature review.

Additionally, prior to conducting a review of this nature, the researcher should form a question (discussed previously; Creswell, 2014). Once a working title is formed, it will be easier to form a tentative research question. Based on the previous example, a good question to pose under the working title of "An ethnography: Preschool education teachers' early childhood literacy knowledge" would be, "What is the knowledge base of preschool education teachers regarding early childhood literacy?" A question of this nature would allow the researcher to investigate the knowledge base and understanding of the teacher-participants.

After a question is formed, there are various recommended sequences to conducting the literature review. Creswell (2014) recommends a 7-step process:

1. Identify a few key words. You can begin by selecting some of the terms used in your working title. Initial readings about your topic area may also yield a few useful key words.
2. Go to the library and search both onsite and online sources using the key words you have identified.
3. Try to acquire a minimum of 50 resources either in the form of articles or books that support your topic area.
4. Narrow the number of resources down to the most relevant.

5. Once you have identified the most useful literature, form a literature map, or a visualization (of your choosing), of the types of research you have so that you can begin categorizing it.
6. Write summaries of the articles that you know you will use. These summaries will start to form the first written draft of the literature review portion of your article. While you are engaged in this process, it is recommended that you begin a citation or reference list using the guidelines of the American Psychological Association (APA, 2020).
7. Construct your literature review in written form. It should be organized according to themes or relevant concepts. It should not be organized by authorship of the articles you are reviewing.

There are certain criteria related to the organization and completeness of a background literature review. McMillan (2012) provides several criteria that guide the researcher in both critiquing and creating a strong literature review:

1. A review of the literature should cover all previous research thoroughly and adequately.
2. A review of the literature should describe the results of other research studies. It should not simply report opinions of others on a specific topic.
3. A review of the literature should be current. The studies that are included should be recent. If the majority of the studies cited are from the 1980s in a paper written in 2017, that literature review would not be considered current.

4. A review of the literature should both summarize and analyze the included studies. When an author includes a study in the literature review, they should not just report findings but also discuss their quality and value to the current study.

5. A review of the literature should be organized by most relevant topic. In other words, paragraphs should cover overall issues and include a few articles in each paragraph to illuminate that issue. The review of the literature should not be organized into paragraphs that simply report on each article that has been chosen for the review of the literature

6. When summarizing articles, talk about minor studies minimally and go into more detail on the major studies that have been conducted on your topic area.

7. There should be a clear reason to conduct the research project based on the studies described in the review of literature.

8. The theoretical background of the study should be well described in a review of the literature. All strong research projects identify and describe the guiding theory that helps to shape the purpose and overall design of the study. The review of literature should clearly describe this aspect of the project.

Table 5–2 contains excerpts from a research project that studied how typically developing siblings of children with autism spectrum disorder mediated social interaction for the sibling with the communication impairment (Abendroth,

2011). These excerpts provide examples of how resources are woven into the introduction/review of the literature portion of a published research article to accomplish several of the previously recommended criteria.

As noted earlier, this chapter addresses several types of literature reviews. The one just described serves the purpose of providing background to a research project. The following sections apply primarily to narrative reviews, systematic reviews, meta-analysis, best-evidence synthesis reviews and clinical practice guidelines, though some aspects of the following section of this chapter may be adapted for background literature reviews.

Formulating Questions for Literature Reviews

It should be noted that this section applies to literature reviews that are research in and of themselves, or literature reviews such as narrative review, systematic review, best evidence synthesis, and so forth. For these types of literature reviews, formulating a question is the first step in the process. This involves determining the type of question, background or foreground. *Background questions* ask for general information about a condition or process—who, what, when, and so forth. *Foreground questions* focus on specific information about clinical decisions or recommendations. Background questions are usually asked because of the need for basic information.

The first step in evidence-based practice and systematic reviews is formulation of clinical guidelines questions. Two methods for formulating clinical

Table 5–2. Example of Review of the Literature Criteria

Indicating the theoretical and conceptual background of the study:

Human beings depend on social interaction during childhood to facilitate cognitive development, construct a working knowledge of the world, and condition cultural expectation in young children (Bruner, 1983; Tomasello, 1990). This is the case from earliest childhood through later language and cognitive development.

Discussing previous research and need for the study:

Previous research on siblings of children with autism spectrum disorder has largely examined the efficacy of a particular intervention involving a typically developing sibling rather than the strategies employed by that sibling (e.g., Bauminger, 2007; Tsao & Odom, 2006; Wolfberg, 2003).

Consequently, previous researchers have not exhaustively evaluated typically developing siblings' natural attempts at mediation for a child with autism spectrum disorders.

Demonstrating a clear reason to conduct that study:

Previous research on siblings of children with ASD has largely examined the efficacy of a particular intervention involving a TD sibling rather than the strategies employed by that sibling (e.g., Bauminger, 2007; Tsao & Odom, 2006; Wolfberg, 2003). Consequently, previous researchers have not exhaustively evaluated typically developing siblings' natural attempts at mediation for a child with ASD.

Source: Abendroth, K. J. (2011) Sibling mediation of children with autism spectrum disorders. *Journal of Interactional Research in Communication Disorders, 2*(1), 85–100.

questions have been described in the literature: PICO and PESICO. Each letter in the acronyms stands for a specific component.

PICO stands for population, intervention, comparison, and outcome. Descriptions for each component are listed in Table 5–3.

This term was first described in 1995 by Richardson et al.. PICO has been used in evidence-based medicine and has been adopted for use in speech-language pathology and audiology. The adequacy and stability of PICO was evaluated by Huang et al. (2006). It was reported that

PICO primarily focused on questions and was less suitable for clinical questions related to diagnosis, prognosis, and etiology. A web-based tutorial for understanding PICO and answering questions as well as accessing and assessing the evidence was developed by LaRue et al. (2009). PICO can be used to answer clinical questions such as the following:

1. What intervention was studied?
2. What outcome is measured?
3. What is studied?
4. Who are the researchers?
5. What are the results?

Table 5–3. Description of PICO Components

Component	Description
Patient Population	**Patient population or disorder of interest** Age Gender Ethnicity
Intervention	**Intervention or range of interventions** Exposure to disorder Prognostic factors Risk(s)
Comparison	**Comparison of intervention** No disorder Placebo or no intervention Prognosis Absence of risk factor(s)
Outcome	**Outcome of interest** Risk of disorder Accuracy of diagnosis Rate of occurrence of adverse outcome

Source: From *Evidence-Based Practice* (pp. 25–37), by R. Nolan, E. Fine-out-Overholt, and P. Stephenson, In B. A. M. Melynk and E. Fineout-Overholt (Eds.), 2005, Philadelphia, PA: Lippincott Wilkins & Wilkins.

6. What is the final analysis/practical application?

PESICO was described by Schlosser et al. (2007). The six components of PESICO are person, environments, stakeholders, intervention, comparison, and outcomes. Table 5–4 summarizes the PESICO framework.

There are differences between PICO and PESICO. PICO is the more frequently used framework for formulating questions. PESICO has two additional components: environments and stakeholders. It may be that PICO does not include these two components because it is based on a medical model that focuses less on environmental and stakeholder issues (Schlosser et al., 2007). See the Schlosser et al. (2007) article for detailed PESICO examples.

The templates described in this section are especially useful when conducting literature reviews for the purpose of finding the best available evidence for practice in speech-language pathology or audiology and writing systematic reviews of literature. It should be noted that PICO and PESICO frameworks were not initially designed to inform background

Table 5–4. PESICO Framework

Component	Description
Person or problem	Age
	Gender
	Ethnicity
	Risk
	Diagnosis or classification
	Sensory status
	Motor status
	Cognitive status
	Communication competence
Environments	Current
	Future
	Communication
Stakeholders	Direct (person)
	Secondary (others)
	Perception of problem
Intervention	Treatment or intervention options
Comparison	Comparison of options
Outcomes	Effectiveness (acquisition, generalization maintenance of skills)
	Efficiency
	Communication partners
	Self-determination
	Quality of life
	Stakeholders

Source: From "Asking well-built questions for evidence-based practice in augmentative and alternative communication," by R. W. Schlosser, R. Kuol, and J. Costello, 2006, *Journal of Communicative Disorders, 40*, pp. 225–238.

literature reviews (discussed earlier). However, it should be noted that they can be adapted for this purpose if necessary.

Narrative Reviews

Traditional *narrative reviews* are nonsystematic reviews of the literature. At one time, narrative reviews were the most prevalent approach to synthesizing the speech-language pathology and audiology literature. However, this has changed in recent years. Systematic reviews are much more prevalent (e.g., Fisher 2017; Rudolph, 2017). There are three major disadvantages of narrative reviews: (1) the sources and identification of studies are not described; (2) the search terms are not specified; and (3) the criteria for including and excluding studies are not specific (Schlosser, 2000). In addition, narrative reviews do not provide a detailed description of each study. Typically, narrative literature reviews are at risk for subjectivity in selecting, evaluating, and interpreting studies.

A more systematic alternative to narrative review has been developed called the scoping review (Arksey & O'Malley, 2005). The Canadian Institutes of Health research defined the scoping review as "an exploratory project that systematically maps the literature available on a topic, identifies key concepts, theories, sources of evidence and gaps in research." Overall, the scoping review examines the information that is available on a topic and helps to determine if a full systematic review should be initiated; it also summarizes the findings. Ultimately, the scoping review identifies gaps that may exist in the available research on a specific topic (Arksey & O'Malley, 2005). Overall, the scoping review is a more systematic and specific variation of a narrative review.

Systematic Reviews

Melnyk and Fineout-Overholt (2015) define *systematic reviews* as "a scientific approach to summarize, appraise, and communicate the results and implications of several studies that may have contradictory results" (p. 126). Systematic reviews are the basis of evidence-based practice (Pring, 2004). These reviews are a source of evidence to guide practice and identify the need for further research (Bannigan et al., 1997). In addi-

tion, systematic reviews have the potential for facilitating the transfer of research evidence into clinical practice and for helping readers understand generalization and consistency of research findings (McCauley & Hargrove, 2004). Parts of a systematic review are listed in Table 5–5.

Table 5–5. Systematic Review Template

Abstract
- Purpose
- Method
- Conclusion

Introduction
- Background/Need
- Purpose/Question

Method (Source Selection)
- Inclusion Criteria
- Exclusion Criteria

Sources
- Electronic databases
- Key words

Total Number of Sources Identified
- Number of sources excluded
- Number of sources included

Discussion
- Quantitative analysis
- Qualitative analysis

Conclusion
- Criterion-based recommendations
- Limitations
- Clinical Implications
- Future Research

References

Tables
- Table 1 Reference levels
- Table 2 Evidence table (appraisal summary of studies)

It should be noted that a challenge often encountered in systematic reviews is a type of literature referred to as gray literature (Hartling et al., 2005). Gray literature includes unpublished studies or services that are not published in peer-reviewed journals (Portney & Watkins, 2009). Gray literature is difficult to locate or retrieve by using electronic databases. The gray literature is heterogeneous and varies substantially in design and quality. Gray literature should be explicitly identified and reported as such in the written portion of any systematic review.

Additionally, a systematic review can be a method for locating, appraising, and synthesizing evidence (Petticrew, 2001). A number of steps are involved in preparing a systematic review, as summarized in Table 5–6. The initial steps are related to finding evidence and later steps focus on using evidence. These are essentially the same steps involved in the development of meta-analysis and evidence-based guidelines.

The last step of conducting a systematic review is writing a report. The report should be concise, conform to standards for professional writing, and provide a critical analysis/synthesis of current information related to the topic. Additionally, the report should identify gaps in knowledge and research needs. It should not simply list what research has been done on the topic. The report should provide the confirming and contradictory evidence about possible explanations of findings (APA, 2020; DePoy & Gitlin, 2011).

There are several reasons for undertaking a systematic review. Among them are to (1) summarize large amounts of information; (2) provide decision-makers with synthesized information; (3) explain consistency and inconsistency of data; (4) identify conflicts; (5) increase power and precision in estimates of risk or effect size; (6) identify gaps in knowledge; and (7) improve treatment (Seers, 1999).

Systematic reviews vary in quality and should be critically appraised. Some systematic reviews are misleading because the quality of the review is poor or biased. In other words, a systematic review may not present accurate analysis/synthesis of research reports. Criteria for evaluating and making recommendations about systematic reviews are presented Table 5–7. Melynk and Fineout-Overholt (2015) suggest a rapid checklist for appraising a systematic review, which consists of three questions: (1) Are the results of the review valid?; (2) What were the results?; and (3) Will the results assist me in caring for clients?

Systematic reviews are available from the websites of the Academy of Neurologic Communication Disorders and Sciences, American Academy of Audiol-

Table 5–6. Steps in Conducting a Systematic Review

Problem Formulations
Information search and retrieval
• Search terms (Key words)
• Search electronic and manual
– Level of evidence
Analysis and synthesis of evidence
• Grades for recommendation of use
Report results

Source: From *Foundation of Clinical Research*, by L. G. Portney & M. P. Watkins, 2009, Upper Saddle River, NJ: Pearson; and *Research in Education*, by J. H. McMillian & S. Schumacher, 2010, Boston, MA: Pearson.

Table 5–7. Criteria for Evaluating Systematic Review

Grade Recommendations	Criterion
A. Good evidence for inclusion	There is good peer-review evidence supporting consideration of use for the treatment
B. Fair evidence for inclusion	There is fair peer-review evidence supporting consideration of use for the treatment
C. Insufficient evidence	There is insufficient peer-review evidence for inclusion supporting consideration of use for treatment although recommendations for use are possible on other grounds
D. Fair evidence for exclusion	There is fair peer-review evidence supporting that the treatment should be excluded from consideration of use
E. Good evidence for exclusion	There is good peer-review evidence supporting that the treatment should be excluded from consideration

Source: From "Evidence-Based Practice in Schools: Integrating Craft and Theory with Science and Data," by L. M. Justice and M. E. Fey, 2004, *ASHA Leader, 9*(4–5), pp. 30–32. Copyright 2004 by American Speech-Language-Hearing Association. All rights reserved. Reprinted with permission.

ogy, American Speech-Language-Hearing Association (ASHA), and the Cochrane collections. These reviews can also be located by manual searches of professional journals. Systematic reviews have been published in a variety of journals in speech-language pathology and audiology. ASHA's National Center of Evidence-Based Practice in Communication Disorders (N-CEP) has made available systematic reviews of several areas of research in the field of speech-language pathology and audiology. Additionally, ASHA has developed guidelines to help in the critical appraisal and application of systematic reviews such as the criteria described in Tables 5–7 and 5–8.

Systematic reviews regarding speech-language treatment have been criticized. Pring (2004) believes many researchers do not follow appropriate procedures for clinical outcomes research. In addition, many studies on which systematic reviews are based have methodological problems and often fail to adequately describe treatment, thereby making it impossible to evaluate or compare different types of treatment.

Garrett and Thomas (2006) responded to Pring's (2004) "Ask a Silly Question: Two Decades of Troublesome Trials" by stating that systematic reviews using qualitative and/or statistical methods for combining studies can be completed within or across any phase of outcome research. Furthermore, systematic reviews can be informative because they help bring together what is, and what is not, known and suggest treatments that may be beneficial or in need of further research.

Pring (2006) replied to Garrett and Thomas (2006) by stating that "systematic reviews are essential to evidence-based practice" (p. 208). Three advantages of

Table 5–8. Examples of Outcomes From Systematic Reviews

Criteria	Yes	No
Did the review address a focused clinical question?		
Were tables used to show key features and to facilitate comparisons of studies?		
Were the criteria used to select articles for inclusion appropriate?		
Is it unlikely that important relevant studies were missed?		
Was the validity of the included studies appraised?		
Were assessments of the studies reproducible?		
Were the results similar from study to study?		
Are the results of a systematic review clear?		
Are the results precise?		
Can the results be applied to my client care?		
Were all clinically important criteria considered?		
Are the benefits worth the harms and costs?		
Were potential conflicts of interest disclosed?		

Sources: Adapted from *Systematic Review* (pp. 85–101), by K. Seers, In M. Dawes, P. Davies, A. Gray, J. Marx, K. Seers, and R. Snowball (Eds.), 1999, New York, NY: Churchill Livingstone; and "Making Sense of an Often Tangled Skein of Evidence," by the Editors, 2005, *Annals of Internal Medicine, 142*(12), pp. 1019–1020.

systematic reviews were identified by Pring: (1) they can provide an overall effect size for treatment of a client group; (2) where different types of treatment have been provided, systematic reviews can compare the effect sizes to determine which treatment is more effective; and (3) the influence of experimental design on the overall effect size can be determined. Furthermore, methodological problems associated with systematic reviews "serve as a further reminder that primary research must be both systematic in its development and rigorous in its procedures" (Pring, 2006, p. 110).

It should be noted that a valuable resource when searching for quality systematic reviews is the Cochrane Collaboration. This organization prepares, maintains, and disseminates systematic reviews. The Cochrane Collaboration requires that systematic reviews address specific decision points; objectives; criteria for considering studies; types of studies; types of participants; types of intervention; types of outcome measures; search strategy; methods for selection of studies; awareness of methodological quality; data management; and data synthesis (Douglas et al., 2004).

Differences Between Narrative and Systematic Reviews

There are major differences between a regular narrative review of the literature and a systematic review. Narrative reviews may lack the objectivity, rigor, and comprehensiveness of systematic reviews (Johnson, 2006). Systematic reviews use more specific search strategies and criteria for inclusion and exclusion. These and other differences are compared in Table 5–9. Overall, systematic reviews are considered superior to narrative reviews for synthesizing research (Meline, 2006).

Meta-Analysis

Meta-analysis is a systematic review in which a statistical summary is provided. It is a relatively recent approach to quantitative synthesis of previous studies which should not be confused with traditional reviews of the literature. In other words, meta-analysis is a statistical approach for combining studies on the same topic to determine the efficacy of a procedure or treatment (Haynes & Johnson, 2009).

Steps in developing and completing a meta-analysis are listed in Table 5–10.

Table 5–9. Differences Between Narratives and Systematic Reviews

Feature	Narrative Review	Systematic Review
Question	Broad, general question	Focused or hypothesis to be tested
Sources and Search	Usually unspecified, risk for bias; do not usually attempt to locate all relevant literature	Comprehensive sources; specific search strategy
Selection	Usually unspecified risk for bias	Criterion-based selection, uniform application; limit selection bias
Appraisal	Variable; do not consider differences in study method or quality	Rigorous systematic critical appraisal; investigate potential biases and sources of heterogeneity
Synthesis	Qualitative	Quantitative
Inferences	Sometimes evidence-based; do not differentiate between sound and unsound studies	Usually evidenced-based; base conclusions on most methodologically sound studies

Sources: From "Systematically Reviewing the Evidence," by M. Law and I. Phillip, 2002. In M. Law (Ed.). *Evidence-Based Rehabilitation* (pp. 109–126). Thorofare, NJ: Slack Incorporated; "Systematic Reviews: Synthesis of Best Evidence for Clinical Decisions," by M. D. Cook, C. D. Murlow, and R. B. Haynes, 1997. *Annals of Internal Medicine, 126*(5), pp. 376–380; and "Systematic Reviews for Astronomy to Zoologoy: Myths and Misconceptions," by M. Petticrew, 2011. *British Medical Journal, 322*, pp. 98–101.

Table 5–10. Steps of a Meta-Analysis

- Selection of a research hypothesis
- Definition of eligibility criteria for inclusion and exclusion
- Development of a search strategy
- Identification of studies for inclusion
- Conversion of study statistic to common effect-size metric
- Complete summary effect and interpret its meaning

A preliminary step in meta-analysis is selection of a model of analysis. There are two analysis models: fixed effects and random effects. *Fixed effects* analysis is appropriate when most of the primary studies obtained are reasonably homogeneous. *Random effects* analysis is appropriate when primary studies have random samples or are heterogeneous (Robey, 1999; Robey & Dalebout, 1998).

Meta-analyses can provide evidence, especially if it includes several randomized controlled trials (RCT), although it is influenced by the evidence available in the literature (Golper et al., 2001). The highest evidence ratings are assigned to meta-analysis studies of RCTs (ASHA, 2004a). Thus, RCTs are considered the gold standard for evidence, but they are not infallible (Hartling et al., 2005).

Meta-analyses can provide information about treatment results if it includes an average effect size that is considered clinically important and provides evidence that statistical power is adequate to detect and affect. Maxwell and Satake (2006) define *effect size* as "the degree to which the null hypothesis is false" (p. 511). That is, meta-analyses provide an average effect size to estimate whether a null hypothesis can be rejected, or the treatment has no influence on outcome.

Some meta-analyses have instigated criticism in speech-language pathology. For example, Johnston (2005) voiced concerns about the meta-analysis of treatment for children with developmental speech and language delay/disorder by Law et al. (2004). These concerns were related to limitations in content, exclusion of practice sections, focus on very young children, and lack of sufficient attention to duration or methods of treatment. Law et al. (2005) replied that "one person's narrowing is another person's strength" (p. 118). The concern about lack of information about treatment was valid.

To address some of the issues that may arise in utilization of meta-analyses, Maxwell and Satake (2006) developed a worksheet for meta-analysis review that is shown in Table 5–11. Another approach for reviewing meta-analysis is a series of questions, which are presented in Table 5–12. Critical review of meta-analysis reporting is important because of limitations associated with this type of analysis. Among these limitations are invalid primary studies, overemphasis on statistical significance, heterogeneous data, overestimation of treatment effectiveness, concern with entire population rather than individuals, and technical skill required for meta-analysis (Law & Philip, 2002; Maxwell & Satake, 2006; Robey, 1999). Furthermore, meta-analysis may or may not have specific criteria for selection of studies. The criteria for inclusion and evaluation of studies may not be as specific as the criteria should be. Ultimately, it should be noted that meta-analysis reviews warrant critical appraisal.

Table 5–11. Meta-Analysis Review

Check one: ☐ Assessment article   ☐ Intervention article

Reference:

_____

_____

Purpose Statement:

_____

_____

Number of Studies: _____

1	2	3	4	5
Seems inappropriate No rationale		Appropriate Limited rationale		Appropriate Useful rationale

Comments: _____

Time Range for Inclusion: _____

1	2	3	4	5
Seems inappropriate No rationale		Appropriate Limited rationale		Appropriate Useful rationale

Comments: _____

Types of Designs Included: Check all applicable:

☐ Large randomized controlled trials
☐ Small randomized controlled trials
☐ Repeated randomized single-case designs
☐ Non-randomized study with control group(s)
☐ Single-case design using alternating treatments or multiple baseline methods
☐ Case control study
☐ Case reports

1	2	3	4	5
Seems inappropriate No rationale		Appropriate Limited rationale		Appropriate Useful rationale

Comments: _____

Criteria for Inclusion in Meta-Analysis:

_____

Comments: _____

continues

113

Table 5–11. *continued*

Variables Studied:

Comments: _____

Main Points/Strategies Found to be Effective:

Comments: _____

Effect Size:

_____

Comments: _____

Interpretation of Results:

1	2	3	4	5
Interpretation beyond data		Some extension of interpretation beyond data		Data related tied to past research

Comments: _____

Credibility of Source:

1	2	3	4	5
Source unknown self-published/reported		Trade journal or edited publication		Peer-reviewed professional journal

Comments: _____

Source: Meta-analysis review. From *Research and Statistical Methods for Communication Sciences and Disorders (p. 485)*, by D. L. Maxwell and E. Satake, 2006, p. 485. Clifton Park, NY: Thomson Delmar Learning. Copyright 2006 Thomson Delmar Learning. Adapted with permission.

Table 5–12. Criteria for Meta-Analysis Studies

- Was the method for accumulating results from individual studies clear and appropriate?
- Were the methods for combining study effects appropriate?
- Were the data tested for heterogeneity and an appropriate statistic model utilized for the analysis?
- Were the data inspected for possible moderate variables?
- Were interpretation and conclusions consistent with the results?
- Were implications for future research discussed?

Source: From *Research in Communication Sciences and Disorders*, by T. Meline, 2006, Columbus, OH: Pearson Merrill. Reprinted with permission.

Best-Evidence Synthesis

Best-evidence synthesis is an alternative to meta-analysis. It is a review of both qualitative and quantitative studies that are selected according to specific criteria (McMillan, 2012). Best-evidence synthesis utilizes the strongest evidence to support conclusions. This means that it does not only include gold standard randomized control trials or "high-quality" research in the review (Slavin et al., 2009).

For example, if a review of available research on approaches to phonological disorders revealed that there were no randomized control trial studies available, a best-evidence synthesis would proceed and include lower-tiered studies such as case studies and quasi-experimental studies in its review of the evidence. In contrast to a meta-analysis, best-evidence synthesis will produce conclusions based on BEST evidence available and will acknowledge the fact that not enough evidence has been generated upon which to draw conclusions (Slavin et al., 2009)

Clinical Practice Guidelines

The types of literature review discussed in this chapter are ways of ensuring that the speech-language pathologist or audiologist is utilizing the best evidence available to guide their steps—either for conduction of research or for everyday treatment of individuals with swallowing or communication impairment. There is a specific type of literature review called a clinical practice guideline (CPG). It should be noted that most practice guidelines are a combination of clinician experience, expert opinion, and research evidence (Cook et al., 1997). However, CPGs provide a more scientific, evidence-based way to approach the process of finding the best clinical practice for clients (Hargrove et al., 2008).

It should be noted that all practice guidelines are not equal. Some are based on expert opinion/consensus and/or evidence-based practice. The former are variable from high quality and credible to low quality—that is, biased and even deceptive and misleading—the latter are explicit statements that assist speech-language pathologists, audiologists, and their clients to make informed decisions about appropriate care for specific speech-language or hearing problems. Furthermore, practice guidelines should be current, that is, developed, reviewed, or revised within the last 5 years (Johnson, 2006). Some practice guidelines may be outdated and need to be updated because of advances in clinical practice (Shojania et al., 2007).

Determining when to develop guidelines should be considered carefully because of the number of resources, skill, and time required (Slutsky, 2005). Criteria used to develop guidelines include the following:

- Potential to change outcomes or costs
- Availability of evidence on which to develop guidelines
- Topic clinically important
- Topic complex enough to initiate debate about recommendations
- Variation between actual and appropriate care
- No existing or relevant guidelines available to use
- Evidence available to support evidence-based development

■ Recommendations acceptable to potential users
■ Implementation of guidelines feasible

Evidence-based guidelines are based on the best available evidence and professional judgment. Melnyk and Fineout-Overholt (2015) describe evidence-based practice guidelines as specific recommendations based on a rigorous review of the best available evidence on a particular topic. ASHA has also defined practice guidelines as part of its preferred practice patterns for speech-language pathology and audiology (ASHA, 2004b). These guidelines "define generally applicable characteristics of activities directed toward individual patients/clients and that addresses structural requisites of the practice, processes to be carried out, and expected outcomes" (ASHA, 2004b).

There are three types of clinical practice guidelines based on evidence: traditional clinical practice guidelines (TPG), systematic reviews (SR; previously described in this chapter), and evidence-based practice guidelines (EBCPGs; Hargrove et al., 2008). Differences between these clinical practice guidelines are listed in Table 5–13.

There is a hierarchy of clinical practice guidelines with traditional-narrative reviews being the lowest rank (meeting the fewest criteria). Traditional reviews met only two of seven criteria. According to Hargrove et al. (2008):

Evidence-based reviews differ from systematic reviews primarily in the quality of the evidence that is considered. Systematic reviews generally only consider higher-quality evidence, whereas evidence-based practice guidelines consider evidence from a

Table 5–13. Difference Between TCPs, SRs, and EBCPGs

Evidence Criteria	TCP	SR	EBCPG
Based on a comprehensive, methodical review of the literature	No	Yes	Yes
Based on the consensus of a panel of experts	No	Yes	Yes
Can include expert opinion	Yes	No	Yes
Identifies evidence that supports recommendations	No	Yes	Yes
Evaluates the quality of the literature used to support the recommendations	No	Yes	Yes
Expertise of the expert or group of experts is disclosed	No	Yes	Yes
Can include case studies, retrospective, nonrandomized research designs	Yes	No	Yes

Source: "Procedures for using clinical practice guidelines," by P. Hargrove and M. Griffer, 2008, *Language Speech, Hearing, and Services in Schools, 39,* 289–302.

variety of levels, including case studies and even expert opinions. (p. 290)

This information is useful in making decisions about using and recommending clinical practice guidelines. The National Evidence-Based Center of ASHA (2011) uses the Appraisal of Guidelines for Research and Evaluation (AGREE) for evaluating and recommending systematic reviews. These reviews are highly recommended, recommended with reservations, or not recommended.

The Academy of Neurologic Communication Disorders and Sciences (ANCDS) has developed evidence-based practice guidelines (EBPG). These EBPGs focus on five areas: aphasia, acquired apraxia, cognitive dysarthria, and communication disorders related to traumatic brain injury and dementia.

Obviously, there is some variation in reporting clinical practice guidelines. Some practice guidelines do not meet the criteria for systematic review and are narrative rather than systematic. There may be limited information about the outcome measures used as well as the literature search strategy or key words used and no inclusion/exclusion criteria for the studies reviewed. Thus, it is important for speech-language pathologists and audiologists to critically appraise practice guidelines. Finding appropriate guidelines depends on being able to critically evaluate the reliability of a guideline because guidelines do not always confirm the best practice (Slutsky, 2005). Criteria for evaluating guidelines include validity, reliability and reproducibility, clinical applicability, clinical

flexibility, clarity, documentation, development by a multidisciplinary program, and plans for review. Additional information about practice guidelines is provided in Chapter 13.

Summary

There are several types of literature reviews with which graduate students and practicing professionals should be familiar. Reviews of the literature or background literature reviews serve to introduce and define the purpose of a research project. Narrative reviews unsystematically review available research and are utilized infrequently in the fields of speech-language pathology and audiology. Systematic reviews and meta-analysis reviews are being utilized more frequently in recent years and provide a rigorous, systematic review of quality research in the fields of speech-language pathology and audiology.

A major aspect of evidence-based practice and literature reviews is the formulation of a question. Two strategies for formulating questions are available for use: PICO and PESICO. Finally, clinical practice guidelines (CPGs) are a useful a tool utilized in the fields of speech-language pathology and audiology that not only present available research on a topic but make recommendations for practice. It is often difficult to make sense of the information on a specific topic, and the various types of literature reviews presented here can assist graduate students and practicing professionals in accomplishing that goal.

DISCUSSION QUESTIONS

1. Discuss the purposes of a review of the literature.
2. Outline the steps for performing and organizing any type of literature review.
3. What are the differences between narrative and systematic reviews?
4. What are the major components of a systematic review?
5. Define meta-analysis and discuss its use in speech-language pathology and audiology.
6. What are the steps in conducting a meta-analysis?
7. What is a best-evidence synthesis?
8. Explain the importance of practice guidelines.
9. How are practice guidelines developed?
10. Outline a hierarchy for clinical practice guidelines.
11. What is the difference between systematic review and an evidence-based clinical practice guideline?
12. How can clinical practice guidelines be used for making clinical decisions?
13. Why should the use of clinical practice guidelines be encouraged?
14. Describe PICO. Describe PESICO. What are the differences between PICO and PESICO?
15. What are the differences between clinical practice guidelines, systematic reviews, and evidence-based clinical practice guidelines?

References

Abendroth, K. J. (2011) Sibling mediation of children with autism spectrum disorders. *Journal of Interactional Research in Communication Disorders, 2*(1), 85–100.

American Psychological Association. (2020). *Publication manual for the American Psychological Association* (7th ed.).

American Speech-Language-Hearing Association. (2004a). *Evidence-based practices in communication disorders: An introduction.* http://www.asha.org/members/desk ref-journal/deskref/default

American Speech-Language-Hearing Association. (2004b). *Preferred practice patterns for the profession of speech-language pathology.*

American Speech-Language-Hearing Association. (2011). *Clinical practice guidelines.* http://www.asha.org/member/guidelines .aspt

Arksey, H., & O'Malley, L. (2005). Scoping studies: Towards a methodological framework. *International Journal of Social Research Methodology, 8*(1), 19–32.

Bannigan, K., Droogan, J., & Entwistle, V. (1997). Systematic reviews: What do they involve? *Nursing Times, 93*(18), 54–55.

Cook, D. J., Mulrow, C. D., & Haynes, R. B. (1997). Systematic reviews: Synthesis of best evidence for clinical decisions. *Annals of Internal Medicine, 126*(5), 376–380.

Creswell, J. W. (2003). *Research design*. Sage.

Creswell, J. W. (2014). *Research design: Qualitative, quantitative and mixed methods approaches* (4th ed.). Sage.

DePoy, E., & Gitlin, L. N. (2011). *Introduction to research*. Mosby.

Douglas, J., Brown, L., & Barry, S. (2004). The evidence base for the treatment of aphasia after stroke. In S. Riley, J. Douglas, & J. Oates (Eds.), *Evidence-based practice in speech pathology*. Whurr.

Fisher, E. L. (2017). A systematic review and meta-analysis of predictors of expressive-language outcomes among late talkers. *Journal of Speech, Language, and Hearing Research, 60*(10), 2935–2948.

Garrett, Z., & Thomas, J. (2006). Systematic reviews and their application to research in speech and language therapy: A response to T. R. Pring's "Ask a silly question: Two decades of troublesome trials" (2004). *International Journal Language Communication Disorders, 41*(11), 95–105.

Golper, L. A., Wertz, R. T., Fratteli, C. M., Yorksten, K., Meyers, K., Katz, R., & Wambaugb, J. (2001). Evidence-based practice guidelines for the management of communication disorders in neurologically impaired individuals. *ANCDS Practice Guidelines*, 1–12.

Hargrove, P., Gruffer, M., & Lund, B. (2008). Procedures for using clinical practice guidelines. *Language, Speech, and Hearing Services in Schools, 39*, 289–302.

Hartling, L., McAlister, F. A., Rowe, B. H., Ezekowitz, J., Frierson, C., & Kiassen, T. P. (2005). Challenges in systematic reviews of therapeutic devices and procedures. *Annals of Internal Medicine, 142*(12), 1100–1111.

Haynes, W. O., & Johnson, C. E. (2009). *Understanding research and evidence-based practice in communication disorders*. Pearson.

Huang, X., Lin, J., & Dummer-Fushman, D. (2006). Evaluation of PICO as a knowledge representation for clinical questions. *AMJA Annual Symposium Proceedings*, 355–363.

Johnson, C. J. (2006). Getting started in evidence-based practice for childhood speech language disorders. *American Journal of Speech-Language Pathology, 15*, 20–35.

Johnston, J. R. (2005). Re: Law, Garrett, & Nye (2004). The efficacy of treatment for children with developmental speech and language delay/disorder: A meta-analysis. *Journal of Speech, Language, and Hearing Research, 4*(5), 1114–1117.

LaRue, F. M., Draus, P. S., & Klem, M. (2009). A description of a web-based educational tool for understanding the PICO framework in evidence-based practice. *Computer Information in Nursing, 27*, 44–49.

Law, J., Garnett, Z., & Nye, C. (2004). The efficacy of treatment for children with developmental speech and language delay/disorder. A meta-analysis. *Journal of Speech, Language, and Hearing Research, 47*(4), 924–943.

Law, J., Garnett, Z., & Nye, C. (2005). The specificity of a systematic review is the key to its value: A response to Johnson (2005). *Journal of Speech, Language, and Hearing Research, 48*(5), 1118–1120.

Law, M., & Philip, I. (2002). Systematically reviewing the evidence. In M. Law (Ed.), *Evidence-based rehabilitation* (pp. 109–126). Slack.

Maxwell, D. L., & Satake, E. (2006). *Research and statistical methods in communication sciences and disorders*. Thomson-Delmar Learning.

McCauley, R. J., & Hargrove, R. (2004). A clinician's introduction to systematic reviews in communication disorders. *Contemporary Issues in Communication Sciences and Disorders, 31*, 173–181.

McMillan, J. H. (2012). *Educational research: Fundamentals for the consumer*. Pearson.

Meline, T. (2006). Selecting studies for systematic review: Inclusion and exclusion criteria. *Contemporary Issues in Communication Sciences and Disorders, 33*, 21–27.

Melnyk, B. M., & Fineout-Overholt, E. (2015). *Evidence-based practice in nursing and health care* (3rd ed.). Lippincott Williams & Wilkins.

Mertens, D. M. (2005). *Research and evaluation in education and psychology*. Sage.

Mertens, D. M. (2014). *Research and evaluation in education and psychology* (4th ed.). Sage.

Petticrew, M. (2001). Systematic reviews from astronomy to zoology: Myths and misconceptions. *British Medical Journal, 332,* 98–101.

Portney, L. G., & Watkins, M. P. (2009). *Foundations of clinical research*. Pearson.

Pring, T. (2004). Ask a silly question: Two decades of troublesome trials. *International Journal of Language Communication Disorders, 39*(3), 285–302.

Pring, T. (2006). Systematic reviews require a systematic approach to therapy research: A reply to Garrett and Thomas (2005). *International Journal of Language Communication Disorders, 41*(11), 107–110.

Richardson, W., Wilson, M., Nishikawa, J., & Hayward, R. (1995). The well-built clinical question: A key to evidence-based decisions. *ACP Journal Club, 123,* A112–A113.

Robey, R. R. (1999). A meta-analysis of clinical outcomes in the treatment of aphasia. *Journal of Speech, Language, and Hearing Research, 41*(1), 172–187.

Robey, R. R., & Dalebout, S. D. (1998). A tutorial on conducting meta-analysis of clinical outcome research. *Journal of Speech, Language, and Hearing Research, 41,* 1227–1241.

Rudolph, J. M. (2017). Case history risk factors for specific language impairment: A systematic review and meta-analysis. *American Journal of Speech-Language Pathology, 26*(3), 991–1010.

Schlosser, R. W. (2000). Synthesis efficacy research in AAC. In R. W. Schlosser (Ed.), *The efficacy of augmentative and alternative communication* (pp. 230–259). Academic Press.

Schlosser, R. W., Koul, R., & Costello, J. (2007). Asking well-built questions for evidence-based practice in augmentative and alternative communication. *Journal of Communication Disorders, 40,* 225–238.

Seers, K. (1999). Systematic reviews. In M. Dawes, P. Davies, A. Gray, J. Marx, K. Seers, & R. Snowball (Eds.), *Evidence-based practice* (pp. 85–100). Churchill, Livingstone.

Shojania, K. G., Simpson, M., Anscni, M. T., Doucette, S., & Moher, D. (2007). How quickly do systematic reviews go over date? *Annals of Internal Medicine, 147,* 224–233.

Slavin, R. E., Lake, C., & Groff, C. (2009). Effective programs in middle and high school mathematics: A best-evidence synthesis. *Review of Educational Research, 79*(2), 839–911.

Slutsky, J. (2005). Using evidence-based practice guidelines: Tools for improving practice. In B. M. Melnyk & E. Fineout-Overholt (Eds.), *Evidence-based practice in nursing and health care* (pp. 221–235). Lippincott Williams & Wilkins.

6

Measurement

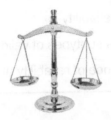

LEARNING OBJECTIVES

Upon completion of this chapter, the reader will be able to:

- Define nominal, ordinal, interval, and ratio levels of measurement
- Provide an example of each level of measurement
- Describe differences in the levels of measurement
- Define validity and reliability
- Describe the various subtypes of validity and reliability
- Discuss the importance of reliability and validity in research

Scales of Measurement

Measurement of relevant variables is important in any research project. Scales of measurement provide a means of assigning numbers to events or objects according to prescribed rules, and preparing numerical data according to these rules permits the use of statistical treatment. Four scales or levels of measurement are used to categorize data. In hierarchical order, they are **nominal**, **ordinal**, **interval**, and **ratio scales** (Table 6–1).

Measurement scales may be based on clearly observable events or subjective impressions. An example of a precise, clearly observable scale is the metric ruler, which is composed of millimeters and centimeters. An example of a scale based on subjective impressions is a scale of listener clarity for different regional dialects. This kind of scale might be constructed simply by asking a group of subjects to assign numbers (scale values) to each dialect in a survey. The lowest number might represent the least clear dialect and the highest number the clearest dialect. Scales that attempt to quantify a relationship between subjective (psychological) sensations and physical quantities are called *psychophysical scales*. Hearing scientists have used both simple and complex scales of measurement to quantify various loudness-intensity and pitch-frequency relationships.

Nominal Level of Measurement

The nominal (lowest) level of measurement classifies an event or object into a category. Examples of such categories may include gender, ethnicity, individu-

Table 6–1. Four Scales of Measurement Used to Categorize Data

Scale of Measurement	Definition	Example
Nominal	Named or counted data; classification of labeling	Color label: male or female
Ordinal	Ranked data; possesses properties of nominal scale	Heaviest-lightest Sweetest-sourest Tallest-shortest
Interval	Equal intervals; no meaningful zero; possesses properties of ordinal and nominal scale	Temperature
Ratio	Equal intervals; true meaningful zero; possesses properties of all other scales	Age, IQ, weight; many personality and educational tests

Source: From *Research and Evaluation in Education and Psychology* (p. 304), by D. M. Mertens, 2005, Thousand Oaks, CA: Sage Publications. Reprinted by permission of Sage Publications, Inc.

als who do and do not stutter, individuals with and without a history of voice problems, hearing sensitivity (normal or abnormal), etiology of hearing loss (conductive, sensorineural, or mixed), and language development (normal or abnormal). A subject is measured at this level by assigning the individual to one of the established categories. Other variables are coded numerically (e.g., 1 = normal, 2 = abnormal, etc.). The numbers assigned represent differences and are not used mathematically for addition, subtraction, multiplication, or division functions which would be meaningless at this level.

According to Portney and Watkins (2009), nominal categories are mutually exclusive; that is, no object or person can logically be assigned to more than one category. Use of the nominal data category also assumes that the rules for classifying a set of attributes are exhaustive; that is, every subject can be accurately assigned to only one category. For example, classifying blood type would follow these rules.

Nominal scales represent the simplest type of measurement scales. They are constructed by placing various scale items into different *categories*, but no attempt is made to order the items. Many studies dealing with the perception of loudness and pitch use nominal scales of measurement. For example, these scales address our ability to discriminate between two auditory stimuli. The question asked in these studies is, "What is the smallest physical (acoustic) difference between two auditory stimuli that the listener can detect?"

For example, if studying loudness discrimination, the following would be addressed:

■ Various pairs of auditory stimuli differing only in their intensities (with frequency the same) would be presented to the listener.
■ Many different combinations would be presented and listeners would have to make judgments for each pair: Do the stimuli sound equally loud? Do the stimuli sound different in loudness?
■ Listeners would have two choices from which to choose, and they assign one of the choices to each pair to which they listen (e.g., yes/no, same/different).

Ordinal Level of Measurement

The ordinal level of measurement shows the position of one variable relative to another, but intervals between variables are not equal. Examples of variables at the ordinal level include college classification (freshman, sophomore, junior, or senior), teacher ranks (instructor, assistant professor, associate professor, or professor) and severity of a disorder (mild, moderate, or severe). Examples of the ordinal categories for the variable of hearing sensitivity include normal, mild, moderate, and severe. As with the nominal level of measurement, variables at the ordinal level are frequently coded numerically (e.g., 1 = freshman, 2 = sophomore, 3 = junior, and 4 = senior). However, mathematical or numeric operations (addition, subtraction, multiplication, and division) remain meaningless with ordinal measures. *Nonparametric* statistical methods (methods not requiring certain assumptions about the data) are used to examine ordinal data.

Ordinal scales of measurement are somewhat more complex than nominal scales, because the scale items are arranged in order with respect to some common feature. Therefore, ordinal scales may be constructed by procedures requiring the subject to rank order various items presented. For example, in a study of listener "clarity" for 10 accented English speech stimuli, each of the 10 accents could be presented to subjects, and they are asked to rank each accent from 1 to 10, with "10" being the *most clear* accent and "1" the least clear accent. No two accents could occupy the same rank. This is an ordinal scale of measurement because items would be arranged in order with respect to clarity of accent. However, it would be impossible to determine *absolute differences* between accents using this type of scale. Thus, it could not be determined whether the accent ranked "10" was actually twice as "clear" as the accent ranked "5," or that the accent ranked "5" was five times as "clear" as the accent ranked "1," and so on (Lass & Donai, 2023).

Ordinal scales of loudness and pitch sensation may be constructed in much the same manner as the previous example of clarity of accents of English. For example, a study could be designed to rank listeners' perceived loudness discomfort with noise produced by various types of aircraft as they fly over homes adjacent to an airport. Six different planes might be considered for study and placed in rank order from "1" to "6," with "6" representing the plane whose loudness was most uncomfortable to hear and a rank of "1" representing the plane with the least uncomfortable noise level. As in the previous example, no two planes could share the same rank. Since the scale of measurement is ordinal, it would only be possible to determine the

relative ranks among aircraft. However, it would not be possible to determine from this scale whether one plane sounded twice as uncomfortable as another plane or planes or to determine any other ratio among individual aircraft (Lass & Donai, 2023).

Interval Level of Measurement

Interval scales are used when there are equal intervals between values but no absolute zero. For a numeric operation to yield meaningful results, it is necessary to have equal intervals between adjacent numerical values. For example, the difference between 3 and 5 should be the same as the difference between 28 and 30, or 41 and 43, or 79 and 81, and so on. In both interval and ratio levels of measurement, there are constant differences in data entries.

According to Portney and Watkins (2009), the interval scale does not allow for comparison of absolute magnitude of an attribute, because an absolute is not zero (as in ordinal measurement). Examples of variables at the interval level include the following:

1. numerical ratings of vocal quality on a 5- or 7-point interval scale;
2. numerical ratings reflecting attitudes of individuals who stutter based on a 5-point Likert-type rating scale; and
3. standard or scaled scores on a language test or IQ scores.

Parametric statistics are used if the following criteria are met: (a) the subjects represent a "normal" population distribution; (b) the sample is sizable, usually more than 30; and (c) information is derived using the interval or ratio level of measurement (Orlikoff et al., 2022). Thus, parametric statistical methods are used to examine equal interval data.

Ratio Level of Measurement

Ratio scales are interval scales with an absolute zero. Thus, it is assumed that the attribute being measured may not be present. This measure is more frequently appropriate for studies involving natural science than for studies in areas of social science. However, if the dependent variable is the frequency of events (such as frequency of moments of stuttering), has time measures (such as the latency period between seeing a printed word and saying it), involves a measured distance (such as measurement of the space constituting a velopharyngeal gap during phonation in patients with velopharyngeal incompetence), and so on, the ratio level may be appropriate. Height, weight, chronologic age, hearing level in decibels, and fundamental frequency of a complex wave are additional examples of variables that can be measured at the ratio level (Lass & Donai, 2023).

The differences between interval and ratio measurements are that multiples are meaningful at the ratio level (e.g., a 6-mm velopharyngeal gap is twice as large as a 3-mm gap), and the units of the variables measured at the ratio level can be changed by simple multiplication (e.g., feet are converted into inches by multiplying by 12). These properties do not hold true for measurements at the interval level. For example, a person with an IQ of 100 is not twice as intelligent as someone with an IQ of 50. All numbers at the ratio level of measurement have mathematical properties, thus allowing parametric statistics to be employed to examine ratio and interval level data (Lass & Donai, 2023).

Ratio scales of measurement contain all properties of nominal, ordinal, and interval scales. That is, they are capable of

1. *classification* (like nominal scales);
2. *ordering* (like ordinal scales); and
3. determination of *exact differences* (like interval scales).

In addition, ratio scales also have the property of determining exact ratios between scale items. Since ratio scales have *true zero points*, numbers on ratio scales reflect actual ratios between items. An example of a ratio scale of measurement is the common metric ruler. On a metric ruler, 8 mm is exactly twice as long as 4 mm, and 50 m is exactly half as long as 100 m. The exact ratio between any two scale items can be derived on a ratio scale because it has a nonarbitrary *absolute zero point*. For example, 0 mm is the total absence of distance ("zero distance"). Ratio scales represent the most precise scale type (Lass & Donai, 2023).

In summary, in ratio scales, variables are treated as categorical (e.g., gender, age, disorder) or quantitative (e.g., height, weight, IQ, frequency of occurrence). It is important that categories for variables be classified so that each subject fits into only one category. Quantitative variables usually are measured in discrete units (e.g., frequency, pounds, milliseconds, and millimeters), and these units must be carefully recorded as the data are collected. Table 6–2 shows hypothetical data for vocal fundamental frequency utilizing all types of measurements.

Table 6–2. Hypothetical Data for Fundamental Frequency Utilizing All Types of Measurements

Subject	Ratio Measure	Interval Measure	Ordinal Measure	Nominal Measure
A	220	4	3	High
B	198	5	2	Medium
C	137	8	1	Low
D	235	3	4	High

Source: From *Foundations of Clinical Research: Application to Practice* (2nd ed., p. 56), by L. G. Portney and M. P. Watkins, 2000, Upper Saddle River, NJ: Pearson Education. Copyright 2000, Pearson Education, Inc. Adapted by permission.

Validity of Measurement

When analyzing the accuracy of the results of a study, the investigator objectively attempts to answer questions of validity and reliability. When assessing the *validity* of a study, the primary question involves determining whether the obtained information contributes to answering the research question (Orlikoff et al., 2022). For example, if the investigator identifies phonatory quality using a Visi-Pitch analysis with an inappropriate frequency range for some of the subjects, perturbation data might be questioned.

Hegde (1994) differentiates between the validity of the data defining the dependent variables and the validity of the experiment itself. Accuracy of the information about the phonation attributes of the subjects is an example of establishing the validity of data defining the dependent variable(s). The design of a study—including control methods for observing, collecting, and recording data and control of the variables that might have an impact on the outcome of the study—contributes to the validity of the experiment. For example, consistent tracking of relevant phonatory habits and phonatory attributes of all subjects would contribute to the validity of the experiment.

Both internal and external validity are important to establish when analyzing the results of a research study. To establish **internal validity**, the experimenter determines if the experimental manipulation really made a difference (Kerlinger, 1973) by ensuring that extraneous factors that could influence the results are carefully controlled (Orlikoff et al., 2022). To establish internal validity, the design of a study should effectively rule out all variables that might affect the dependent variable so that it can be concluded that the independent variable was ultimately responsible for any change in the dependent variable (Doehring, 1988).

Portney and Watkins (2009) cited several factors that affect internal validity. Some of these are the effectors of prior events: maturation, attrition, testing effects by repeated testing, instrumentation, statistical regression (regression toward the mean), compensatory rivalry, and resentful demoralization of respondents receiving fewer desirable treatments. In summary, internal validity involves answering the question of whether the experimental treatments actually made a difference in the study (Isaac & Michael, 1987).

For the voice study cited previously, internal validity could be established by demonstrating voice improvement using Visi-Pitch data and a comparison of pre- and postexperimental perceptual analyses of the quality of subjects' voices. In addition, internal validity could be further established by reporting that (a) the Visi-Pitch equipment was properly set and calibrated; (b) subjects with phonatory disorders related to preexisting laryngeal conditions were not selected; (c) all perceptual judgments were made by the same speech-language pathologists whose perceptual judgments were calibrated to the same criteria in training sessions administered by the experimenter; (d) all subjects received the same training in identifying poor vocal habits and establishing good vocal habits; and (e) all received the same medical diagnosis and treatment.

External validity is the extent to which the results of a study satisfy representativeness or generalizability (Kerlinger, 1973) or can be generalized to the population as a whole (Orlikoff et al., 2022). Practical clinical use of findings is determined by establishing external validity. The extent to which effects of independent variables on dependent variables apply to the natural setting must be determined to establish external validity (Doehring, 1988). Hegde (1994) cites effects of treatment dur-

ing a study and knowledge of expected results by subjects as factors that may influence the external validity of a study. Isaac and Michael (1987) concluded that questions about external validity involving what populations, settings, treatment variables, and measurement variables to which an effect can be generalized may not be completely answerable. The researcher must attempt to control all variables as well as possible.

For the voice study, establishing external validity could be done by showing that (a) the individuals selected for the study were typical in age, sex, and occupation to those generally reported in the literature as having chronic voice problems related to vocal abuse and/or inflammatory laryngeal conditions; (b) standard treatment information was given to all subjects about identification and reduction of vocal abuses; (c) typical medical management was used for the conditions' diagnoses; and (d) it was established that the data provided by the Visi-Pitch and pre- and postperceptual analyses by examiners are typical of that collected by certified speech-language pathologists in varied clinical settings.

Three types of validity should be considered when using a test or questionnaire to measure an individual's knowledge or attitudes. These are content validity, criterion-related (including predictive and concurrent) validity, and construct validity. **Content validity** concerns whether the substance or content of a measure adequately represents the universe of content of the attribute being measured or how well the content of the attribute being measured or how well the content of a test reflects the subject matter from which conclusions will be drawn (Isaac & Michael, 1987; Kerlinger, 1973; Portney & Watkins, 2009). Kerlinger (1973) further explained that content validation is basically judgmental in that each item is judged for its pertinence or applicability to the property or characteristic being measured.

Orlikoff et al. (2022) further described content validity as a subjective means of logically explaining and evaluating test items to determine how well they reflect the characteristics to be measured. Content validity is concerned with adequately assessing all the aspects of the behaviors to be measured. For example, to assess IQ, the research usually assesses quantitative and verbal abilities, because both have been shown to correlate with intelligence. In another example, the content validity of a test of language development would be determined by identifying the important behaviors that reflect good or poor language performance, then determining whether the content of the test items reflects those behaviors or skills.

Orlikoff et al. (2022) define *criterion-related validity* as a test of whether a test (or measure) correlates with a known indicator (validating criterion) of the behavior (characteristic) being measured. Two types of criterion-related validity include concurrent and predictive validity (Kerlinger, 1973). Kerlinger (1973) further described concurrent criterion-related validity as involving the ability to check a currently administered measuring instrument against an outcome occurring now. Predictive criterion-related validity involves the ability to check a currently administered measuring instrument against a future outcome. For example, future achievement is predicted by aptitude tests (predictive), and present (concurrent) and achievements are predicted by achieve-

ment tests. Present and future ability to learn and solve problems are predicted by IQ tests (Kerlinger, 1973). Therefore, it is difficult to separate the predictive and concurrent components of criterion-related validity.

Criterion-related validity involves a test's ability to predict current or future performance. This may involve using correlation measures to compare test scores with criteria known to identify the same skills as the proposed test (Isaac & Michael, 1987). In fact, criterion-related data may be collected concurrently with the test to ascertain whether the test involves criteria-related procedures (Isaac & Michael, 1987).

The major difficulty in establishing criterion-related validity is determining whether criteria exist to predict a specific skill or performance, such as teaching effectiveness. The question of what constitutes appropriate criteria to measure teaching effectiveness has long been proven to be very controversial.

Construct validity involves scientific inquiry by testing a hypothesized relationship and validating a test and the theory behind it (Kerlinger, 1973). By investigating the qualities that a test measures, the degree to which the concepts or theory behind the test account for performance on the test may be determined (Isaac & Michael, 1987). Thus, construct validity is concerned with the extent to which a test or questionnaire measures what it is supposed to measure by reflecting the theory, behavior, or characteristic to be measured (Orlikoff et al., 2022). The scores on a test are correlated with other accepted measures of the same behavior. If subjects' scores on a new test are strongly correlated with their scores on an established test, then construct validity has been established.

Reliability of Measurement

Reliability refers to the consistency of a rater or of a measurement. Several words have been used to define reliability: dependability, predictability, consistency, credibility, and stability. In research, reliability refers to the consistency or correlation among repeated measures or observations. However, reliability does not ensure accuracy or validity. Thus, it is possible that observations can be consistent without being accurate. For example, children's responses to audiometric screening in a noisy environment might very well be consistent but certainly would not be considered accurate or valid indicators of their hearing sensitivity.

Three types of reliability—**intraexaminer (intrareader or intrajudge)**, **interexaminer (interrater or interjudge)**, and **test-retest** reliability—should be assessed when establishing the reliability of the results of a study. Strong intraexaminer reliability implies that in repeated observations of the same subject, the same examiner gets similar results. Intraexaminer reliability is usually not difficult to establish. However, interexaminer reliability implies agreement among different observers measuring the same phenomenon. Interexaminer reliability is considered a crucial measure of objectivity and is a necessary element to subjecting a study to scientific review (Hegde, 2003). Test-retest reliabil-

ity involves how well subjects perform on one set of measurements as compared to their performance on a second evaluation of the same measurements.

The relationship between validity and reliability is shown in Figure 6–1.

Measurement may be very reliable but not very valid (Figure 6–1A). However, a measurement with random error is usually considered neither reliable nor valid (Figure 6–1B). It should be noted that if a measurement has only a small amount of error, then it is possible to have relatively valid and reliable measurements (Figure 6–1C). If a measurement has no variance and is consistently reliable and valid, then the confidence in those measurements is high (Figure 6–1D).

Summary

Measurement of variables includes the control of factors that may influence reliability and validity. The level of measurement may be nominal, ordinal, interval, or ratio. It is important that the level of measurement used fits the study so that appropriate analysis of the data can be used. Moreover, it is important for all researchers to understand that validity and reliability are separate concepts but are interrelated. Various types of factors may influence internal and external validity as well as different forms of reliability.

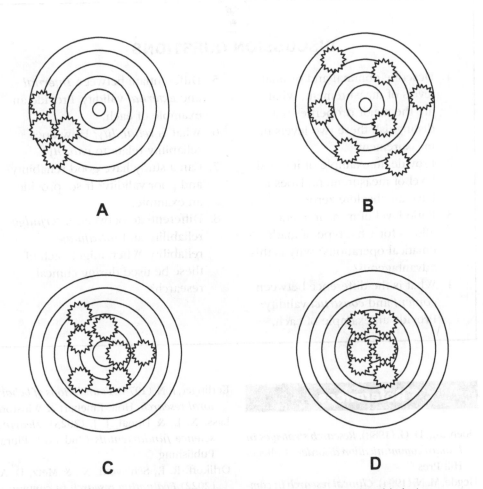

Figure 6–1. Representation of targets to illustrate the relationship between reliability and validity. **A.** Scores are highly reliable, but not valid, demonstrating systematic error. **B.** Scores are neither reliable nor valid, demonstrating random error. **C.** Reliability had improved but is still low; scores are somewhat valid. **D.** Scores are both reliable and valid. From *Foundations of Clinical Research: Applications to Practice* (3rd ed., p. 80), by L. G. Portney and M. P. Watkins, 2009, Pearson Education. Copyright 2009 Pearson Education, Inc. Adapted by permission.

DISCUSSION QUESTIONS

1. Describe nominal and ordinal levels of measurement. What are the major properties that distinguish these two levels of measurement?

2. Provide an example of interval level of measurement. Does it have an absolute zero?

3. Ratio level of measurement allows for what type of mathematical operations? Why is this advantageous?

4. What is the difference between *content* and *construct* validity? Provide an example of each.

5. Differentiate between *internal* and *external* validity. Provide an example of each.

6. What is *reliability*? How does reliability relate to *validity*?

7. Can a study have good reliability and poor validity? If so, provide an example.

8. Differentiate between *interjudge* reliability and *intrajudge* reliability. When might each of these be used during clinical research?

References

Doehring, D. G. (1988). *Research strategies in human communication disorders*. College-Hill Press.

Hegde, M. N. (1994). *Clinical research in communicative disorders* (3rd ed.). Pro-Ed.

Hegde, M. N. (2003). *Clinical research in communicative disorders* (4th ed.). Pro-Ed.

Isaac, S., & Michael, W. B. (1987). *Handbook in research and evaluation*. Edits Publishers.

Kerlinger, F. N. (1973). *Foundations of behavioral research*. Holt, Rinehart & Winston.

Lass, N. J., & Donai, J. J. (2023). *Hearing science fundamentals* (2nd ed.). Plural Publishing.

Orlikoff, R. F., Schiavetti, N., & Metz, D. A. (2022) *Evaluating research in communication disorders*. Pearson Education.

Portney, L. G., & Watkins, M. P. (2009). *Foundation of clinical research: Applications to practice* (3rd ed.). Prentice-Hall Health.

7

Research Design and Strategy

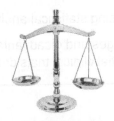

LEARNING OBJECTIVES

Upon completion of this chapter, the reader will be able to:

- Describe several group designs for between-subjects and within-subjects

- Discuss single-subject designs related to clinical practice

- Describe the basics of sequential clinical trials

- Describe trends in using statistical analysis programs

- Discuss the advantages and disadvantages of group, single subject, and sequential clinical trials designs

Introduction

All types of research have a strategy or design that permits statistical analysis of differences between and within groups of subjects (Doehring, 1988; Maxwell & Satake, 2006; Portney & Watkins, 2009; University of Southern California, 2019). Several types of research were described in previous chapters. Research strategy and design refer to the plans for answering research questions and testing research hypotheses. Some authorities differentiate between these terms; others do not. The strategy or design of a study indicates the methods and procedures used in the investigation. There are essentially two types of research designs: group designs and single-subject designs. **Group designs** include between-subjects designs, within-subject designs, and mixed-group designs. **Single-subject designs** include case studies, within-subject experimental designs, multiple baseline, and multiple treatment designs. Group research designs and single-subject designs are compared in Table 7–1.

Characteristics of a Good Design

Good research design may be described in terms of several characteristics. Understanding that systematic changes are the result of the experiment being conducted involves the use of "the researcher's ability to manipulate and control variables and measurements, so that rival hypotheses are ruled out as a possible explanation for the observed response" (Portney & Watkins, 2000, p. 153). Essentially,

there are two types of extraneous variables: (a) intrinsic and (b) extrinsic (Polit & Hungler, 1999; Portney & Watkins, 2000). **Intrinsic variables** are variables associated with subjects of an investigation, such as age, gender, socioeconomic status, and marital status. There are a number of ways to reduce intrinsic variability, such as randomization (each subject has an equal chance of being assigned to any group), homogeneity (choosing only subjects who have the same characteristics), blocking (building extraneous variables into the design by using them as independent variables), using the subject as his or her own control, and analysis of covariance (selecting a covariate and adjusting scores statistically to control for differences on the extraneous variable; Portney & Watkins, 2009). **Extrinsic variables** are variables associated with the research situation or environment. These variables are related to the place and time the research was conducted and adherence or not to the research specification or protocols. The most effective method of controlling external factors is directly related to the consistency of conditions under which an investigation is performed; that is, the conditions under which data are collected should be as similar as possible for every subject.

The second characteristic of good research design is that it should be appropriate for the question(s) being asked. Third, the design should not result in data that are biased. A fourth characteristic of good research design is precision, which can be accomplished using a well-described protocol. Research designs differ considerably in the sensitivity with which statistically significant results can be detected. A fifth characteristic is the power of the design or its

Table 7–1. Comparison of Group-Research Designs and Single-Subject Designs

Group Designs	Single-Subject Designs
Compare at least 2 groups from a target population	Compare within-subject performance for 1 subject or a small group of subjects.
Minimum number of subjects: 10	Minimum number: 1
Outcome measures collected infrequently; usually only pretest/ post-test.	Performance repeatedly measured over a period corresponding to requirements of design.
Unnecessary to run subjects more than once under each experimental condition.	Necessary to run subject more than once under each experiment.
Little or no subject feedback; emphasis on outcome.	Subject feedback monitored; emphasis on process and outcome.
Inflexible; changes not permitted once intervention is introduced.	Flexible, permits addition or elimination.
Standardized measurement procedures and comparisons between subjects.	Measurement procedures flexible, individualized.
Generalization	Limited generalization.
Expensive	Inexpensive
Statistical procedures well developed.	Statistical procedures relatively new.
Relatively easy to control for order and sequence effects.	Difficult to control for order and sequence effects.

Sources: From "Clinically Relevant Designs for Rehabilitation Research: The Idiographic Model," by K. J. Ottenbacher, 1990, *American Journal of Physical Medicine and Rehabilitation, 69,* pp. 286–292; *Research Design and Evaluation in Speech-Language Pathology and Audiology,* by F. H. Silverman, 1993, Englewood Cliffs, NJ: Prentice-Hall; and "Group Designs in Clinical Research," by G. M. Siegelo and M. A. Young, 1987, *Journal of Speech and Hearing Disorders, 52*(3), pp. 194–199.

ability to detect relationships among variables. According to Portney and Watkins (2000), the power of a statistical test addresses the ability of a test to reject the null hypothesis, that is, "to document a real relationship between independent and dependent variables" (p. 164). The appropriateness of research designs must also be considered relative to the current state of the art. Portney and Watkins (2009) suggest that when important extraneous variables cannot be controlled, a descriptive or correlational design may be more appropriate.

Portney and Watkins (2000) identified six critical questions that should be considered when choosing a specific design:

1. How many independent variables are being tested?

2. How many levels do each independent variable have, and are these levels experimental or control conditions?
3. How many groups of subjects are being tested?
4. How will subjects be selected, and how will they be assigned to groups?
5. How often will observation of responses be made?
6. What is the temporal sequence of interventions and measurements?

Group Designs

Group designs permit comparison of the average or typical performance of a group to other groups or other conditions (Warren, 1986). Several terms are used for this design: between-groups design, between-subjects designs, correlational design, preexperimental design, quasi-experimental design, and true experimental design (Bordens & Abbott, 1988; Portney & Watkins, 2009). Hegde (1999) indicates that the basic method for implementing group designs is to initially have two or more comparable groups that represent the populations from which they were drawn (especially

when the random procedure is used) and at least one of the groups receives a treatment (experimental group) and another group does not (control group).

Between-Subjects Designs

A classic design for exploring cause-and-effect relationships includes the pretest/posttest randomized control group (Patten, 2005). Figure 7–1 illustrates the classic design, which assumes that all groups are equal except that one received an experimental treatment and the other did not. Patten (2005) states that the advantage of using a pretest is that it will allow a researcher to determine how much each group has gained or changed, not just whether they are different at the end of the experiment.

If a researcher is concerned that a pretest might make subjects more sensitive to what is being studied, an alternative is to implement the posttest-only design (Portney & Watkins, 2009). A researcher would have used random assignment of subjects, and the groups would be comparable. The posttest-only design is most successful when the groups are large so the probability of balancing interpersonal characteristics is increased (Portney & Watkins, 2009).

	Group A:	Pretest	Experimental	Posttest
Assign subjects at random to groups	(Experimental group)		Treatment	
	Group B:	Pretest	Control condition	Posttest
	(Control group)			

Figure 7–1. Classic design for cause-and-effect relationship. Adapted from *Understanding Research Methods* (5th ed.), by M. L. Patten, 2005, Pyrczak Publishing.

Multiple control group design is a variation of the single-factor, multiple group design. This design uses multiple control groups, because a single control group is inadequate for assessing the impact of each potentially confounding factor of the dependent variables. Multiple control groups can be included in both parametric and nonparametric designs (Bordens & Abbott, 1988; Portney & Watkins, 2009).

Factorial designs manipulate two or more independent variables; one group in the design accounts for each possible combination of the levels of the independent variables. A factorial design is usually described according to its dimensions so that a two-way or two-factor design has two independent variables and a three-way or three-factor design has three independent variables. These designs can be described as a 2 × 2 design, which would pair two independent variables with two different levels. For example, if a researcher utilized two independent variables (types of speech sample) for connected speech and single word articulation production and manipulated the environment (child's home and another sample in the clinic), this would be designated as a 2 × 2 factorial design. Again, all subjects would be assigned to one of four groups receiving a combination of connected or single-word articulation speech samples in a home or clinic setting. A factorial design has two or more independent variables, which are manipulated simultaneously; it permits analysis of the main *effects* of the independent variables separately and the **interaction effects** of these variables. Each main effect is a single-factor experiment, and the interaction addresses the question of the effect of one variable at different levels of the second variable (Portney & Watkins, 2009).

Multivariate designs involve two or more dependent variables and provide information about the effect of the independent variable on each dependent variable and on a composite dependent variable formed from a weighted combination of the individual independent variables. In a multivariate design, Gutierrez-Clellen and Heinrichs-Ramos (1993) examined the referential cohesion of the narratives of Spanish-speaking children. Pezzei and Oratio (1991) conducted a multivariate analysis of job satisfaction for public school speech-language pathologists. Sawuerwin and Burris (2022) did a multivariate design regarding a course in augmentative and alternative communication.

The validity of between-subjects experimental designs can be confounded or damaged by a variety of sources, such as nonrandomization randomization, experimenter bias, and poor planning and execution of experimental conditions. Confounding can be avoided by randomization, use of blinding, and careful planning and execution of a research protocol. **Double-blinding** is where neither the subjects nor the investigators are aware of the identity of the treatment groups until after data are collected (Portney & Watkins, 2000). **Single-blinding** of a study involves only the investigator(s) not knowing which treatment is used. It is often difficult to offer a placebo for studies involving rehabilitation procedures; therefore, single-blinding is more often used to try new or experimental procedures.

Within-Subjects Designs

In within-subjects designs, every subject in the experiment is exposed to all of the experimental or treatment conditions. Fewer subjects are required for this design than for an equivalent between-subjects design. Sometimes referred to as a repeated measures design, within-subjects designs are a group of designs that incorporate the same basic structure, that is, using the same subjects in all conditions (Bordens & Abbott, 1988; Patten, 2005; Portney & Watkins, 2009). Within-subjects designs are classified or described like between-subjects designs and include two treatments, single-factor, multilevel, factorial, multiple control group, and multivariate designs. Shim et al. (2021) conducted a within-subjects design of the auditory brain response and uncomfortable loudness level in ears with and without tinnitus.

The advantages of within-subjects designs include fewer subjects required, matching of subject factors, and power in detecting effects of dependent variables. Disadvantages include less power than equivalent between-subject designs if the dependent variable is only weakly related to subject differences and possible carryover effects when exposure to one treatment influences behavior in a subsequent treatment. Carryover can be reduced by randomizing the order of presentation of levels of the independent variable. More frequently, counterbalancing is used in which individual subjects are exposed to the treatments in different orders. Utilizing treatment order as an independent variable makes it possible to determine whether carryover effects are present and, if so, their magnitude and direction. Despite the advantages of making treatment order an independent variable, there are disadvantages. The primary disadvantage is that every treatment order requires a separate group of subjects who must be tested under every treatment condition. This is expensive in terms of number of subjects and the time

required testing them. Smit et al. (2018) studies different approaches to treatment of children with phonological disorders. Wolfe et al. (2022) did a repeated design study regarding the low-level speech recognition for children with hearing aids.

Mixed-Group Designs

Mixed designs combine within-subjects and between-subjects designs and are used to investigate the effects of treatment for which carryover effects would be a problem while repeatedly sampling behavior across time or trials. Warren (1986) and Portney and Watkins (2009) consider mixed designs both descriptive and experimental. Three advantages of mixed designs are ease of implementation, generalizability of findings, and availability of statistical techniques. Frequent misinterpretation and overinterpretation of the results are the primary disadvantages. Mamo et al. (2021) completed a mixed design study. The purpose of this study was to characterize the communication needs of older adults in group care environments and understand the factors that foster engaged communication.

The nested design is a variation of the mixed-group design that combines within-subjects and between-subjects designs. It involves more than one task for each level of the independent variable. For example, assume that you were conducting an experiment on the ability to write diagnostic reports. The between-subjects factor might be difficulty (low, moderate, and high). Under each level of difficulty, two sets of diagnostic data would be included, with all subjects in each level of difficulty completing both sets of reports. By demonstrating the effect of item difficulty with different tasks, effects are not limited to a specific type of problem. This design is useful when subjects must be tested in groups rather than individually. It also has the advantage of increasing the generality of results (Bordens & Abbot, 1988; Portney & Watkins, 2009).

Clement and Wijner (1994), in a study of vowel contrasts, analyzed their data utilizing a "three-way ANOVA, with factors subject group, vowel, and subject (nested under subject group)" (p. 86). It is important to note that subjects are always nested under subject group. An example of a nested design, with speech-language pathologists nested within states, follows.

A group of six speech-language pathologists—two each from Louisiana, Oklahoma, and Texas—were discussing the treatment of patients with spasmodic dysphonia. The speech-language pathologists from Louisiana decided that Botox injections were the best means of treatment; therefore, their patients were injected with Botox, received no voice management, and were reevaluated 3 months later to determine the amount of improvement. The speech-language pathologists from Oklahoma decided that voice management coupled with Botox injections were the best means of treatment; therefore, their subjects were injected, received voice management for 3 months, and then were reevaluated to determine the amount of improvement. The speech-language pathologists in Texas decided that voice management was the best means of treatment; therefore, their patients received voice management for 3 months and then were reevaluated to determine amount of improvement. All data were then analyzed statistically. Patterson et al. (2022) concluded cluster-randomized and stepped-wedge designs should be considered by researchers as experimental alternatives to individual-randomized trials when testing speech, language, and hearing care interventions in real-world settings.

Advantages and Disadvantages of Group Designs

Advantages and disadvantages of group designs are summarized in Table 7–2 and discussed briefly here. Group designs have several advantages. Statistical procedures for determining reliability are available for group designs. Another advantage is that it is possible to control order or sequence effects because a relatively large number of subjects permits randomization (Portney & Watkins, 2009; Silverman, 1998). Group designs also allow generalization of results from samples of subjects to the population as a whole (Doehring, 1988; Portney & Watkins, 2009). Another advantage is the ability to demonstrate causal relationships (Patten, 2005; Portney & Watkins, 2000).

Despite the advantages of group designs, there are several disadvantages. First is the assumption of homogeneity of group members, that is, that all members of a group respond similarly to an experimental condition. Related to this is subject attrition, which can affect results because loss of group members may disrupt group equivalency (Portney & Watkins, 2009; Warren, 1986). A second disadvantage is related to availability of subjects; in group designs, more subjects may be required than are available (Silverman, 1998). Third, the typical subject may not be typical; in other words, the mean or average of the group may not accurately reflect differences in individ-

Table 7–2. Advantages and Disadvantages of Group Designs

Advantages	Disadvantages
Reliability of data	Assumption of homogeneity of group members
Availability of statistical procedures	Subject attrition
Generalization from sample to population	Availability of subjects
Established population characteristics	Typical subject may not be typical
Control order or sequence of effects	Generalizability of results
	Quantitative information
	Ethical considerations

Sources: From *Research Strategies in Human Communication Disorders*, by D. G. Doehring, 1988, Boston, MA: College-Hill Press; *Research Design and Evaluation in Speech-Language Pathology and Audiology* (4th ed.), by F. H. Silverman, 1998, Needham Heights, MA: Allyn & Bacon; *Language Intervention Strategies in Adult Aphasia* (pp. 66–80), by R. L. Warren, In R. Chapey (Ed.), 1986, Baltimore, MD: Williams & Wilkins; *Understanding Research Methods: An Overview of the Essentials* (5th ed.), by M. L. Patton, 2005, Glendale, CA: Pyrczak; and *Foundations of Clinical Research: Applications to Clinical Practice* (2nd ed.), by L. G. Portney, 2000, Upper Saddle River, NJ: Prentice-Hall Health.

ual performance (Patten, 2005; Portney & Watkins, 2009; Silverman, 1998). Fourth, it may be difficult to generalize results because of the possibility of uncertain validity (Portney & Watkins, 2009; Silverman, 1998). Another disadvantage is related to limitations of quantitative information (Doehring, 1988). Last, there are ethical considerations about group designs because of concern about withholding treatment for research projects (Portney & Watkins, 2009; Warren, 1986).

Single-Subject Designs

Single-subject designs focus on the behavior of one or a few subjects. These designs are also referred to as applied behavioral analysis designs or behavioral analysis, idiographic designs, single-subject experimental designs, single-case designs, intrasubject replication designs, small N-approach, and within-subjects designs. The use of the term is confusing, because it is also used to refer to a variety of group designs (Hegde, 1999). Cardon and Azuma (2011) describe the use of single-subject research designs for individuals with autistic spectrum disorder (ASD). These authors stated that individuals with ASD are a rather heterogeneous group to study; therefore, single-subject research designs may be very helpful when describing the impact of various types of clinical treatment.

It is misleading to consider any design that uses one or a few subjects as a single-subject design. Designs that use single subjects also can be classified as case studies or single-subject designs (Warren, 1986). Single-subject designs are experimental designs that attempt to establish cause-and-effect relations. According to Portney and Watkins (2000), "Single-subject designs are structured around two core elements that distinguish them from a case study or group studies; repeated measurement and design phases" (p. 224). Single-subject designs can be used to study comparison between several types of treatment or between treatment and no treatment (Portney & Watkins, 2000). Bordens and Abbott (1988) described four characteristics of single-subject designs:

1. Individual subjects are observed intensely under each of several treatment conditions; these observations provide a baseline against which any future change induced by the independent variable can be evaluated.
2. All incidental variables that may affect the dependent variable are controlled as rigidly as possible.
3. Each subject is observed under all treatment conditions, and each treatment is repeated at least twice during the course of the experiment. This repetition of intrasubject replication shows the reliability of the findings. Subjects usually remain in each treatment of the experiment until the behavioral measure meets a stability criterion.
4. If more than one subject is used, the additional subjects are included to evaluate the generality of findings across subjects. This intersubject replication establishes whether the results obtained with one subject are similar or dissimilar to those obtained with other subjects. (p. 263)

There are many types of single-subject designs, but two basic categories of single-subject designs known as baseline designs and discrete trials designs have been identified (Bordens & Abbott, 1988; Portney & Watkins, 2009). Baseline designs include designs that manipulate a single independent variable (single-factor designs), those that manipulate two or more independent variables (multifactor designs), and those that measure several dependent variables (multiple baseline designs). In baseline designs, the variable, also known as the target behavior, is measured prior to the experimental treatment of intervention. It includes a baseline condition (A) during which a baseline of subject performance is established and a treatment or intervention condition (B) in which the effect of the treatment or intervention is observed. There are several types of these designs, including AB, ABA, ABAB, ABAC, and BAB (Portney & Watkins, 2009; Silverman, 1998). These symbols are designed as follows:

A = baseline;

B = first treatment or intervention; and

C = second treatment or intervention different from the first.

It includes more than one independent variable and require that different combinations of the independent variable be tested across the study. The effects of the independent variables and their interactions can be assessed. A factorial design may be used or specific combinations may be evaluated (Portney & Watkins, 2000). These designs can be very time consuming, because each treatment is evaluated at least twice for intrasubject replication. Multiple baseline designs involve observation of different behaviors and establishing baselines for each. Thus, several behaviors are observed within the experimental context to provide multiple baselines.

Treatment is considered effective if the level of each behavior changes after the treatment is applied to it.

In **single-subject discrete trial designs**, individual subjects receive each treatment condition of the experiment dozens of times. Each treatment or trial produces one data point for each dependent variable measured. Extraneous variables that could introduce unwanted variability in the dependent measure are rigidly controlled. If possible, the order of treatments is randomized or counterbalanced to control order effects. Intrasubject replication is established by comparing the behavior of individual subjects undergoing the same treatment.

The advantages and disadvantages of single-subject designs are summarized in Table 7–3. Single-subject designs often are frequently used to determine treatment efficacy (Hegde, 1999; Portney & Watkins, 2009). These designs are economical in terms of time, because single-subject research frequently can be conducted during regular clinical hours and during regularly scheduled treatment sessions (Gillam & Gillam, 2006). Furthermore, single-subject designs are similar in form to the design of therapy and are the best, if not the only, appropriate strategy to advance clinical knowledge and make use of evidence-based practice. Table 7–4 provides examples of studies using single-subject designs in communication disorders.

Sequential Clinical Trials

Group studies often require a fixed sample size prior to starting an experiment (Portney & Watkins, 2009). An alternative to group studies and single-subject designs includes sequential clinical trials (SCTs). Instead of waiting until the end of an experiment for data analysis, the

Table 7–3. Advantages and Disadvantages of Single-Subject Designs

Advantages	Disadvantages
Control of error variance	Limited generalization
Establish causal relationships	Control of extraneous variables
Identify individual differences	Control of order and sequence effects
Flexibility	Limited availability of statistical procedures
Small number of subjects (as few as 1)	
Focus on actual behavioral outcomes	
Practical clinical application	
Can be done during scheduled treatments	
Economical	

Sources: From *Research Design and Methods,* by K. S. Bordens and B. B. Abbott, 1988, Mountain View, CA: Mayfield; *Research Design and Evaluation in Speech-Language Pathology* (4th ed.), by F. H. Silverman, 1988, Needham Heights, MA: Allyn & Bacon; and *Foundations of Clinical Research: Applications to Practice* (2nd ed.), by L. G. Portney and M. P. Watkins, 2000, Upper Saddle River, NJ: Prentice-Hall Health.

Table 7–4. Examples of Studies Using Single-Subject Experimental Designs (SSEDs) in Communication Disorders

Author(s)	Topic
Ali et al. (2018)	Outcome of script training in a patient with Broca's aphasia
Gevarter & Zamora (2018)	A review of SSEDs regarding teaching expressive use of speech-generating devices
Wandin et al. (2021)	Communication intervention for expressive language for individuals with Rett Syndrome
Wallace et al. (2022)	A review of studies reporting restorative designed to improve auditory to improve auditory comprehension in people with aphasia
Tabrizi et al. (2022)	Repetition priming as a method for targeting implicit processes in anomia treatment

SCT allows for analysis when each subject is tested and can be stopped at any point, as the evidence is there to determine a significant difference between treatments (Portney & Watkins, 2009). An SCT can be used to compare two treatments such as an "old" or standard treatment to a "new" experimental treatment.

Once the parameters of the study have been adequately defined, then the first eligible subject can be enrolled. The patient is assigned to either the standard or experimental treatment by some randomization process. When the next eligible patient is enrolled, that patient is enrolled in a condition that is the opposite of the first patient.

Portney and Watkins (2000) stated that it is often "convenient to evaluate the relative effectiveness of two treatments by collecting a series of qualitative preferences in favor of one or the other" (p. 205). The preference by the subject is defined on the "basis of clinically meaningful differences between two treatments" (p. 205).

There are four possible outcomes for classifying preference. First, both subjects could indicate "improvement." Second, both subjects could indicate "no improvement" with their treatment. Third, one subject could indicate "improvement" and the other subject could show "no improvement." Fourth, the situation could be reversed in which the first subject showed "no improvement" and the other subject showed "improvement." For further discussion about data collection and analysis, one should consult Portney and Watkins (2009). Table 7–5 describes advantages and limitations for SCTs.

Technologic Applications and Research Designs

Whether using group or single-subject research designs, a researcher should make use of the technology available when conducting data analysis. Group

Table 7–5. Advantages and Limitations for Sequential Clinical Trials (SCTs)

Advantages	Limitations
Fixed sample size not needed to start	Only compare 2 treatments
Can analyze data as subjects complete trials	Do not explore multiple or interaction effects
Subjects can be enrolled once eligible	Control extraneous variables only with randomization of pairs
Statistical technique can be done without computer	If a pair doesn't state preference those data are discarded
Holds much potential in rehabilitation research	Effects of treatment should be soon so time is limited

Source: From *Foundations of Clinical Research: Applications to Practice* (2nd ed.), by L. G. Portney and M. P. Watkins, 2000, Upper Saddle River, NJ: Prentice-Hall Health.

designs usually involve more inferential statistics, because a researcher is interested in making inferences from a sample to a population (Pyrczak, 2004). Descriptive statistics can be used with a variety of research designs (group, single-subject, SCTs) and would include information about, but not limited to, the mean, standard deviation, mode, median, and correlations.

There are many different programs for statistical analysis. These programs can perform a variety of statistical functions. Masuadi et al. (2021) conducted a bibiometric analysis study of 10,596 articles published in PubMed in three 10-year intervals from 1997, 2007 and 2017. This study described the trend and usage of currently available statistical tools. Of the statistical software in the retrieved articles, Statistical Package for Social Sciences (SPSS) was found to be the most common statistical software used (52.1%), followed by Statistical Analysis System (SAS; 12.9%), and Stata (12.6%; IMB Corp., 2022). These researchers also analyzed which research designs were

most associated with a statistical program. SPSS was mostly frequently used with observational (61.1%) and experimental designs (65.3%). Student versions of SPSS (GradPack) including base, standard, and premium editions are available that typically provide sufficient capacity for studies involving numerous variables and data entries.

When utilizing IBM SPSS, it is important that a researcher understand there are many methods that can be used for the collection of data (e.g., pencil-paper, direct observation, etc.), but SPSS assists during the analysis of the data. Initially, all data must be entered into the SPSS program in which the researcher defines the variables to be entered and analyzed.

SPSS supports the researcher by saving data to a file that can be analyzed and graphically displayed in a variety of ways. This includes, but is not limited to, descriptive statistics, t-tests, ANOVA, linear regression, correlations, and multiple linear regressions. There are useful tools to support a researcher when making decisions about statistical analysis in

SPSS, including a tutorial program, statistics coach, and results coach.

A researcher must be mindful that SPSS, or any other statistical analysis program, will only provide support in terms of the calculations and graphically displaying the information (which can be exported to text documents). It is still the responsibility of any researcher or team of researchers to determine which type of design to use and what statistical methods will help answer questions as well as provide an accurate interpretation.

Summary

Group research designs require the formation of two or more groups. Single-subject designs are based on an individual subject's performance under different conditions. Although group designs are often used, they do not meet the practical needs of speech-language pathologists and audiologists to evaluate treatment. These designs were described as if they were mutually exclusive, but this is not so. Some studies use designs that generate both types of data. Different study designs have different strengths and weaknesses. It is important to remember that research designs that are appropriate today may not be in the future. Technology supports the analysis of data used with a variety of research designs but still requires the researcher to make decisions regarding the appropriate application of the technology, data analysis, and interpretation.

DISCUSSION QUESTIONS

1. Distinguish between strategic planning and research design.
2. Distinguish between group and single-subject designs. What are the advantages and disadvantages of each?
3. When would a between-subjects design be appropriate? When would a within-subjects design be used?
4. Why might there be ethical concerns with certain types of research designs?
5. Why should single-subject designs be used by clinicians?
6. Are single-subject designs used by clinicians daily (in some form)? Explain your answer.
7. When would sequential clinical trials be used? Why are SCTs not frequently seen in rehabilitation literature?
8. What is SPSS? How would SPSS help a researcher? When is an SPSS not helpful to a researcher?
9. Explain to your faculty advisor that the program needs to invest in SPSS.
10. Choose one of the single-subject designs listed in Table 7–4. Describe the statistical analysis that was used. What did you find interesting about it?

References

Ali, N., Rafi, M. S., Ghayas Khan, M. S., & Mahfooz, U. (2018). The effectiveness of script training to restore lost communication in a patient with Broca's aphasia. *JPMA. The Journal of the Pakistan Medical Association*, *68*(7), 1070–1075.

Bordens, K. S., & Abbott, B. B. (1988). *Research designs and methods*. Mayfield.

Cardon, T. A., & Azuma, T. (2011). Deciphering single-subject research design and autism spectrum disorders. *ASHA Leader*.

Clement, C. J., & Wijner, F. (1994). Acquisition of vowel contrasts in Dutch. *Journal of Speech and Hearing Research*, *37*, 83–89.

Doehring, D. G. (1988). *Research strategies in human communication disorders*. College-Hill Press.

Gevarter, C., & Zamora, C. (2018). Naturalistic speech-generating device interventions for children with complex communication needs: A systematic review of single-subject studies. *American Journal of Speech-Language Pathology*, *27*(3), 1073–1090. https://doi.org/10.1044/2018_AJSLP-17-0128

Gillam, S. L., & Gillam, R. B. (2006) Making evidence-based decisions about child language intervention in schools. *Language, Speech, and Hearing Services in Schools*, *37*, 304-315.

Gutierrez-Clellen, V. F., & Heinrichs-Ramos, L. (1993). Cohesion in the narrative of Spanish-speaking children: A developmental study. *Journal of Speech and Hearing Research*, *36*(3), 559–567.

Hegde, M. N. (1999). *Clinical research in communication disorders* (4th ed.). Pro-Ed.

IBM Corp. (2022)). *IBM SPSS Statistics GradPack and Faculty Packs* [Computer software]. https://www.ibm.com/products/spss-statistics/gradpack

IBM Corp. (2022). *IBM SPSS Statistics for Windows* (Version 29.0) [Computer software].

Mamo, S. K., Wheeler, K. A., Clark, V. L., & Jacolen, C.S. (2021). A mixed methods study of hearing loss, communication, and social engagement in a group care setting for older adults. *Perspectives of the ASHA Special Interest Groups: SIG 15 Gerontology*, *7*(2), 592–609.

Masuadi, E., Mohamud, M., Almutairi, M., Alsunaidi, A., Alswayed, A. K., & Aldhafeeri, O. F. (2021). Trends in the usage of statistical software and their associated study designs in health sciences research: A bibliometric analysis. *Cureus*, *13*(1), e12639. https://doi.org/10.7759/cureus.12639

Maxwell, D. L., & Satake, E. (2006). *Research and statistical methods in communication sciences and disorders*. Thomson-Delmar Learning.

Ottenbacher, K. J. (1990). Clinically relevant research designs for rehabilitation research: The idiographic model. *American Journal of Physical Medicine and Rehabilitation*, *69*, 286–292.

Patten, M. L. (2005). *Understand research methods: An overview of the essentials* (5th ed.). Pyrczak.

Patterson, C. G., Leland, N. E., Mormer, E., & Palmer, C. V. (2022) Alternative designs for testing speech, language hearing and hearing interventions: Cluster-randomized trials and stepped-wedge designs. *Journal of Speech, Language, and Hearing Research*, *65*(7), 2677–2690.

Pezzei, C., & Oratio, A. R. (1991) A multivariate analysis of the job satisfaction of public-school speech-language pathologists. *Language, Speech, and Hearing Services in the Schools*, *22*(3), 139–146.

Polit, D. F., & Hungler, B. P. (1999). *Nursing research: Principles and methods* (6th ed.). Lippincott.

Portney, J. G., & Watkins, M. P. (2009). *Foundations of clinical research: Applications to clinical practices* (3rd ed.). Pearson.

Portney, L. G., & Watkins, M. P. (2000). *Foundations of clinical research: Applications to clinical practice* (2nd ed.). Prentice Hall Health.

Pyrczak, F. (2004). *Success at statistics: A work text with humor.*

Sawuerwin, A., & Burris, M. M. (2022). Augmentative and alternative communication course design and features: A survey of expert faculty and instructors. *American Journal of Speech-Language Pathology*, *31*(1), 221–238.

Shim, H. J., Cho, Y. T, Oh, H. S., An, Y. H., Kim, D. H., & Kang, Y. S. (2021). Within-subjects comparisons of the auditory brainstem response and uncomfortable loudness levels in ear with and without tinnitus in unilateral tinnitus subject with normal audiograms. *Otology and Neurology*, *42*(1), 10–17.

Siegel, G. M., & Young, M. A. (1987). Group designs in clinical research. *Journal of Speech and Hearing Disorders*, *52*(3), 194–199.

Silverman, F. H. (1993). *Research design and evaluation in speech-language pathology and audiology* (3rd ed.). Prentice Hall.

Silverman, F. H. (1998). *Research design and evaluation in speech-language and audiology* (4th ed.). Allyn & Bacon.

Smit, A. B., Brumbaugh, K. M., Weltsch, B., & Hilers, M. (2018) Treatment of phonological disorder: A feasibility study with focus on outcome measures. *American Journal of Speech-Language Pathology*, *27*(2), 536–552.

Tabrizi, R., Walton, L., Simon, E., & Silkes, J. P. (2022). Repetition priming in treatment of anomia. *American Journal of Speech-Language Pathology*, *31*(1), 48–66. https://doi.org/10.1044/2021_AJSLP-20-00278

University of Southern California. (2019). *Research guides: Organizing your social sciences research paper.* https://libguides.usc.edu/writingguide

Wallace, S. E., Patterson, J., Purdy, M., Knollman-Porter, K., & Coppens, P. (2022). Auditory comprehension interventions for people with aphasia: A scoping review. *American Journal of Speech-Language Pathology*, *31*(5S), 2404–2420. https://doi.org/10.1044/2022_AJSLP-21-00297

Wandin, H., Lindberg, P., & Sonnander, K. (2021). Aided language modelling, responsive communication and eye-gaze technology as communication intervention for adults with Rett syndrome: Three experimental single case studies. *Disability and Rehabilitation: Assistive Technology.* Advance online publication. https://doi.org/10.1080/17483107.2021.1967469

Warren, R. L. (1986). Research design: Considerations for the clinician. In R. Chapey (Ed.), *Language intervention strategies in adult aphasia* (pp. 66–79). Williams & Wilkins.

Wolfe, J., Duke, M., Miller, S., Schafer, E., Jones, C., Rakita, L., . . . Manning, J. (2022). Low-levels speech recognition of children with hearing aids. *Journal of the American Academy of Audiology*, *33*(4), 196–205.

8

Quantitative Research

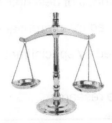

LEARNING OBJECTIVES

Upon completion of this chapter, the reader will be able to:

- Describe characteristics of quantitative research
- Identify various types of quantitative research
- Select an appropriate statistic based on the type of data
- Explain different methods of descriptive statistics
- Describe methods used for inferential statistics
- Interpret data provided by special methods such as meta-analysis
- Evaluate quantitative research

Research can be classified as either qualitative or quantitative. The latter involves investigation of phenomena that lend themselves to precise measurement and quantification, often under controlled conditions that can be subject to statistical analysis (Maxwell & Satake, 2006; Polit & Beck, 2010). Qualitative research (discussed in Chapter 9), conversely, involves delineating themes or patterns in data with less concern for precise measurement of specific variables. This chapter describes various aspects of quantitative research including descriptive and inferential statistics.

Characteristics of Quantitative Research

Quantitative research is a type of research in which objective data are gathered and analyzed numerically (McMillan & Schumacher, 2010). The emphasis is on numbers, measurement, deductive logic, control, and experimentation. Characteristics of quantitative research are shown in Table 8–1 and Figure 8–1.

Advantages and Disadvantages of Quantitative Research

Historically, quantitative research has been the gold standard for research, that is, superior to other types of research. A major strength of quantitative research is its credibility, which is the extent to which the data and conclusions are believable and trustworthy. Other advantages are objectivity, standardization, replication, and limited bias. There is no uniform agreement regarding disadvantages. The disadvantages that have been identified are superficial/oversimplification, unrelated to the real world, too intense, focused only on hard data, and unnatural environment (French et al., 2001).

Quantitative Research Designs

There are major differences in the credibility of nonexperimental and experimental designs. Quantitative designs may be viewed on a continuum. True experimental designs are at one end of the continuum (highest), and nonexperimental studies are at the other end (lowest). *Five major categories of research designs* have been identified: nonexperimental, preexperimental, quasi-experimental, experimental (true experimental), and single subject.

Nonexperimental Designs

Nonexperimental or observational designs are the weakest of all designs because they do not involve randomization, manipulation, or use of control groups. Furthermore, causal relations (i.e., cause-effect relationships) cannot be established (Maxwell & Satake, 2006). This type of research includes descriptive research and correlational studies. The advantages of nonexperimental research are (a) its appropriateness for studying problems not amenable to experimental research and (b) its efficiencies and effectiveness for studying a large amount of information about a problem. The disadvantages are the failure to describe causal relationships

Table 8–1. Qualitative Versus Quantitative Research: Distinguishing Features

Characteristics	Quantitative	Qualitative
Purpose	Explain and predict	Describe and explain
	Conform and validate	Explore and interpret
	Test theory	Build theory
Process	Focused	Holistic
	Known variables	Unknown variables
	Established guidelines	Flexible guidelines
	Predetermined methods	Emerging methods
	Somewhat context free	Context bound
	Detached view	Personal view
Researcher's role	Detached	Observer or participant
Data collection	Statistical analysis	Search for themes and categories
	Stress objectivity	Acknowledgment of subjectivity and bias potential
	Deductive reasoning	Inductive reasoning
Communication of findings	Numbers	Words
	Statistics, aggregated data	Narrative, individual quotes
	Formal voice, scientific style	Personal voice, literary style

Sources: *Practical Research Planning and Design*, by P. D. Leedy & J. E. Ormrod, 2010, Boston, MA: Pearson; and *Research in Education*, by J. H. McMillan & S. Schumacher, 2010, Boston, MA: Pearson.

and faulty interpretation on selection of groups and self-selection.

Nonexperimental research includes descriptive and correlational studies (Polit & Beck, 2010). Descriptive studies provide descriptive information about population parameters and relationships among subjects. Correlational studies describe relationships among variables (DePoy & Gitlin, 2011).

Nonexperimental research is undertaken when (a) a number of independent variables, such as gender and height, are not amenable to randomization; (b) some variables cannot be ethically manipulated; (c) there are practical constraints

to manipulating variables; and (d) avoiding manipulation achieves a more realistic understanding (Polit & Beck, 2010). There are a variety of nonexperimental research designs, which are summarized in Table 8–2.

Preexperimental Designs

Preexperimental designs are sometimes referred to as pseudoexperimental designs because they do not meet at least two of the three criteria for true experiments: randomization, manipulation, or control. Furthermore, preexperimental

Associated terms or phrases
- Positivist*
- Experimental
- Hard data
- Statistical

Key concepts
- Variable
- Operationalized
- Controlled
- Reliable
- Statistically significant
- Replicated
- Hypothesized

Goals
- Test theory
- Establish facts
- Show relationships
- Predict
- Statistically describe

Design
- Structure
- Predetermined
- Formal
- Specific

Sample
- Large
- Representative
- Random selection
- Control group
- Stratified

Data
- Quantities
- Count
- Measures/instruments
- Numbers
- Statistics

Techniques or methods
- Experiments
- Quasiexperiments
- Structured observations
- Structured interviews
- Surveys

Data analysis
- Deduction
- Statistical

Figure 8–1. Characteristics of quantitative research. (*Positivist or postpositivism is based on the assumption that phenomena should be studied objectively; the goal is obtaining a single true reality, or at least within known probabilities.) Adapted from *Educational Research*, J. H. McMillan, 2004, Pearson.

Table 8–2. Nonexperimental Quantitative Research Designs

Name of Design	Description
Case Study	In-depth analysis of single individual, a few individuals, or an institution.
Case control	Retrospective comparison of case and a matched control.
Case series	Three or more cases in a case study.
Cohort	Focuses on specific subpopulation from which different samples are selected at different points in time.
Correlational	Study of interrelationships among variables of interest without any active intervention of inferring causality.
Descriptive	Summarizes status on phenomena, that is, characteristic and/or frequency with which certain phenomena occur.
Ex post facto	Presumed cause that occurred in the past. Also called causal comparison.
Retrospective	Begins with outcome and looks back in time for antecedent caused.
Prospective	Begins with examination of presumed causes and then goes forward in time for its effect.
Natural experiments	Comparison of groups in which one group is affected by a seemingly random event.
Path analysis	Uses correlation of several variables to study causal patterns
Causal comparison	Dependent variable already occurred so its relationship to other variables can only be studied. Also called ex post facto.
Structural equation modeling	Relatively new method, more powerful than path analysis for studying correlations to identify causal patterns.
Surveys	Focuses on obtaining information about activities, beliefs, preferences, attitudes, by direct questioning.
Cross-sectional survey	Survey given at one time.
Longitudinal survey	Same or similar subjects surveyed over time.

Sources: Research and Statistical Methods, by D. L. Maxwell and E. Satake, 2006, Clifton Park, NY: Thomson-Delmar Learning; *Educational Research*, by J. H. McMillan, 2005, Boston, MA: Pearson; and *Nursing Research: Principles and Methods*, by D. F. Polit and C. T. Beck, 2010, Philadelphia, PA: Lippincott Williams & Wilkins.

studies are limited to describing outcomes because appropriate statistical analysis cannot be performed. Thus, the goal of such studies is to explore or describe phenomena rather than explain their causes. Currently, the use of pre-experimental designs is limited due to inadequate control of numerous extraneous variables. Maxwell and Satake (2006) noted that preexperimental designs "give the impression of constituting credible scientific studies but are characterized by numerous sources on invalidity" (p. 204). These designs were described as "fools gold" because of the "misleading impressions of belonging to more rigorous and powerful kinds of experimental methodologies" (p. 203). Schiavetti et al. (2011) point out that these designs are weak in both internal and external validity.

There are *four types* of preexperimental designs: single group pretest only, single group pretest-posttest, time series design, and nonequivalent groups posttest only. These designs are summarized in Figure 8–2.

The weakest of the preexperimental designs is the **one-group postdesign**, which is also known as the single group posttest only or one-shot case study. This design involves study of the presumed effect of an independent variable in one group of subjects by administering a posttest after some treatment.

The **single or one-group pretest-posttest design**, also known as a before-after design, compares pretest and posttest data subsequent to treatment. There is inadequate control for internal and external validity because there is no control group from which to make comparisons.

The **time series design** involves repeated measures before and after treat-

Nonequivalent Groups Posttest Only
$$X\ O_1$$
$$X\ O_2$$

⇩

Static Group Comparison
$$X\ O$$
$$X$$

⇩

Single Group Pretest-Posttest
$$O,\ X,\ O_2$$

⇩

Single Group Posttest Only
$$XO$$

Figure 8–2. Nonexperimental research designs from highest to lowest (O = observation; X = treatment). Adapted from *Educational Research*, J. H. McMillan, 2004, Pearson; and *Research and Statistical Methods*, D. L. Maxwell, D. L., and E. Satake, 2006, Thomson Delmar Learning.

ment using the same instruments with the same or similar subjects over an extended period of time. McMillan (2005) believes this is "a good design for frequently occurring measures of the dependent variable at regular intervals" (p. 218). There is some confusion about the classification of time series designs. This design is classified by some as preexperimental (McMillan, 2005; Mertens 2005) and by others as quasi-experimental (DePoy & Gitlin, 2011; Maxwell & Satake, 2006; Meline, 2006; Polit & Beck, 2010). The next section on quasi-experimental designs provides further information about time series designs.

Nonequivalent groups; posttest-only design has a comparison control group, both of whom are tested after treatment and not before treatment. Another type of preexperimental design is the static group comparison in which the performance of two groups is compared. One group receives treatment, and the other does not.

Quasi-Experimental Designs

These designs are commonly used in speech-language pathology and audiology research (Meline, 2006). Quasi-experimental studies are sometimes referred to as nonrandomized. These designs are also referred to as controlled trials without randomization and are close to true experiments but lack randomization and a control group (i.e., subjects are not randomly assigned to groups). Quasi- or semiexperimental designs combine some of the characteristics of both experimental and nonexperimental research (Kumar, 1996). These designs are used when true experiments are impractical or impossible. Quasi-experiments are not as powerful as true experiments in establishing causal relationships between treatments and outcomes (Polit & Beck, 2010).

The nonequivalent group pretest-posttest design involves the use of two non-randomized comparison groups, both of whom are tested before and after treatment. The most serious threat to validity of this design is that subjects are not randomly assigned to these groups (DePoy & Gitlin, 2011). This design is similar to the nonequivalent groups posttest-only design and static group comparison, except for the addition of a pretest (Maxwell & Satake, 2006; McMillan, 2005).

Another type of quasi-experimental research is the **single time series design**, which is sometimes referred to as inter-rupted time series design. These designs involve repeated data collection over time for a single group (DePoy & Gitlin, 2011). The advantage of this design over the nonequivalent comparison group design, which has single pretest and posttest measures, is the use of several pretest and posttest measures (Maxwell & Satake, 2006). This, however, could threaten validity because administration of several pretest and posttest measures could result in a greater degree of test sensitization. Another disadvantage is the lack of a control group.

True Experimental Designs

True experimental designs or randomized controlled trials (RCTs) are considered by many as the *gold standard*, that is, the strongest of the research designs (Maxwell & Satake, 2006; Polit & Beck, 2010). Randomization, also called random assignment, is the selection of a sample of subjects so that each member of a population has an equal probability of being selected (Polit & Beck, 2010). Random assignment is randomization of subjects to experimental and control groups so that the groups are comparable at the onset of the experiment. Control is the process of holding constant confounding influences of the dependent variable under study. This usually means a control group of subjects who do not receive treatment. These designs can provide information about cause-and-effect relationships among independent and dependent variables.

A **true experimental design** is characterized by manipulation (treatment or intervention), randomizations or random assignment (equal chance of being represented), and control. If a research design does not meet these three criteria, it is probably a quasi-experimental design. There are several types of experimental designs. Some of the more common designs are summarized in Table 8–3. Additional information about experimental designs is available in Blessing and Forester (2012), Isaac and Michael (1987), and Vogt (2006).

Single-Subject Designs

Single-subject designs can be used to study one subject or a small number of subjects for an extended period of time before and after treatment. This design involves a variation of several group designs (repeated measures; time series). Single-subject designs are classified as quasi-experimental (Maxwell & Satake, 2006) or experimental (McMillan, 2005). They have been described as a special application of experimental research. These designs are described in more detail in Chapter 7.

Quantitative Analysis

Quantitative or **statistical analysis** is the organization and integration of quantitative data according to systematic mathematical rules and procedures. Statistical analysis is guided by and dependent upon all previous steps of the research process, including the research problem, study, design, number of study variables, sampling procedures, and number of subjects. Each of these steps should lead to the selection of appropri-

ate statistical analysis (DePoy & Gitlin, 2011). Statistical analysis and statistic warrant definition. Statistical analysis is concerned with summarizing numerical data, assessing its reliability and validity, determining the nature and magnitude and relationships among sets of data, and making generalizations from current to future events (Nicolosi et al., 2004). Statistic, according to Maxwell and Satake (2006), "is a number derived by counting or measuring sample observations drawn from a population that is used in estimating a population parameter" (p. 529). DePoy and Gitlin (2011) described statistic as a "number derived from a mathematical procedure as part of the analytic process experimental type research" (p. 324).

Descriptive Statistics

Descriptive statistics are used to describe and synthesize data. Table 8–4 summarizes the different types of descriptive statistics. The most basic statistic is frequency distribution, which is a systematic arrangement of values from lowest to highest with a count of times each value was obtained.

Graphs can be used to display frequency or relative frequency of percentages. The most frequently used graphs are *histographs* (bar graphs) and frequency *polygons* (line graphs). Other graphs for displaying distributions include pie graphs and trend charts. *Pie charts* are used to represent the proportion of data falling into certain categories in the form of a circle containing segments, which are also called slices, sections, or wedges. These graphs are useful in illustrating percentages in relation to each other and to the whole (Nicol &

Table 8–3. Experimental Designs

Name of Design	Description
Between-subjects	Comparison of groups treated differently on some independent variable.
Counterbalance	Variation of experimental design in which more than one treatment is tested and the order of participation in each treatment is manipulated.
Factorial (ANOVA)	Any design in which more than one treatment factor is investigated.
Latin square	Repeated measures design in which presentation of conditions is counterbalanced so that each occurs in each sequential position of a block.
Parallel	Experiments that generally have at least two randomly assigned independent groups of participants, each of whom receive only one of the treatments (independent variables) under investigation.
Posttest only (after only)	Data collected from subjects only after treatment. Most basic of the experimental designs
Pretest-posttest (before-after)	Data collected from subjects both before and after treatment. Most commonly used true experimental design.
Randomized block	Involves two or more factors (independent variables), only one of which is experimentally manipulated.
Repeated measures (crossover)	One group of subjects is exposed to more than one condition or treatment in random order..
Randomized clinical trial (RCT)	Experimental test of a new treatment, involving random assignment to treatment groups; typically a large and diverse sample. Also known as a phase III clinical trial.
Solomon four group	Uses a before-after design for one pair of experimental and control groups, and after only design for a second pair.
Split plot	Uses both within-subject and between-subject design elements of statistical analysis of treatment effects.
Within-subjects	Comparison within same subjects under circumstances in which they were exposed to two or more treatment conditions.

Sources: Introduction to Research, by E. DePoy and L. N. Gitlin, 2011, Philadelphia, PA: Elsevier Mosby; *Nursing Research: Principles and Methods*, by D. F. Polit and C. T. Beck, 2010, Philadelphia, PA: Lippincott Williams & Wilkins; and *Research and Statistical Methods in Communication Sciences and Disorders*, by D. L. Maxwell and E. Satake, 2006, Clifton Park, NY: Thomson-Delmar Learning.

Table 8–4. Descriptive Statistics

Type of Analysis	Method	Description
Shape of distribution	Skewed	Asymmetric distribution
	Positively skewed	Asymmetric distribution tail points to right (positive) side because frequency of low scores greatly outnumber high scores
	Negatively skewed	Asymmetric distribution; tail points left (negative) side because frequency of high scores greatly outnumbers low scores
	Modality	Describes number of peaks, values with high frequencies.
	Unimodal	Distribution of values with one peak (high frequency)
	Bimodal	Distribution of values with two peaks
	Multimodal	Distribution of values with more than one peak.
	Leptokurtic	Too peaked
	Platykurtic	Too flat
Central tendency	Mode	Value that occurs most frequently
	Median	Point in distribution where 50% above and 50% below; mid-score
	Mean	Arithmetic average
Variability	Range	Difference between lowest and highest score
	Interquartile range	Range of middle 50% of scores
	Semiquartile	Same as interquartile range
	Sum of squares	Difference between each score and the mean
	Variance	Mean of squares deviation from the mean
	Standard deviation	Square root of the variance; indicates average deviation of scores around the mean

continues

159

Table 8–4. *continued*

Type of Analysis	Method	Description
Bivariable	Contingency table	Two-dimensional table that illustrates frequencies of responses for two or more nominal or quantitative variables
	Correlation	Describes relationship between two or more variables
	Pearson's product moment correlation	Uses interval or ratio data; yields a score between −1 and +1
	Spearman's rho	Uses ordinal data; yields a score between −1 and +1; preferable to product moment for numbers under 20 nonparametric equivalent of Pearson *r*
	Kendall's tau	Used with ordinal data; yields a score between −1 and +1; preferable to *rho* for numbers under 10
	Point biserial	To examine relationship between a nominal variable and an internal level measure; yields lower correlation than *r* and much lower than *r* big
	Phi coefficient	Describes the relationship between two dichotomous variables
	Terrachoric correlation coefficient	Used when both variables are artificial dichotomies
	Cramer's *V*	Describes relationship between nominal level data; used when contingency table to which it is applied is larger than 242
	Contingency coefficient	Two dichotomous variables on a nominal scale; closely related to chi square
	Multiple correlation	One single variable and some combination of two or more other variables
	Partial correlation	Two variables studied; influence of their or several other variables held constant. Also called first order–correlation

Sources: Foundation of Clinical Research, by L. G. Portney and M. B. Watkins, 2009, Upper Saddle River, NJ: Prentice-Hall Health; *Handbook in Research and Evaluation*, by S. Isaac and W. B. Michael, 1987, San Diego, CA: Edits Publishers; *Nursing Research: Principles and Methods*, by D. F. Polit and C. T. Beck, 2010, Philadelphia, PA: Lippincott Williams & Wilkins; *Reading Statistics and Research*, by S. W. Huck, 2004, Boston, MA: Pearson; and *Research and Statistical Methods*, by D. L. Maxwell and E. Satake, 2006, Clifton Park, NY: Thomson-Delmar Learning.

Pexman, 2003). They are also referred to as pie charts, pie diagrams, cake charts, circle graphs, percentage graphs, or 100% graphs. An example of a pie chart is in Figure 8–3. The pie on the right is an exploded pie chart that emphasizes the proportion of time devoted to research (Bordens & Abbott, 1988). The major advantage of pie charts is that people typically think of as a circle encompassing 100%. A trend chart also can be used to illustrate frequencies or percentages of change in a dataset that is organized in a developmental or temporal order. A trend chart is shown in Figure 8–4.

Shapes of Distributions

Data can be described relative to shape. Several shapes have been described and are illustrated in Figure 8–5 and defined in Table 8–4. Some distributions occur so frequently that they have special names. The **normal curve** or **normal distribution** is a symmetrical bell-shaped curve that has a concentration of scores in the middle of the distribution with fewer scores to the right and left sides of the

distribution (Figure 8–6). An important characteristic of the normal curve is that predictable percentages of the population are within any given portion of the curve (Leedy & Ormrod, 2010). About two-thirds (68.2%) of the population fall within plus or minus one standard deviation of the mean, 96% fall within plus or minus two standard deviations of the mean, and 99% of the population fall within plus or minus three deviations of the mean.

Central Tendency

Measures of central tendency provide statistics that indicate an average or typical value of a set of scores. There are three measures of central tendency, **mode**, **median**, and **mean**, which are described in Table 8–4.

Variability

Measures of variability or dispersion are the degree of dispersion or the difference among scores. These measures include the **range, interquartile range,**

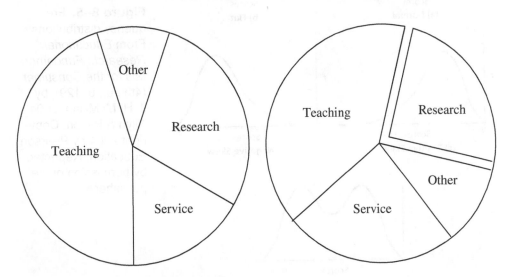

Figure 8–3. Pie chart and exploded pie chart.

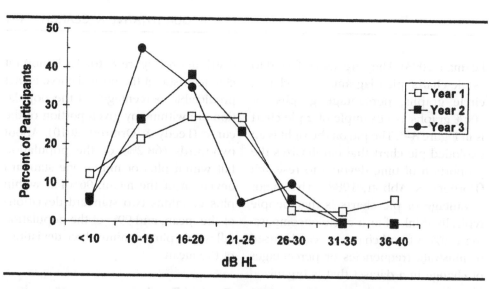

Figure 8–4. Trend chart showing distribution of average hearing levels for children with OME in years 1, 2, and 3. Data are presented according to hearing level (HL) categories in decibels (db). Four-frequency (500, 1000, 2000, and 4000 Hz) average values displayed were derived by categorizing each participant's mean hearing levels across each study year. Reprinted by permission from "Effects of Otitis Media With Effusion in the First 3 Years of Life," by J. S. Gravel and I. F. Wallace, I. F., 2000, *Journal of Speech, Language, and Hearing Research, 43*, p. 638. Copyright 2000 by American Speech-Language-Hearing Association. All rights reserved.

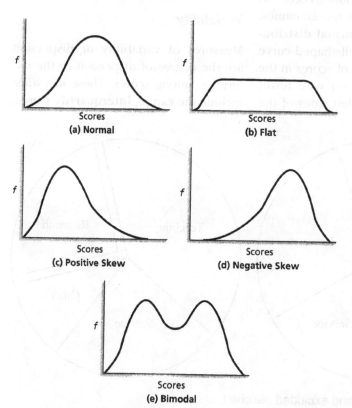

Figure 8–5. Frequency distributions. From *Educational Research: Fundamentals for the Consumer* (4th ed., p. 129), by J. H. McMillan, 2004, Allyn & Bacon. Copyright 2004 by Pearson Education. Reprinted by permission of the publisher.

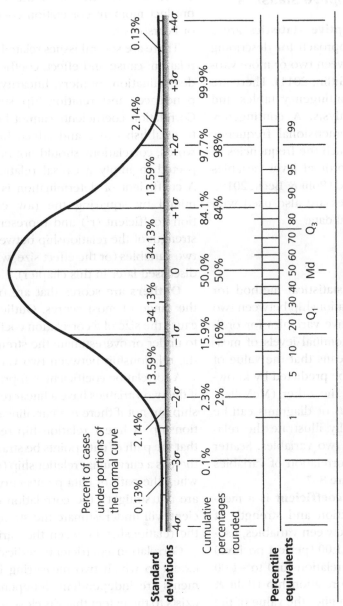

Figure 8–6. Normal distribution curve. From Test Service Notebook #148. Copyright 1980 by Harcourt Assessment, Inc. Reproduced with permission. All rights reserved.

Source: Seashore, H. G. (1980). Methods of expressing test scores. In *Test service notebook 148.* Courtesy of The Psychological Corporation.

sum of squares, variance, and the **standard deviation**. See Table 8–4 for definitions of these measures.

Bivariate Descriptive Statistics

Bivariate descriptive statistics are a data reduction approach for describing relationships between two or more variables (DePoy & Gitlin, 2011). There are two methods: contingency tables and correlational analysis. A contingency table is a two-dimensional frequency distribution in which the frequencies of two nominal or ordinal level variables are cross-tabulated (Polit & Beck, 2010). Contingency tables are also used with nominal or ordinal data.

Correlation

Correlation is a statistical method for measuring the relationship between two or more quantitative variables for ordinal, interval, or nominal levels of measurement. This means that the value of one variable can be predicted by knowing the value of the other (McMillan, 2005). *Scatter plots* or diagrams can be used to graphically illustrate the relationship between two variables. Scatter plots indicating correlation of variables are shown in Figure 8–7.

A **correlation coefficient** is a measure of the direction and strength of the relationship between variables, usually ranging from 1.00 (perfect positive) through zero (no relationship) to –1.00 (perfect negative) relationship (Polit & Beck, 2010). The higher the value of the coefficient, the stronger is the relationship. Correlation coefficients between 0.10 and 0.30 are considered small or low relationships, 0.40 to 0.60 are considered moderate relationships, and 0.70

and above are considered high or strong relationships. There are several types of correlation coefficients, as summarized in Table 8–4. The most frequently used correlation coefficient is the Pearson product moment correlation coefficient or Pearson's r.

There are several issues related to correlation: cause and effect, coefficient of determination, outliers, linearity, independence, and relationship strength. Correlation coefficients cannot be used to establish cause and effect. In other words, correlations should not be interpreted to imply a causal relationship. A coefficient of determination is determined by squaring the raw correlation coefficient (r^2) and represents the strength of the relationship between the two variables (or the effect size, which is discussed later in this chapter).

Outliers are scores that are outside the range of most scores. Outliers can cause the size of a correlation coefficient to under or overestimate the strength of the relationship between two variables.

A correlation coefficient is appropriate if the two variables have a linear relationship but not if there is a curvilinear relationship. A linear relationship requires that the path of data points be straight. If there is a curvilinear relationship (occurs when the path of data points curve and are not straight), the correlation coefficient will underestimate the strength of the relationship between the variables.

Correlation coefficients indicate the extent to which two measuring instruments are independent. Independence exists to the extent that r is close to zero, that is, high correlations suggest lack of independence, whereas low correlations imply independence (Huck, 2004). There are no widely accepted criteria for describing the strength of the relationship

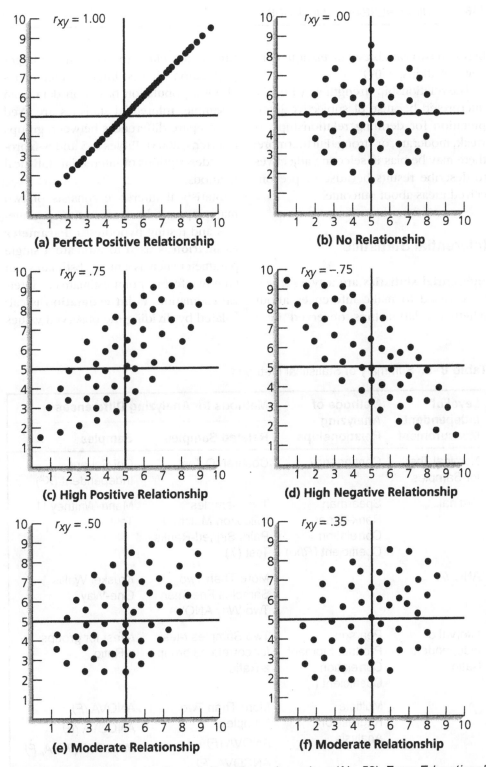

Figure 8–7. Scatter plots of correlations for various sizes ($N = 50$). From *Educational Research: Fundamentals for the Consumer* (4th ed., p. 135), J. H. McMillan, 2004, Allyn & Bacon. Copyright 2004 by Pearson Education. Reprinted by permission of the publisher.

between two variables (correlation; Portney & Watkins, 2009)

The relationship strength may be misinterpreted because of subjective interpretation for defining relationships as weak, moderate, or strong. Furthermore, there may be bias in selecting adjectives to describe results because of preconceived ideas about outcome.

Inferential Statistics

Inferential statistics are a type of statistics used to make inferences about whether relationships observed in a

sample are likely to occur in the larger population, that is, infer characteristics about a population based on data from a sample. Inferential statistics are used to compare differences between groups (Mertens, 2005). Tables 8–5 and 8–6 provide descriptions of inferential statistical methods.

Statistical inference consists of two major approaches: estimating parameters and testing hypotheses. **Parameter estimation** is used to estimate a single parameter such as a mean. Estimates can take two forms: point estimates or interval estimation. **Point estimation** is calculated by dividing the observed values

Table 8–5. Summary of Statistical Methods

Level of Independent Measurement	Methods of Analyzing Relationships	Methods for Analyzing Differences	
		Related Samples	**Samples**
Nominal Test for Samples	Contingency	Cochran Q Test	Chi Square Independent (X^2)
Ordinal	Spearman Rank-Order Correlation Coefficient (*Rho*)	Two Samples Wilcoxon Matched Pairs Signed-Ranks Test (*T*)	Mann-Whitney U Test
ANOVA		More Than Two Samples Friedman Two-Way ANOVA	Kruskel-Wallis One-Way
Interval or Independent Ratio	Pearson Product-Moment Correlation Coefficient (*r*)	Two Samples *t*-test for correlated groups z-Ratio	*t*-Test for groups z-Ratio
	Multiple Regression Analysis	More Than Two Samples ANOVA (*F*) ANCOVA (*F*) MANOVA (*T², A, F*)	ANOVA (*F*) ANCOVA (*F*) MANOVA (*T², A, F*)

Source: Evaluating Research in Communication Disorders, by N. Schiavetti and D. E. Metz, 2002, Boston, MA: Allyn & Bacon. Reprinted with permission.

Table 8–6. Inferential Statistics

Parametric Statistics	
ANOVA	Comparison of three or more treatment groups or conditions or the simultaneous manipulation of two or more independent variables
ANCOVA	Used to compare two or more treatment groups while controlling effect of one or more extraneous variables (covariables)
Factor Analysis	Used to examine structure within a large set of variables and to determine underlying dimensions that exist within that set of variables
Pearson's r	Determine relationship between two variables
Structural equation models	Examines correlation among a number of variables to identify possible causal relationships. Includes methods such as path analysis and confirmatory analysis
t-test	Used for comparing two means. Also called student t-test
Nonparametric Statistics	
Chi square	Compares observed frequencies within categories to frequencies expected by change. Computed for nominal, ordinal, inferential, or ratio data
Fishers exact t-test	Used with small samples to test significance of difference in proportions
Kendall's tau	Measure of association or ordinal measuring
Kruskal-Wallis	Compares more than two independent groups representing levels of one independent variables; nonparametric counterpart of ANOVA
Mann-Whitney U test	Compares two independent groups; nonparametric counterpart of t-test
McNemar test	Used for nominal level measures to correlated samples: For Chi square test
Median test	Compares median values of two independent groups to determine if groups are from populations with different medians
Odds ratio	Estimate of relative risk by a case control study
Phi coefficient	Used to estimate relationship between two dichotomous variables
Spearman's rho	Correlation coefficient indicates magnitude of relationship between ordinal level measures
Wilcoxon signed rank test	Compares two correlated samples (repeated measures); nonparametric counterpart of t-test

Sources: Foundation of Clinical Research, by L. G. Portney and M. P. Watkins, 2009, Upper Saddle River, NJ: Prentice-Hall Health; and *Nursing Research: Principles and Methods*, by D. F. Polit and C. T. Beck, 2010, Philadelphia, PA: Lippincott Williams & Wilkins.

from the sample by the size of the sample, that is, a single statistic to estimate the population parameter. Point estimation is described as an educated guess on the basis of the sample data about the unknown value of the population. **Interval estimation** is a statistic that indicates the upper and lower limits of a range of values within which the parameter has a given probability of occurring, that is, the confidence intervals or the range of values within which a population parameter is estimated to lie. *Confidence intervals* are used to indicate the degree of confidence to which the data reflect the population's mean (Mertens, 2005). Confidence limits are the upper and lower limits of the confidence level (Polit & Beck, 2010).

Huck (2004) provided four cautionary statements about point and interval estimation. First, the second of two numbers separated by a plus and minus sign may or may not be the numerical value of the estimated standard error. Second, sample data permit estimation of the standard error, not definitive determination of the standard error. Third, the sample statistic will always be located between the upper and lower limits of the confidence interval but will not always be located halfway between the interval's end points. Fourth, estimation requires that the data used for inference come from a random sample.

Hypothesis Testing

Hypothesis testing is concerned with making objective decisions based on statistical analysis of differences between groups or relationships of values. The **null hypothesis** states that there is no difference or no relationship between variables, that is, the statistical hypothesis (Portney & Watkins, 2009). Conversely, the **alternative hypothesis** states that there is a significant difference or relationship between variables. Rejection of the null hypothesis.

There are two types of errors in testing hypothesis: rejecting a true null hypothesis (Type I) or accepting a false null hypothesis (Type II). Conversely, there are two possible correct decisions: accepting a true null hypothesis and rejecting a false null hypothesis. Figure 8–8 summarizes these decisions.

A *Type I error* occurs if the null hypothesis is rejected when it should not have been, namely, that a relationship exists when it does not. A *Type II error* is when the null hypothesis is not rejected when it should have been rejected, namely, that no relationship exists when it actually does exist (Polit & Beck, 2010).

The risk of being wrong is rejecting the null hypothesis (Type I error) and is called the *level of significance* or *limit of confidence* (Schiavetti et al., 2011). The level of significance is indicated with the small letter p (probability) or by the Greek letter α (alpha). The most frequently used levels of significance are 0.05 and 0.01. This means that the probability of making a Type I error is 0.05 (5 chances in 100) or 0.01 (1 chance in 100). This means at the 0.01 level the null hypothesis would be rejected when it should have not been in only 1 out of 100 samples.

The level of significance is affected by three factors (McMillan, 2005): (a) the differences between the groups being compared—the greater the difference, the smaller is the p-value; (b) the degree of sampling and measurement error—the lower the error, the smaller is the p-value; and (c) the sample size—the p-value will

Status of null hypothesis

	Null hypothesis is true	Null hypothesis is false
Accept null hypothesis	Correct decision	Type II error
Reject null hypothesis decision	Type I error	Correct decision

Figure 8–8. Hypothesis decisions. Reprinted with permission from *Evaluating Research in Communicative Disorders*, by N. Schiavetti and D. E. Metz, 2002, Allyn & Bacon.

be smaller for a very large sample, that is, if a small sample size is used.

One- and Two-Tailed Tests

A *one-tailed (directional) test* of statistical significance is one in which only values at one extreme (tail) of a distribution are considered when testing significance (Polit & Beck, 2004). A one-tailed test may be appropriate if there is a strong basis for a directional hypothesis, which is a hypothesis that makes a specific prediction about the direction and nature of the relationship between two variables. An example of a directional hypothesis would be predicting poorer (decreasing) speech recognition scores as the signal-to-noise ratio (ratio of level of speech to noise) decreases (i.e., poorer speech recognition with increasing noise). The use of one-tailed tests is controversial because differences found with two-tailed tests are more rigorous than those found with a one-tailed test (Schiavetti et al., 2011). However, Ludbrook (2013) suggests one-tailed tests to be appropriate when the directionality of the alter-

native hypothesis is specified a priori (before the experiment is conducted).

Two-tailed (nondirectional) tests are usually preferred, particularly in studies not specifying a directional hypothesis. These tests involve both ends of the sampling distribution (both tails) to determine improbable values (Polit & Beck, 2010). Two-tailed tests are more strict than one-tailed tests; that is, a greater difference between groups is required when using a two-tailed test compared to a one-tailed test. Conversely, a smaller difference may not be significant with a two-tailed test but may be significant with a one-tailed test.

Parametric and Nonparametric Statistics

Parametric (distribution bound) statistics involve the estimation of at least one parameter: the use of interval or ratio measures, normal distribution, and a fairly large sample. The sample has a central high point and is not seriously skewed, that is, leptokurtic. Parametric statistics are more powerful (more sensitive to differences and relationships) than nonparametric statistics and are usually preferred. **Nonparametric statistics** are sometimes called distribution-free statistics because they do not involve rigorous assumptions about the distribution. They are used most often with nominal or ordinal measures. Tables 8–5 and 8–6 list parametric and nonparametric statistical methods.

Between- and Within-Subject Tests

There are **between-subject tests** (test for independent groups) for comparing separate groups of subjects and **within-subject tests** (test for dependent groups) for comparing a single group of subjects under different conditions or at different points in time (Polit & Beck, 2010). An example of a between-subject (independent group) test would be comparing performance on a sentence recognition task between two groups: one group with normal hearing and one group with hearing loss. An example of a within-subject (dependent group) test would be measuring sentence recognition among thirty individuals with hearing loss using three different hearing aids. Each subject produces a word recognition score obtained listening to speech through each type of hearing aid, resulting in three scores for each subject. There is no between-subject (independent group) comparison in this example.

Steps in Hypothesis Testing

The steps of hypothesis testing are basically the same starting with stating a hypothesis and ending with a decision about the hypothesis. The sequence of these steps is illustrated in Figure 8–9. They are described as follows:

State hypothesis

⇩

Select test statistic

⇩

Establish level of significance

⇩

Choose sample size

⇩

Select one-tailed or two-tailed test

⇩

Compute test statistic

⇩

Calculate degrees of freedom

⇩

Obtain tabled value for statistical test

⇩

Compare test statistic with tabled value

⇩

Make decision about hypothesis
(Reject or fail to reject the null hypothesis)

Figure 8–9. Steps in hypothesis testing. From *Nursing Research: Principles and Methods*, by D. F. Polit and C. T. Beck, 2004, Lippincott Williams & Wilkins; and *Research in Communication Sciences and Disorders*, by T. Meline, 2006, Pearson Education

1. *State the hypothesis.* The null hypothesis is a statement of no difference between or among groups or conditions. The alternative hypothesis is a hypothesis that is different from the one being tested and usually different from the null hypothesis (Polit & Beck, 2010).

2. *Select the test statistic.* The following factors are usually considered: type of groups (independent, dependent, repeated measures, matched groups, randomized blocks, or mixed groups); the number of independent and dependent variables; the scale of measurement; and whether parametric tests are appropriate. DePoy and Gitlin (2011) developed a series of seven questions to consider in selecting appropriate statistical tests. These questions are presented in Table 8–7.

3. *Establish level of significance.* The level of significance for accepting or rejecting the null hypothesis is established before analyzing the data. The level of significance is usually set at 0.05 or less.

4. *Choose sample size.* The sample size influences the power of a statistical test. A larger sample usually results in a more powerful test of the null hypothesis (Meline, 2006). Small samples are at greater

Table 8–7. Guidelines for Selecting a Statistical Test

1. What is the research question?
   - Is it about differences?
   - Is it about degrees of a relationship between variables?
   - Is it an attempt to predict group membership?
2. How many variables are being tested, and what types of variables are they?
   - How many variables do you have?
   - How many independent and dependent variables are you testing?
   - Are variables continuous or discrete?
3. What is the level of measurement? (Interval level can be used with parametric procedures.)
4. What is the nature of the relationship between two or more variables being investigated?
5. How many groups are being compared?
6. What are the underlying assumptions about the distribution of a measurement in the population from which the sample was selected?
7. What is the sample size?

Source: Introduction to Research, by E. DePoy and L. N. Gitlin, 2011, Philadelphia, PA: Elsevier. Reprinted with permission.

risk for a Type II error, that is, accepting the null hypothesis when it is false (due to a lack of statistical power associated with small sample sizes).

5. *Select a one- or two-tailed test.* Consider the previously noted discussion on one- versus two-tailed tests.

6. *Compute test statistic.* Calculate a test statistic using a computational formula or a computer. The test statistic is a standard score such as z- or t-statistic (Meline, 2006). The test statistic is computed using the formula in Figure 8–10.

7. *Calculate degrees of freedom.* Degrees of freedom are the number of values within a distribution that are free to vary, given restrictions on the data; often the number of subjects (i.e., *n*) minus 1 (or *n* – 1; Portney & Watkins, 2009).

8. *Obtain tabled value for the statistical tests.* All test statistics have theoretical distributions. By examining these distributions, it can be determined whether obtained values of the test statistic are beyond the range of what is probable if the null hypothesis is true. A table is consulted for the appropriate test statistic to obtain the critical value corresponding to the degree of freedom and significance level (Polit & Beck, 2010).

9. *Compare the test statistic with the tabled value.* If the test statistic is smaller than the tabled value,

the results are nonsignificant. If the computed value is larger, the results are statistically significant. Note: current statistical software programs perform steps #8 and #9.

10. *Make decisions about the hypothesis.* The final step involves making a decision about rejecting or not rejecting the null hypothesis. If the null hypothesis is rejected, the alternative hypothesis is supported but not proven (Meline, 2006).

Evaluating Inferential Statistics

McMillan (2005) suggested eight criteria for evaluating inferential statistics. These criteria were as follows: (a) basic descriptive statistics are needed to evaluate the results of inferential statistics; (b) inferential analyses refer to statistical, not practical or clinical, significance; (c) inferential statistics do not indicate external validity; (d) inferential statistics do not indicate internal validity; (e) the results of inferential tests depend on the number of subjects; (f) appropriate statistical tests should be used; (g) the level of significance should be interpreted correctly; and (h) be cautious of statistical tests with small numbers of subjects in one or more groups or categories.

Multivariate Statistics

The preceding statistical procedures were univariate or bivariate because one or two dependent variables were analyzed.

$$\text{Test Statistic} = \frac{(\text{statistic}) - (\text{parameter})}{\text{standard error of the statistic}}$$

Figure 8–10. Computation of the test statistic.

Multivariate statistics analyze all the dependent variables in a single procedure; this is important in understanding the relationship between dependent variables (McMillan, 2005). Multivariate statistical procedures are being used more often in speech-language pathology and audiology research to study complex relationships among three or more dependent variables. Most outcomes in speech-language pathology and audiology are fundamentally multivariable regardless of whether or not the study is designed for multivariable statistics.

Commonly used multivariable statistical procedures are multiple regression, analysis of covariance (ANCOVA), discriminate analysis, and factor analysis. Multiple regression analysis is the most widely used multivariable statistical procedure (Polit & Beck, 2010). These and other multivariable statistical procedures are summarized in Table 8–8.

Meta-Analysis

Meta-analysis statistically combines the results of two or more studies, that is, conclusions are made about other researchers' statistical analyses. It is a specialized quantitative synthesis of the results of existing research. The major advantages of meta-analysis are (a) increased statistical power by increasing sample size, (b) improved estimated effect, (c) resolution of uncertainty about conflicting results, and (d) improved generalizability of findings.

Effect size is an important concept in meta-analyses. The **effect size** is a standardized scale-free measure of the relative size of the effect of an intervention or strength of relationship (Turner & Bernard, 2006). Effect sizes are interpreted in two ways: (a) common benchmarks of small, medium, and large; or (b) by comparing reported effect size to those reported in prior studies of a similar nature. Schuele and Justice (2006) suggest that authors should report and interpret effect size, and currently it is widely accepted that these values should be included in peer-reviewed publications. Effect sizes should be disassociated from statistical significance due to the fact that statistical significance provides information related to how likely the results of a study are due to experimental manipulation (or conversely due to chance), whereas effect sizes provide information regarding the strength of the results or relationships under study. As such, it is possible to find statistical significance but have a small effect size, which is important when considering the practical or clinical significance (how this outcome may inform clinical decision-making). Statistical significance without an effect size measure limits the conclusions that can be drawn from the study. There are several methods for determining effect size, which are described by Maxwell and Satake (2006) and Turner and Bernard (2006). The statistical methods used in meta-analyses vary widely and depend, in part, on the research designs used in the studies being analyzed (Leedy & Ormrod, 2010). For example, correlated studies require different meta-analytic procedures than do experimental studies. For further discussion regarding meta-analyses, see Chapter 5.

Table 8–8. Multivariable Statistics

ANCOVA (analysis of covariables)	Extension of ANOVA; used to compare the means of two or more groups
Canocial correlation	Analyzes relationship between two or more independent variables and two or more dependent variables
Discriminary analysis	Used to determine if a set of variables can predict group membership
Factor analysis	Procedure for reducing a large set of variables into a smaller set of variables with common characteristic or underlying dimensions
Hierarchical multiple regression	Prediction variables are entered into the equation in steps that are prespecified
Hoxelling's T^2	Extension of t-test: comparison of two groups
LIS-REL (linear structural relations analysis	Another approach to causal modeling; does not have as many assumptions and restrictions as path analysis; uses maximum likelihood estimation
Logistic regression	Based on maximum likelihood estimation; used to predict categorical dependent variables
MANOVA (multivariable analysis of variables)	Extension of ANOVA; used to test significance of differences between means of two or more groups on two or more dependent variables considered simultaneously
MANOVA (multivariable analysis of covariables)	Controls extraneous variables (covariables) when there are two or more dependent variables
MCA (multiple classification analysis)	Supplement to ANCOVA; provides information about adjusted means of groups on a dependent variables after removing effect of covariables
Multiple regression	Method for predicting a continuous dependent variable on basis of two or more independent variables
Multiple classification analysis	Variant of multiple regression and ANCOVA; yields group means by the dependent variables adjusted for effects or covariants
Multiple correlation coefficient	Summarizes degree of relationship between two or more independent variables and a dependent variable
Path analysis	Regression-based procedure for testing causal models
Simultaneous multiple regression	All predictor variables are entered into the equation simultaneously. Also called direct or standard multiple regression
Stepwise multiple regression	All prediction variables are entered into the regression equation at the same time
Survival analysis	Used when dependent variables represent a time interval between an initial event and a terminal event

Source: Nursing Research: Principles and Methods, by D. F. Polit and C. T. Beck, 2004, Philadelphia, PA: Lippincott Williams & Wilkins.

Summary

In this chapter, quantitative research was discussed relative to design and analysis. Quantitative research uses procedures for collection of data that can be subjected to statistical analysis. There are several types of quantitative research designs: nonexperimental, pre-experimental, quasi-experimental, single subject, and experimental. Major differences between these designs are related to control, manipulation, and intervention (treatment). Quantitative analysis can be classified as descriptive statistics, inferential statistics, multivariable statistics, and meta-analysis. Guidelines for evaluating quantitative research were also discussed.

DISCUSSION QUESTIONS

1. Define quantitative research.
2. Why is quantitative considered to be the sole standard for research?
3. Why must one be cautious when interpreting results from a quasi-experiment?
4. Compare the between-subjects, within-subjects, and single-subject designs.
5. What are the strengths and limitations of single-subject design?
6. What are the major characteristics of single-subject design? How can it be used in speech-language pathology and audiology research?
7. Why is it important to graph data?
8. What factors would affect your decision about which measure of central tendency to choose?
9. Compare parametric and nonparametric statistics.
10. What is the difference between cross-sectional and longitudinal studies?
11. What are the advantages and disadvantages of quantitative research?
12. Why is it necessary to use descriptive statistics? Inferential statistics?
13. How is the null hypothesis used in inferential statistics?
14. What is the difference between Type I and Type II errors?
15. What is the difference between parametric and nonparametric statistics?
16. What are the major characteristics of quantitative research?
17. What are the major characteristics of qualitative research?
18. What is the difference between quantitative and qualitative research?
19. Why is randomization an important consideration in choosing a statistical test?
20. What can be done when the basic assumptions for parametric inferential statistics are not met?
21. How can quantitative research be evaluated?

References

Blessing, J. D., & Forester, J. G. (2012). *Introduction to research and medical literature for health professionals*. Jones & Bartlett.

Bordens, K. S., & Abbot, B. B. (1988). *Research design and methods*. Mayfield.

DePoy, E., & Gitlin, L. N. (2011). *Introduction to research*. Elsevier.

French, S., Reynolds, F., & Swain, J. (2010). *Practical research*. Butterworth-Heinemann.

Gravel, J. S., & Wallace, I. F. (2000). Effects of otitis media with effusion on hearing in the first 3 years of life. *Journal of Speech, Language, and Hearing Research, 43*, 631–644.

Huck, S. W. (2004). *Reading statistics and research*. Pearson.

Isaac, S., & Michael, W. B. (1987). *Handbook in research and evaluation*. Edits Publishers.

Kumar, R. (1996). *Research methodology: A step by step guide for beginners*. Sage.

Leedy, P. D., & Ormrod, J. E. (2010). *Practical research: Planning and design*. Pearson.

Ludbrook, J. (2013). Should we use one-sided or two-sided P values in tests of significance? *Clinical and Experimental Pharmacology and Physiology, 40*, 357–361.

Maxwell, D. L., & Satake, E. (2006). *Research and statistics methods*. Thomson-Delmar Learning.

McMillan, J. H. (2005). *Educational research*. Allyn & Bacon.

McMillan, J. H., & Schumacher, S. (2010). *Research in education*. Pearson.

Meline, T. (2006). *Research in communication science and disorders*. Pearson.

Mertens, D. M. (2005). *Research and evaluation in education and psychology*. Sage.

Nicol, A. M., & Pexman, P. M. (2003). *Displaying your findings*. American Psychological Association.

Nicolosi, L., Harryman, E., & Krescheck, J. (2004). *Terminology in communication disorders: Speech-language-hearing* (5th ed.) Lippincott, Williams & Wilkins

Polit, D. F., & Beck, C. T. (2004). *Nursing research: Principles and methods*. Lippincott Williams & Wilkins.

Polit, D. F., & Beck, C. T. (2010). *Nursing research: Principles and methods*. Lippincott Williams & Wilkins.

Portney, L. G., & Watkins, M. P. (2009). *Foundation of clinical research*. Prentice Hall.

Schiavetti, N., Orlikoff, R. T., & Metz, D. E. (2011). *Evaluating research in communicative disorders* (7th ed.). Allyn & Bacon.

Schuele, C. M., & Justice, L. M. (2006). The importance of effect sizes in the interpretation of research. *ASHA Leader, 11*(10), 14–15, 26–27.

Turner, T. M., & Bernard, R. M. (2006, Spring). Calculating and synthesizing effect size. *Contemporary Issues in Communication Science Disorders, 33*, 42–55.

Vogt, W. P. (2006). *Quantitative research methods for professionals in English and other fields*. Pearson Education.

9

Qualitative Research

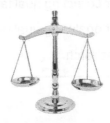

CHAPTER OUTLINE

LEARNING OBJECTIVES

Upon completion of this chapter, the reader will be able to:

- Describe qualitative research
- Discuss the major issues surrounding qualitative research
- Explain qualitative research designs
- Describe methods for collecting qualitative data
- Describe methods for analyzing qualitative data
- Critique qualitative research

Qualitative research is "a variety of analytic procedures designed to systemically collect and describe authentic, contextualized, social phenomena with the goal of interpretive adequacy" (Damico & Simmons-Mackie, 2003, p. 132). In the field of speech-language pathology and audiology, qualitative research can be a valuable resource in helping practitioners understand complicated real-life phenomena and establish functional, contextualized speech and language therapy and audiological treatment.

Qualitative research is often starkly contrasted with quantitative or experimental research. For example, qualitative research is often described as nonnumerical, while quantitative research is described as numerical. Further, qualitative research is at times described as subjective, while quantitative research is described as objective. While these statements may hold some truth, discussion of these differences does not help us understand the nature of qualitative research. In fact, this type of comparison creates a false dichotomy (Damico & Simmons-Mackie, 2003). A stark comparison does not provide us with an understanding of the relationship between quantitative and qualitative research. It also does not help us understand that qualitative research is simply attempting to ask different questions in different ways. One type is not inferior to the other, with both offering different pieces of information regarding a topic or problem. Ultimately, it is more accurate and beneficial to recognize that qualitative research often merges interpretive description with numerical data to form a clear picture of a phenomenon (Damico & Simmons-Mackie, 2003). This process can be initiated to support quantitative studies and can also be fully integrated into the research plan to cre-ate mixed methods studies, which are discussed in the next chapter.

Traditionally, research in speech-language pathology and audiology was dominated by quantitative methods. This trend was apparent in both textbooks and scholarly journals. Although most studies continue to be quantitative, a greater number of qualitative studies have been published in recent years. Damico and Simmons-Mackie (2003) identified some reasons for this trend: (a) increasing recognition of a need to focus on complexity of communication in the context in which it occurs; (b) concentration of consumer-based issues, that is, efficacy, clinical outcomes, and impact of services on quality of life; (c) response to social and economic conditions and trends; (d) social diversification; and (e) recognition of the relationship between clinical practice and research.

It is important to note that qualitative research is an essential part of establishing evidence-based practice (EBP). Often the first stage of EBP involves qualitative methods (Johnson, 2006). Therefore, the purpose of this chapter is to describe the characteristics of qualitative research, qualitative research design, data collection and analysis, and evaluation of qualitative research.

Characteristics of Qualitative Research

The primary characteristic of qualitative research is that it focuses on understanding real-life events or situations. Qualitative research is concerned with subjective, narrative information and is typically obtained under less structured conditions than quantitative research (Portney

& Watkins, 2009). Qualitative research involves insight into the participant's personal experiences, the possibility of unexpected findings, understanding of individual needs and requirements, and continued development of the therapeutic relationship (French et al., 2001).

Other characteristics of qualitative research have been described (Creswell, 2014; McMillan & Schumacher, 2010). The following are some of these characteristics.

Natural setting. Individuals who conduct qualitative research collect data from natural environments, such as classrooms, homes, playgrounds, or therapy rooms. It is necessary to collect data for qualitative studies in natural, everyday environments because one of the goals of qualitative research is to richly describe how or why human behavior occurs. This is more difficult in an unnatural, lablike environment.

Researcher as key instrument. The qualitative researcher collects data via personal interaction, observation, and video recording, among other methods. The researcher is typically present and does not rely on questionnaires or surveys. This is necessary because qualitative research relies on accurate interpretation of the researcher's perception and experience with the participants and setting. The researcher must be present if this is to occur.

Multiple sources of data. Qualitative researchers, under almost any tradition of inquiry (case study, ethnography, etc.), utilize several different types of data. They may collect interviews, journal entries, or participant observation for analysis. The researcher then codes the data to examine for themes or categories that can be organized to reveal a higher level of understanding of the topic under investigation.

Emergent design. Qualitative research seeks to deeply understand a particular topic. Therefore, the specific procedures and design should not be fixed or predetermined, rather they should be emergent. As data are collected, further questions will be revealed that need to be answered by additional means of data collection. The qualitative research project may take multiple turns and change data collection methods several times before the questions it poses are answered.

Participant view. Throughout an entire qualitative research project, the investigator is interested in how participants view the topic of interest. Qualitative research is highly concerned with uncovering and making sense of the participants' personal experiences. Therefore, ensuring that the researcher is not superimposing only his or her own views and is taking the perspective of the participant is vital in qualitative research.

A further description of qualitative research can be seen in some basic criteria set forth by Simmons-Mackie and Damico (2003):

- Social phenomena are studied. Qualitative research is concerned with social, human interaction.
- Data collection is contextualized and authentic. Qualitative research data collection must take place in the original, natural context that is the subject of inquiry. It should not be recreated in a lab or clinic room.
- Data collection is systematic. Qualitative research is inherently flexible and emergent. However, each data collection technique utilized should be defensible and clearly explained.
- Results are well described. When a researcher is studying social phenomena, it is not advantageous

to simply use numerical data that can reduce and simplify behavior into broad categories. Rather, it is necessary to also thoroughly describe the social behavior under investigation so that inherently rich, complex meaning can be derived. Any numerical data resulting from the investigation should align with thick, rich, narrative description and interpretation of the researcher.

Issues in Qualitative Research

Qualitative research presents specific advantages to researchers who are willing to embrace complexity, rather than control variability. As mentioned previously, the primary advantage of qualitative research is its focus on phenomena that occur in natural settings. For example, Damico and Simmons-Mackie (2003) have studied aphasia treatment via video transcripts of actual therapy sessions in both individual and group settings and have revealed significant therapeutic implications for clinicians who treat individuals with aphasia.

In addition, qualitative research may bridge the gap between research and clinical practice and involve studying these phenomena in all their complexity (Maxwell & Satake, 2006). There is often a large gap between what the research says about what we should do in therapy and what we actually do in the treatment room, and qualitative research can provide support for this problem. For example, Page and Howell (2015) studied the nature of the clinical practice of speech-language pathologists (SLPs) who treated individuals with aphasia.

They worked from the premise that little is known about the actual, current practices of speech-language pathologists who work with individuals with aphasia (Page & Howell, 2015). Given that there is often a gap between research evidence and practice, the researchers sought, via interviews, to establish a theory regarding the state of current practice in aphasia treatment. The study revealed that SLPs had a process of establishing the best therapy plan for their clients that involved creating a relationship with them as they developed treatment strategies. It also revealed that SLPs do, in fact, struggle to implement evidence-based practice in the treatment of individuals with aphasia, and that this struggle is often due to time constraints (Page & Howell, 2015). This study provided some relevant information to researchers explaining why the gap between research and practice exists.

It is important to note that even though there has been an increase in use of qualitative methods in the last few years, qualitative research is often seen as inferior to quantitative research. This may occur because even well-designed nonexperimental studies rank low on any hierarchy of evidence-based practice, below quasi-experimental designs, randomized controlled studies, and meta-analyses. This conception of a hierarchy in strength of research, which permeates both publication and peer review, fails to consider that researchers are asking and answering different questions when they select qualitative or more experimental methods. That question, more than anything else, centers on whether the researcher feels comfortable embracing the complexity of social phenomena or seeks to restrict it to a few isolated variables.

In any discussion of advantages and disadvantages of qualitative research, there are concerns with reliability, validity, and generalizability in qualitative research, and whether or not there is enough power or strength in the results of a qualitative study. It is true that the best research method is the one that is most appropriate, singly or combination, to the problem and will produce credible information. Qualitative studies should be designed from this perspective—not from the perspective that one research paradigm is superior to the other.

Despite the advantages of qualitative research, there are limitations. First is perceived issues with credibility, which is based primarily on the concepts of validity and reliability (McMillan, 2005). It is important to note here that because the focus of qualitative research is entirely different than quantitative research, the concepts of validity and reliability mean different things in the context of qualitative research. We discuss the issue of generalizability next and revisit the issues of validity and reliability later in this chapter.

One of the weaknesses mentioned by many is that qualitative research is not (a) randomized or (b) controlled or (c) involves manipulation of variables (the three criteria for experimental research) and, therefore, is often not applicable to a wider population. This perspective of qualitative research is based on a view of generalization that is rooted in probability theory—the idea that predictions can be made or extrapolated from a smaller set of data if the data are randomized, controlled, and include manipulated variables (Damico & Ball, 2010). However, Damico and Ball propose two additional perspectives of generalizability that help explain the rel-

evancy and the generalizability of qualitative research in the field of speech-language pathology and audiology. The first type is analytic generalization. This view purports that qualitative research methods study the underlying human processes of the behavior in question. Therefore, results of these analyses are applicable to a wider population because they were derived from basic, systematic human processes that are common to all humans (Damico & Ball, 2010). In other words, generalizability is not determined by high statistical probabilities, but rather, via a deep understanding of the fundamental entities of which human social behavior is comprised (Damico & Ball, 2010).

The second type of generalizability is **case-to-case transfer**. Case-to-case transfer occurs when a reader consumes a published qualitative study and decides to apply the findings to a client he or she is seeing. In this case, the reader of the research is responsible for making the decision regarding generalization, rather than the researcher. It is, therefore, important for the researcher to engage in thorough, rich, thick description of the topic under investigation to ensure later application of the result is valid and warranted.

Qualitative Research Designs

There are a wide variety of qualitative research designs or traditions of inquiry. Tesch (1990) listed 46 different qualitative designs. It should be noted that there is often a great deal of overlap between these designs (Damico & Simmons-Mackie, 2003). There are a few research designs that are relatively common in the field of speech-language pathology and audiology, and those designs are discussed in this chapter. These include case study, ethnography, ground theory, phenomenology, and conversation analysis. Other designs—such as critical theory, heuristic, life history, and narrative—are less common. These designs differ in several ways: purpose, focus, data collection, and analysis. Table 9–1 provides a summary of qualitative designs.

Case Study

One of the most frequently used qualitative research designs is the case study. A case study is a retrospective research method involving detailed analysis of one or more individuals, groups, institu-

tions, programs, or other entities (McMillan, 2012; Polit & Beck, 2010; Tetnowski, 2020). A case study may be an expansion of an earlier case study. Typically, a case study is a detailed qualitative analysis of a single entity and utilizes various qualitative data collection methods. Case studies, however, may be quantitative and occasionally combine quantitative and qualitative methods (McMillan, 2012).

Case studies have several purposes. Among these purposes are understanding unusual patients and conditions, providing examples of creative or innovative treatments, generating and testing theory, and providing implications for further research (Portney & Watkins, 2009). It should be noted that there has been an increase in the use of case studies in the field of speech-language pathology and audiology.

Table 9–1. Summary of Qualitative Designs

Design	Description
Case study	A detailed qualitative analysis of a single entity. Utilizes various qualitative data collection methods.
Ethnography	Studies complex and contextually sensitive aspects of social interaction and culture. Allows the researcher to investigate aspects of social action or patterns of human behavior in a natural, original context.
Phenomenology	Focuses on the subjective, lived experiences of individuals. Typically conducted via interviews that are loosely structured with open-ended questions.
Grounded theory	A general methodology for developing theory that is grounded in data systematically gathered and analyzed.
Conversation analysis	Created to reveal how individuals accomplish social action within conversation. Involves detailed analysis of video transcripts.

Source: Damico, J. S., & Simmons-Mackie, N. N. (2003). Qualitative research and speech-language pathology: A tutorial for the clinical realm. *American Journal of Speech-Language Pathology,* 12(2), 131–143.

The following is an example of how a case study can be utilized to understand issues in our fields. Daniels (2012) studied one school-age child who stuttered. This child had previously been treated using speech modification techniques only (an approach that focuses only on "fixing" nonfluent speech). The child was admitted for treatment at a university clinic. Over three semesters, speech modification techniques were taught as well as strategies for how to manage emotions that surround stuttering. This study was necessary due to the fact that many approaches to stuttering focus only on modifying the stuttering behavior while ignoring a widely proven fact that stuttering is the result of many factors, one of which involves psychosocial aspects. Addressing emotions within therapy is widely recommended. Since there is a disparity between the recommendations of research and actual practice, a case study that demonstrates the benefit of such an approach was warranted. This study found that successful therapy outcomes were achieved with a broad therapeutic focus that included both stuttering modification and strategies that help the child who stutters overcome the psychosocial barriers he or she encounters (Daniels, 2012).

This case study is an example that demonstrates how this design can be used to explain the impact of a specific therapeutic approach on one person or group. It is just one way that case studies can be used in the field of speech-language pathology or audiology.

Ethnography

Ethnography was born in the field of anthropology, which is the study of the aspects of life that make us human. It has been adapted by various disciplines such as psychology and education, and it is not used the same by every field (Damico & Simmons-Mackie, 2003). At its core, ethnography is a research design that studies complex and contextually sensitive aspects of social interaction and culture (Damico & Simmons-Mackie, 2003). This research design allows the researcher to investigate aspects of social action or patterns of human behavior in a natural, original context. Additionally, ethnography gives the researcher an opportunity to utilize various forms of data collection such as observation, interviewing, and collection of artifacts as needed (Damico & Simmons-Mackie, 2003). Therefore, it is a natural, often very useful tool to study communication disorders. Finally, ethnography is driven by discovery (Damico & Simmons-Mackie, 2003). When discovery is part of the decision-making process, the researcher changes the approach to data collection methods based on the themes that emerge from analysis. For example, if data collected from interviews indicates that the participants should be observed in their natural environment, the researcher can change course and include that type of data in the collection plan.

Cohen (2011) utilized ethnography to explore and describe teacher-student interaction in classrooms wherein children with specific learning difficulties were learning English as a second language. This study had the aim of understanding how second-language learning was facilitated within the social interaction in a classroom. The researchers spent time observing in the classroom, recording those observations and videotaping (for later transcription). Analysis of the data collected revealed that teachers had the most success in the classroom when they deviated from a traditional initiate-response-feedback style and instead used a style of questioning and facilitation that promoted participation and opportunities for learning (Cohen, 2011). In this example, ethnography was employed by utilizing various forms of data collection to study the culture of a classroom in order to explain intricate interaction patterns. The results of this ethnographic study yielded important information that practicing speech-language pathologists can utilize.

Ethnography holds promise for the field of speech-language pathology and audiology as the call for more functional, real-world treatment options increases. Ethnography has the potential to thoroughly explain human behavior in context, so its ability to describe the impact of treatment, the nature of therapeutic relationships, and the real lives of individuals with communication disorders is significant.

Phenomenology

Phenomenological research focuses on the subjective, lived experiences of individuals (Mertens, 2014). This research is typically conducted via interviews that are loosely structured with open-ended questions. These interviews are intended to reveal the thoughts, feelings, and overall perceptions individuals have of a particular phenomenon (Mertens, 2014) It should be noted that the researcher is not concerned with any form of objective reality that exists outside of the person being interviewed (Mertens, 2014). Rather, that person's lived experience is the sole focus of a phenomenological project.

Fencel and Mead (2017) conducted a phenomenological study to investigate how speech-language pathology interns perceived the relationship with their supervisor while in graduate school. Graduate students were interviewed to record their perceptions of what contributed to a positive or negative relationship with a graduate supervisor. Results indicated that respect, clear expectations, constructive feedback, positive praise, and structured clinical guidance contributed to a positive relationship. However, a lack of these attributes contributed to a negative supervisor/supervisee relationship (Fencel & Mead, 2017). This study utilized interviews to investigate graduate students' lived experiences in order to understand how they perceived their relationships with their supervisors. This is an example of how phenomenology can be used to provide useful information to guide the quality of clinical teaching in our field.

Grounded Theory

Grounded theory research was created for the purpose of bringing a more systematic approach to the field of qualitative research. Grounded theory can be best described as "a general methodology for developing theory that is grounded in data systematically gathered and analyzed" (Strauss & Corbin, 1994, p. 273). The key characteristic of grounded theory is that there is no theoretical orientation stated at the outset of the project. Rather, theory emerges as data are collected and analyzed (Mertens, 2014).

As in the case of previously discussed qualitative designs, data are collected through various methods. These data are then analyzed using procedures that have been specifically developed to reveal aspects of the theory that the researcher goes on to generate and explain (Simmons-Macke & Damico, 2003). The analytic process is a transactional one wherein the researcher observes the data and codes the data in a way that allows for comparisons to be made between various datasets. Then, the researcher asks a variety of questions about the data (Damico & Simmons-Mackie, 2003). The answers to these analytic questions then lead the researcher to be able to ask generative (or productive) questions that link and describe the different sets of data that have been collected (Damico & Simmons-Mackie, 2003). Another term for this type of data analysis procedure is the constant comparative method (Damico & Simmons-Mackie, 2003; Mertens, 2014). The constant comparative method gave rise to what we now call triangulation in a general sense (Damico & Tetnowski, 2014). Triangulation involves uncovering and interpreting themes from the coded data, and then collecting more data from additional, different sources by way of confirming interpretation (Damico & Tetnowski, 2014). This continues in a cyclical, iterative process until conclusions are credible and sound. The final product of grounded theory research is a new theory that is based on or "grounded" in the data.

For example, Marshall et al. (2017) explored the experiences of parents of children with language delays who were navigating various intervention systems. The researchers sought to understand, via interviews with 20 parents, what primary issues arise in this sometimes very complicated process. The results revealed that parents must demonstrate advocacy and engagement throughout a rigorous process of recognizing the delay, getting assessment results, and finally enrolling in the needed services for their children (Marshall et al., 2017). This rigorous process presented many challenges for the parents, and the study ultimately concluded with a recommendation that program planners should facilitate a more streamlined, timely response to the issues faced by these parents (Marshall et al., 2017). These results were grounded in the words of the individuals. That is, the conclusions were directly tied to the statements produced by the parents in the interviews (Marshall et al., 2017). Grounded theory was used in this case to investigate how professionals could better assist parents of individuals with disabilities.

Conversation Analysis

Conversational analysis (CA) is a qualitative research design that was created to reveal how individuals accomplish social action within conversation (Goodwin, 1995). According to Damico and Simmons-Mackie (2003), CA "is intended to determine and understand how speakers produce their own behaviors in conversation and how they interpret the conversational behaviors of others." In order to achieve this goal, CA uses methodologies that assist the researcher in determining the interactional devices a speaker uses to accomplish a communicative goal within a conversation. Goodwin used CA to reveal how an individual with aphasia achieved success in conversation (Goodwin, 1995). He found that the speaker used his limited vocabulary (which included the words *and, yes,* and *no*) as well as several other interactional devices such as gestures and collaboration with a fluent speaker to maintain competency within conversation (Goodwin, 1995)

Damico and Simmons-Mackie (2003) report that there are three basic assumptions of conversation analysis:

- All aspects of social action have organized patterns of stable, identified structural features.
- Conversation tends to be sequentially organized. In other words, speakers will respond or produce an utterance based on what the previous speaker did or said.
- CA must be grounded empirically during the data analysis and data interpretation portion of the research project. Researchers must utilize a specific set of procedures to analyze the data, and any decisions that are made based on that data are grounded or directly derived from the data.

Conversation analysis has been used extensively to understand how individuals with aphasia negotiate meaning in conversation. This can be especially helpful when trying to design plans for therapy that focus on real-life interaction. Damico and Simmons-Mackie (2003), in particular, studied how engagement is facilitated in group therapy. Engagement is an essential component of therapy, especially in a group, because some individuals may not participate as frequently if they are not confident or fluent, thereby missing out on the therapeutic impact of group therapy. Damico and Simmons-Mackie (2009) videotaped group therapy sessions and transcribed them. They then studied those transcripts using conversation analysis procedures to reveal that clinician behaviors were important aspects of engaged group

therapy with individuals with aphasia. Clinicians' body orientation, mirroring, and shared laughter, among other things, played a significant part in establishing engagement (Damico & Simmons-Mackie, 2009).

In this example, the researchers utilized the data methodology of conversation analysis to reveal how engagement was achieved in the moment-to-moment interaction in the conversational, informal dynamic of a group session. This is one of the ways in which conversation analysis can be used to reveal the intricacies of interaction that help individuals accomplish social action. Since speech-language pathology is highly interested in helping individuals communicate to their fullest potential, conversation analysis is a valuable tool in the study of communication disorders.

Data Collection Procedures

Qualitative research is inherently emergent. Therefore, data collected to answer the questions posed in a qualitative research project must be ongoing, interactive, and flexible. As data are collected, data are analyzed, and more data are then collected, if necessary. This section discusses general guidelines that should be in place prior to data collection as well as describes specific types of data collection. More discussion regarding data analysis is provided in the following section.

When a qualitative researcher begins a study, he or she must first set general, flexible boundaries for the study, collect information through various data collection methods that are further discussed in this section and, if necessary, create a protocol for recording and keeping a permanent record of the data (Creswell, 2014). When creating general boundaries, selection of participants or site of data collection is necessary (Creswell, 2014). It is also necessary to choose the participants or site that will best answer the question. This is in contrast to quantitative research wherein random selection of participants is valued in order to fulfill the requirement of generalizability (that if participants are selected randomly, there is greater likelihood that the results will be applicable to others). Rather, a solid qualitative research design selects participants in order to best understand the problem at hand.

A common issue that arises in qualitative research is the question of how many participants to include in the study (Creswell, 2014). There are no set criteria for numbers of participants in qualitative research. However, the recommendation is to follow a general rule of thumb: phenomenological studies typically have 3 to 10 participants, grounded theory usually has 20 to 30, ethnography investigates one single cultural group (children with autism, internationally adopted children, etc.), and case studies can include anywhere from one to five cases (Creswell, 2014). Another way of thinking about numbers of participants comes from the grounded theory literature (Charmaz, 2014), and this is the idea of saturation. When a researcher stops getting fresh, new information from the data, he or she has likely collected enough (Creswell, 2014). The researcher has reached a level of saturation in the amount of data collected and can move on to interpretation.

A variety of methods for collecting qualitative data have been identified: observation, interviews, qualitative documents, and qualitative audio and visual information. Furthermore, multiple versions of methods are often used for any single study (Damico & Simmons Mackie, 2003; Silverman, 2014).

Data collection and analysis occur in overlapping phases. While there is a significant amount of flexibility in qualitative research, there are five general phases of data collection: (a) planning, (a) beginning data collection, (c) basic data collection, (d) closing data collection, and (e) completion. Phases 2 through 4 involve actual data collection. The last phase (e) focuses on data analysis, including development of tables and figures (McMillan & Schumacher, 2010). These phases help give structure to the data collection process, but it is not necessary to strictly follow these phases.

Observation

Observation is comprehensive because it is continuous and total (McMillan, 2012). Observations can vary in the degree of structure from totally unstructured to highly structured (French, 2001). In **unstructured observation**, there is no attempt to manipulate the situation. Events are observed as they occur naturally and encompass the entire situation. **Semi-structured observation** is concerned with some aspects of the situation more than others. In **structured observation**, what to observe is decided in advance, and there is an observational schedule. A single observation may involve all of these methods of observation. Unstructured and semistructured observations tend to be time consuming and labor intensive. These methods are most frequently associated with qualitative research.

There are several types of observational methods, which are based on the degree of participation and involvement of the researcher, ranging from complete participation at one end to complete observer at the other end (McMillan, 2012). A **participant observer** is when the researcher is an active participant in the activity being studied, that is, the researcher participates as a member of the group and is not identified as the researcher. According to Meline (2004), participant observation "is more demanding than direct observation because the researcher must acclimate to the situation and become an accepted member in the scene" (p. 79). A complete observer or **passive participant** is detached from the group being studied and is identified as the researcher.

Observation as a data collection technique is particularly well suited to speech-language pathology and audiology. Speech-language pathologists and audiologists are in an advantageous position to observe the behaviors and activities of clients and their families. Moreover, speech-language pathologists and audiologists, if trained, may be very reliable observers. Many speech, language, and hearing problems are well suited to an observational approach.

There are, however, disadvantages, including possible ethical consideration, distorted behavior of the person being observed if the observer is conspicuous, a high refusal rate, and observer bias (Polit & Beck, 2010). Creswell (2004) believes "first and foremost the researcher has an obligation to respect the rights, needs, values, and desires of the informant(s)" (p. 201). Observation is vulnerable to observation bias for a number of reasons (Polit & Beck, 2010). Among these reasons are emotions, prejudices, attitudes, and values of observers; personal interest and commitment; preconceived ideas about what is to be observed; and inappropriate decisions about data collection.

Interviewing

Interviewing is the most common method of data collection in qualitative research (Llewellyn, 1996). The **interview** is a form of data collection in which questions are asked orally and participants' responses are recorded (Maxwell & Satake, 2006). Interviews are conducted face-to-face, by telephone, or electronically. Some general guidelines for interviewing are provided in Table 9–2.

Additional information about interviewing can be found in French et al. (2001), Haynes and Pindzola (2016), Shipley

Table 9–2. Guideline for Conducting Qualitative Interview Research

• Identify questions in advance
• Make interviews representative of the group
• Obtain written permission
• Establish and maintain rapport
• Focus on actual rather than abstract or hypothetical
• Do not put words in people's mouths
• Record responses verbatim
• Keep your reaction(s) to yourself
• Remember you are not necessarily obtaining the facts
• When conducting a focus group, consider group dynamics

Source: Adapted from *Practice Research*, by P. D. Leedy and J. E. Ormrod, 2005, Upper Saddle River, NJ: Pearson.

and McAfee (2009), and Stein-Rubin and Adler (2012).

Interviews have both advantages and disadvantages. Advantages are related to rapport with the participants, which can enhance motivation and results in obtaining information that might not otherwise be obtained; clarification of participants' questions; follow-up on leads or probing; use with many different types of persons (illiterate or too young to read or write); and higher return of results (McMillan, 2012). Face-to-face interviews also have additional advantages, such as observation of nonverbal behavior, and a tendency to reduce no and unknown answers or neutral responses. The disadvantages of interviews are cost, time, small sample size, possible subjectivity, or the training and experience of the interviewer. It is important that questions not be leading or suggest a specific response (McMillan, 2012).

Interviews may be structured, semistructured, or unstructured. *Structured interviews* are often used in telephone interviews (Maxwell & Satake, 2006). Structured interviews have the advantage of efficient use of time and allow some flexibility (Llewellyn, 1996). *Semistructured interviews* are predetermined, but the participants are not predetermined. Rather, the questions are open-ended but specific, which permits individual responses. *Unstructured interviews* are sometimes referred to as informal conversation or in-depth interviews, because they are open ended and flexible. This type of interview is especially useful for understanding individual behavior over time. The disadvantages of unstructured interviews are the time involved and resources needed to analyze the data obtained.

Focus Groups

Focus groups are a method of interviewing a group of individuals about a specific topic or issue. The same format used for individual interviews is used for focus groups: structured, semistructured, or unstructured. The advantages of focus groups are that multiple responses can be obtained in a relatively short period of time, observation of interaction between focus group members, and some people feeling more comfortable talking in a group than alone (Leedy & Ormrod, 2010). Disadvantages are related to possible domination of the group by one or more members. Furthermore, if the facilitator of the focus group is not skilled in group processes and interviewing methods, this will adversely affect the responses of others (Law, 2002).

Analyzing Qualitative Data

As data are being collected, the data *analysis* portion of the study can begin. It is important to note again that data analysis is an integral part of data collection. As the data are collected, it is necessary to start the analysis process so that further data collection can be modified, if needed. If, for example, a study involving interviewing is being conducted, it is advisable to read over and code the first interview as the interviews are being collected to help shape the content of the subsequent interviews (Creswell, 2014).

Data collection, in qualitative research, can lead to a copious amount of information and potential details to unravel. It is easy as a novice (or even seasoned) qualitative researcher to get lost in the wealth of information and struggle to focus on the most relevant aspects of the data. Then, it becomes necessary to go through a process of "winnowing" the data (Creswell, 2014). This involves choosing to only look at the aspects of data that are most relevant to the questions and purpose of the qualitative study. It should be noted that this is in contrast to quantitative research, wherein all data are necessary to fulfill the requirements of the study, and missing data are replaced if at all possible (Creswell, 2014).

There are a variety of methods of analyzing qualitative data ranging from objective and systematic to subjective and interpretive (Maxwell & Satake, 2006). One helpful step-by-step process seen in the literature by Creswell (2014) is the following:

Step 1. *Data collected should be prepared and organized for analysis*. This involves transcribing interviews, videos of therapeutic interaction, typing up observation field notes, and so on.

Step 2. *Look at all of the data*. This will assist the researcher in getting an overall picture of the information. When an overall picture is achieved, it is then possible to reflect on specific issues that may need to be areas of focus.

Step 3. Begin the *coding* process. Coding is a process wherein all of the individual units of data are assigned a name of some type. For example, when coding transcripts, each utterance or conversational turn would be given an interpretive label. The researcher then takes

those individual codes and brackets them into larger chunks or units of meaning to derive a broad theme for interpretation.

Step 4. The coding process leads to *description* of the setting or participants. This description arises from the broad categories or themes that are generated from the coding process. When each theme is thoroughly and richly described, a detailed picture of the participants or setting will emerge. All description should include quotes and many examples from the data to back up any narrative description. This ensures that the broader themes stay tied to the original data.

Step 5. *Decide how themes and description of those themes will be represented in the finished product*. Most researchers rely on narrative writing to share the findings of a qualitative study. This narrative is often supported by tables or graphs that represent the data.

Step 6. The final step in data analysis is to *interpret the data*. This is accomplished by asking and answering the questions: "What does this mean?" or "What lessons can be learned from this investigation?"

Validity and Reliability

In any discussion of data analysis in qualitative research, it is necessary to address the issues of validity and reliability. Similar to the issue of generalizability discussed earlier in this chapter, validity and reliability do not mean the same things in qualitative research as in quantitative research. Rather, in qualitative research, validity indicates that the researcher has ensured accuracy of findings by implementing specific, necessary procedures. Additionally, qualitative research reliability indicates that the researcher has maintained consistency of approach across all researchers involved and methodologies utilized (Creswell, 2014).

To ensure that a qualitative study is valid, Creswell (2014) describes eight strategies:

1. **Triangulation.** The researcher should utilize multiple forms of data collection to verify the meanings of the themes that emerge from data analysis. If each theme is backed up by multiple examples and data points, it will have much stronger validity.

2. Member checking. This is accomplished by taking some of the descriptions of the themes that were established back to the participants for discussion of their accuracy. Member checking is often done in interviews, wherein the final results of a study are presented and discussion is held to establish whether or not the findings are accurate and realistic.

3. Rich, thick description. The researcher should provide highly detailed description to the point that readers may feel that they are in the setting or know the participants. Providing descriptions of different viewpoints and perspectives is also very helpful. By thoroughly describing the setting, participants, and findings, it is

possible to achieve a higher level of validity in qualitative research.

4. Be clear about author bias. One characteristic of qualitative research is that it is interpretive. Therefore, the writer/researcher will inevitably integrate his or her own experience and perspective as they are interpreting the results. It is necessary, from the beginning of the study, for the researcher to be reflective and to write clearly about his or her own theoretical orientation and background. This will help the consumer of qualitative research to be aware of the overall perspective of the researcher and how it influences the outcome of the study.

5. Present contradicting evidence. In most every qualitative study, there will be data that do not agree with one or more of the themes the researcher has established. This is common and realistic. Therefore, it is necessary for the researcher to be honest about these issues. Reporting contradicting evidence will increase the validity of the study.

6. Spend a significant amount of time in the field. When a researcher spends a lot of time with the participants in the setting under investigation, it increases his or her understanding of the entire larger picture. This ultimately will lead to more accurate, realistic interpretation of findings and, thus, validity of the study.

7. Peer debriefing. It is helpful to share the written product and findings with a peer. This will give the researcher a perspective other than his or her own to ensure that the findings resonate with a wider audience. This also ensures validity of interpretation.

8. External auditor. The researcher should also consider asking someone completely external to the project (has had no part in constructing the study or collecting the data) to review every aspect of the study. This will help identify weaknesses and clarify interpretation.

Additionally, ensuring reliability, which is the concept that the research design is consistent across researchers and methodologies, is essential in qualitative research. There are several ways to ensure reliability of a qualitative study (Gibbs, 2008):

■ Checking transcripts to ensure that there are no obvious mistakes in transcription.
■ Constantly comparing data that have been coded to ensure that there is no drift in the meaning of the codes that have been assigned (this refers only to unintended drift; constant comparison may also result in purposeful adjustment of codes or their meaning based on new information from the incoming data; cf. Srivastava & Hopwood [2009]).
■ Conducting regular meetings between those doing the coding to ensure interpretation and meaning are being maintained.
■ Ensuring intercoder agreement by cross-checking codes through a process of comparing results that have been interpreted independently.

Data analysis in qualitative research is an intense, often long process that can yield deep, useful, and wide-reaching results. If done appropriately, following the previously described guidelines, it is possible to achieve outcomes in a qualitative study that are generalizable, valid, and reliable.

Criteria for Evaluation of Qualitative Research

Qualitative research requires different criteria for evaluation because of differences in design and data. Several authors have described criteria for evaluation of qualitative research (Creswell, 2014; French et al., 2001; Leedy & Ormrod, 2010; Silverman, 2014; Trochim, 2001). A checklist for evaluation of qualitative research by Silverman (2014) is as follows:

■ Are the methods of research appropriate to the nature of the question being asked?
■ Is the connection to an existing body of knowledge or theory clear?
■ Are there clear accounts of the criteria used for the selection of cases for study and of the data collection and analysis?
■ Does the sensitivity of the methods match the needs of the research question? Were the data collection and record keeping systematic?
■ Is reference made to accepted procedures of analysis?
■ How systematic is the analysis?
■ Is there adequate discussion of how themes, concepts, and categories were derived from the data?
■ Is there adequate discussion of the evidence for and against the researcher's arguments?
■ Is a clear distinction made between the data and the researcher's interpretation?

This checklist is one of many that can be utilized to critique qualitative research. However, it is key to this process to remember that the specific design and data collected must be well suited and specific enough to investigate the phenomenon in question.

Summary

Qualitative research is a valuable way to approach complex issues worthy of study in the fields of speech-language pathology and audiology. The increasing popularity of qualitative research in speech-language pathology and audiology is evident in the growing number of qualitative studies reported in the past few years. In speech-language pathology, the demand for real-life, functional therapy outcomes is high. Due to the fact that the main focus of qualitative research is to richly describe complex phenomena as they occur in a natural context, this approach to research is vital to the further development of the fields of speech-language pathology and audiology.

DISCUSSION QUESTIONS

1. Define and describe qualitative research.
2. What are the reasons for the increase in qualitative research?
3. Compare qualitative and quantitative research.
4. List and briefly describe qualitative research designs.
5. How are data collected for qualitative research?
6. Explain observer participation and involvement.
7. What are the advantages and disadvantages of interviews?
8. What is the difference between structured and unstructured interviews?
9. How can focus groups be used to collect data?
10. Describe the advantages and disadvantage of focus groups.
11. How can qualitative data be analyzed?
12. What are the criteria for evaluation of qualitative data?
13. What are the characteristics of qualitative research?

References

Cohen, I. (2011). Teacher-student interaction in classrooms of students with specific learning disabilities learning English as a foreign language. *Journal of Interactional Research in Communication Disorders, 2*(2), 271–292.

Creswell, J. W. (2004). *Research design*. Sage.

Creswell, J. W. (2014). *Research design: Qualitative, quantitative and mixed methods approaches* (4th ed.). Sage.

Damico, J., & Tetnowski, J. (2014). *Triangulation*. In *Encyclopedia of social deviance* (pp. 751–754). Sage.

Damico, J. S., & Simmons-Mackie, N. N. (2003). Qualitative research and speech-language pathology: A tutorial for the clinical realm. *American Journal of Speech-Language Pathology, 12*(2), 131–143.

Damico, J. S., & Ball, M. J. (2010). Prolegomenon: Addressing the tyranny of old ideas. *Journal of Interactional Research in Communication Disorders, 1*(1), 1–29.

Daniels, D. E. (2012). Treatment of stuttering in a school-age child: A description of a single case-study. *Perspectives on Fluency and Fluency Disorders, 22*(2), 88–96.

Fencel, J. A., & Mead, J. S. (2017). A qualitative study describing positive and negative supervisor-student clinician relationships in speech-language pathology. *Perspectives of the ASHA Special Interest Groups, 2*(11), 17–22.

French, S., Reynolds, F., & Swain, J. (2001). *Practical research*. Butterworth-Heinemann.

Gibbs, G. (2008). *Analyzing qualitative data*. Sage.

Goodwin, C. (1995). Co-constructing meaning in conversations with an aphasic man. *Research in Language and Social Interaction (Special Issues of Construction), 28*, 233–260.

Haynes, W. O., & Pindzola, R. H. (2016). *Diagnosis and evaluation in speech pathology*. Allyn & Bacon.

Johnson, C. J. (2006). Getting started in evidence-based practice for childhood speech-language disorders. *American Journal of Speech-Language Pathology, 15*, 20–35.

Law, M. (2002). *Evidence-based rehabilitation*. SLACK.

Leedy, P. D., & Ormrod, J. E. (2010). *Practical research*. Pearson.

Llewellyn, G. (1996). Qualitative research. In F. Stein & S. K. Cutler (Eds.), *Clinical research in allied health and special education* (pp. 411–424). Singular Publishing.

Marshall, J., Adelman, A., Kesten, S. M., Natale, R. A., & Elbaum, B. (2017). Parents' experiences navigating intervention systems for young children with mild language delays. *Journal of Early Intervention, 39*(3), 180–198.

Maxwell, D. L., & Satake, E. (2006). *Research and statistics methods in communications*. Thomson-Delmar Learning.

McMillan, J. H. (2005). *Educational research: Fundamentals for the consumer*. Pearson.

McMillan, J. H. (2012). *Educational research: Fundamentals for the consumer* (6th ed.) Pearson.

McMillan, J. H., & Schumacher, S. (2010). *Research in education* (7th ed.). Pearson.

Meline, T. (2004). *Research in communication science and disorders*. Pearson.

Mertens, D. M. (2014). *Research and evaluation in education and psychology* (4th ed.). Sage.

Page, C., & Howell, D. (2015). Current clinical practice of speech-language pathologists who treat individuals with aphasia: A grounded theory study. *Journal of Interactional Research in Communication Disorders, 6*(1), 1–2.

Polit, D. F., & Beck, C. J. (2010). *Essentials of nursing research*. Lippincott Williams & Wilkins.

Portney, L. G., & Watkins, M. P. (2009). *Foundation of clinical research*. Prentice Hall.

Silverman, D. (2014). *Doing qualitative research* (4th ed.). Sage.

Simmons-Mackie, N., & Damico, J. S. (2003). Contributions of qualitative research to the knowledge base of oral communication. *American Journal of Speech-Language Pathology, 12*(2), 144–154.

Srivastava, P., & Hopwood, N. (2009). A practical iterative framework for qualitative data analysis. *International Journal of Qualitative Methods, 8*(1), 76–84.

Stein-Rubin, C., & Adler, R. T. (2012). Counseling and the diagnostic interview for the speech-language pathologist. In C. Stein-Rubin & R. Fabus (Eds.), *A guide to clinical assessment and professional report writing in speech-language pathology.* Delmar.

Strauss, A., & Corbin, J. (1994). Grounded theory methodology—An overview. In K. D. Norman & S. L. Y. Vannaeds (Eds.), *Handbook of qualitative research.* Sage.

Tesch, R. (1990). *Qualitative research. Analysis types and software tools.* Falmer Press.

Tetnowski, J. A. (2020). A case study of fluency in a preschool child. In J. Nollen & S. M. Molfenter (Eds.), *Speech-language pathology casebook.* Thieme. https://shop.thieme.com/Speech-Language-Pathology-Casebook/9781626234871

Trochim, W. M. (2001). *The research methods knowledge base.* Atomic Dos.

10

Multimethod Research

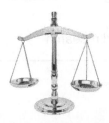

LEARNING OBJECTIVES

Upon completion of this chapter, the reader will be able to:

- Describe the sequences for combining qualitative and quantitative research
- Discuss designs used in multimethod research
- Discuss the advantages and disadvantages of multimethod research
- Evaluate multimethod research

Multimethod or mixed method research combines quantitative and qualitative research methods to ideally use the best of both methods. According to Creswell and Clark (2007), "the use of quantitative and qualitative approaches in combination provides a better understanding of research problems than either approach alone" (p. 5). Speech-language pathologists and audiologists should understand multimethod research because a significant amount of clinical research combines quantitative and qualitative research methods. For the purpose of this chapter, the terms multimethod and mixed method research are used interchangeably and refer to the use of both quantitative and qualitative techniques as part of a research study.

Characteristics of Multimethod Research

Multimethod or mixed method research is a growing trend resulting from discussion and controversy regarding quantitative and qualitative research. These discussions gave rise to a new approach in order to solve some of the issues that arose. Multimethod research combines both quantitative and qualitative features in design, data collection, and analysis (McMillan, 2012; Mertens, 2014). The steps in multimethod research, from determining the feasibility of the study through data collection to reporting the results, are shown in Figure 10–1. Similar steps have been described by Creswell (2014), McMillan (2012), and McMillan and Schumacher (2010).

Creswell (2014) further describes and defines mixed method research in a comprehensive sequence of points:

- Collection of both quantitative and qualitative research
- Analysis of both types of data
- Data collection and analysis conducted with rigor
- The two forms of data are either connected, merged, or embedded
- The procedures are integrated into a new, distinct mixed methods design that has a distinct timing of data collection and a specific emphasis on either qualitative or quantitative research (equal versus unequal)

Additionally, a number of publications describe methods for combining research (Creswell, 2009; Mertens, 2014; Polit & Beck, 2010; Tashakkori & Teddlie, 2010). The *Handbook of Mixed Methods in Social and Behavioral Research* (Tashakkori & Teddlie, 2010) and *Designing and Conducting Mixed Methods Research* (Creswell & Clark, 2007) are comprehensive publications about issues related to combining quantitative and qualitative research. Additionally, there are a number of journals that emphasize mixed method research specifically, such as *Field Methods*, the *International Journal of Multiple Research Approaches*, and *Journal of Mixed Methods Research*. The increased singular focus of these journals on mixed methods indicates a significant shift and increased use of mixed method research in academia.

Despite the increasing popularity of mixed method research, there is considerable debate (Adamson et al., 2004). These two methods of research are different, and the results may be reported separately. Also, it may be difficult to combine quantitative and qualitative methods because of technical problems or conflicts between theoretical perspectives about research (Morgan, 1998).

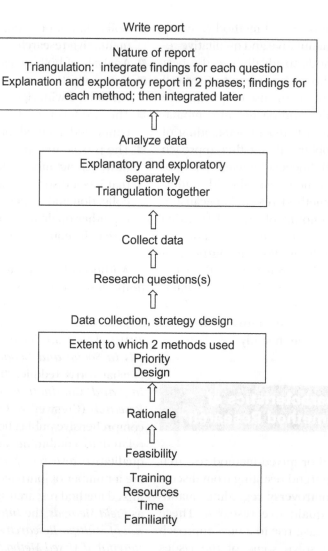

Figure 10–1. Steps in conducting multimethod research. Adapted from *Educational Research*, by J. H. McMillan, 2005, Merrill/Prentice Hall.

Until recently, research in speech-language pathology and audiology has been dominated by quantitative studies. However, qualitative studies gained considerable attention during recent years. Another trend is the blending of quantitative and qualitative data. Multimethod studies are now published in a greater number of speech-language pathology and audiology journals.

Advantages and Disadvantages of Multimethod Research

There are both advantages and disadvantages in multimethod research. The major advantage is that by combining qualitative and quantitative methods, the weaknesses of one may be reduced or avoided; that is, there is the potential for one to offset the other's weaknesses (Polit & Beck, 2010).

There are other advantages to multimethod research, such as (a) providing comprehensive data analysis, both objective (quantitative) and subjective (qualitative); (b) permitting study of both process and outcome; (c) allowing for different types of research questions; (d) compensating for use of a single type of research method; and (e) enhancing credibility of findings (Abusabha & Welfel, 2003; McMillan & Schumacher, 2010). In addition, a multimethod approach may lead to theoretical insight that might be possible without combining methods.

Different methods are more appropriate for different phases of research; that is, qualitative methods are appropriate for exploration of hypothesis generation and quantification is needed later for verification. Multiple and complementary types of data can improve the validity of results. When there are conflicting findings, careful review of the discrepancies between qualitative and quantitative data can provide new insights and enhance theoretical understanding.

There are also disadvantages and limitations in combining qualitative and quantitative research. Depoy and Gitlin (2011) believe mixed method research should not be viewed with skepticism and as nontraditional because of its in-consistency. Polit and Beck (2010) identified five limitations: (a) cost, (b) biases, (c) research training, (d) analytic challenges, and (e) publication biases. First, multimethod research is usually expensive. Second, there are extreme preferences; some prefer quantitative research, whereas others prefer qualitative research. Third, training can

be a challenge be-cause multimethod research requires knowledge and understanding of both qualitative and quantitative research. Furthermore, many training programs offer training in only one method or the other, but not both. Fourth, there are analytic challenges related to combining numeric (quantitative) and narrative (qualitative) data and resolving and interpreting inconsistent or contradictory results. In addition, writing the report and formatted conclusions can be challenging (McMillan & Schumacher, 2010). The fifth limitation is a possibility of publication biases. Some journals prefer qualitative research; however, typically more journals prefer quantitative research. There is also the possibility of a mismatch or bias between the theoretical perspectives of the reviewers and the authors—that is, quantitative researchers serving as reviewers for qualitative research (Belgrave et al., 1998). According to Meline (2006), "it is somewhat popular to indicate that research has both components, even though one of the two methods is only used superficially" (p. 288). Other issues identified by Tashakkori and Teddlie (2003) are related to overreliance on one method alone and the need for an alternative to mixed methods designs. The former involves going beyond mixing at the method level only. The latter suggests that mixed studies go beyond the mixing of methods to include combining other stages of the research cycle. Related to the disadvantages are several myths and misunderstandings that Creswell and Clark (2007) identified. The more common myths are that (a) multimethod research is just qualitative research, (b) it is a method that has always been used, and (c) multimethod research is universally accepted. Acceptance ranges from minimal to major/most (Table 10–1).

Sequencing

Typically, multimethod research is sequential. An explanatory design may be the most common type of mixed methods research. Quantitative data are collected first, and qualitative data are collected in the second phase—that is, qualitative follows quantitative. Another type of mixed methods research is an explanatory design in which qualitative data are collected first and then followed by a quantitative phase—that is, quantitative follows qualitative. The other type of multimethod study is the triangulation design in which both qualitative and

Table 10–1. Levels of Acceptance for Mixed Methods Studies

Major Acceptance	
_____	Special issue of a journal focusing on the use of mixed methods in the profession
_____	Publication of mixed methods studies in top professional journals
_____	Course on mixed methods research as part of graduate training programs
Moderate Acceptance	
_____	Leaders in the profession advocate for use of mixed methods research
_____	Workshops on mixed methods research forums dedicated to the profession
_____	Funding agencies supporting mixed methods research
_____	Methodological discussions of mixed methods in journals devoted to the profession
Minimal Acceptance	
_____	Awareness within the profession of qualitative research
_____	Publication of actual mixed methods studies in professional journals
_____	Graduate students using mixed methods in dissertation research
_____	Discussions in journals about need for mixed methods
_____	Mixed methods research discussed at professional conferences

Source: From *Designing and Conducting Mixed Methods Research*, J. W. Creswell and V. L. R. Clark, 2007, Thousand Oaks, CA: Sage Publications. Copyright 2007 by Sage Publications, Inc. Reprinted by permission of Sage Publications, Inc.

quantitative data are collected simultaneously (McMillan, 2012). Mixed methods research can also be described relative to the stage in which the methods occur (Tashakkori & Teddlie, 2010).

In equal-status (equivalent) mixed methods designs, both quantitative and qualitative methods are used about equally. Dominant–less dominant mixed methods designs refer to studies in which one method is dominant and a small part of the study evolves from the other method. Qualitative and quantitative data are collected and analyzed simultaneously in parallel/simultaneous mixed methods designs.

Research Designs

The choice of research methods is frequently associated with a specific theoretical orientation (Adamson et al., 2004). There are, however, specific criteria for selection of appropriate mixed method designs (Creswell, 2009). These criteria are related to (a) implementation for data collection (concurrent or sequential), (b) priority or equal weight given to quantitative or qualitative approach, (c) phase of research in which the two methods are combined, and (d) identification of theoretical orientation used in the study.

A checklist of questions may help in designing a mixed methods study. Such a checklist is presented in Table 10–2. Mixed method designs have been described in various ways. This chapter discusses three designs and later describes advanced designs that integrate the three basic designs described in this section. We describe convergent, explanatory, and exploratory designs in this section, with attention to detail in the areas of overall description, data collection, data analysis, and interpretation.

Convergent parallel mixed method design is the most common of all the mixed method designs (Creswell, 2014). This type is conducted by implementing both qualitative and quantitative methods simultaneously. The data are then analyzed separately and compared to identify whether or not there is agreement (Creswell, 2014). There are some issues with data analysis. Two types of data analysis are suggested. The first is to analyze the data side-by-side in an effort to compare and discuss. The second is to convert the qualitative data into quantitative data (via Likert scales, etc.) The two forms of data are then merged into table or graph format to present in visual form (Creswell, 2014).

In convergent parallel mixed method designs, after data are collected, analyzing involves searching for either convergent or divergent findings between the two types of data (Creswell, 2014). When divergence occurs, it is very important to report on it and to explain it rather than ignore it.

An example of convergent parallel mixed method design can be found in a study wherein the researchers investigated aspects of driver safety in older adults in order to establish an intervention program for older drivers (Classen et al., 2008). The researchers used the national crash dataset numbers along with interviews that acquired the participants' perspectives, goals, and needs in order to be safe drivers (Creswell, 2014).

The second type of mixed methods research is explanatory sequential mixed methods design (Creswell, 2014).

Table 10–2. Checklist for Designing a Mixed Method Study

Is the basic definition of mixed methods research provided?	Yes	No
Does the reader have a sense for the potential use of a mixed methods strategy?	Yes	No
Are the criteria identified for choosing a mixed methods strategy?	Yes	No
Is the strategy identified, and its criteria for selection given?	Yes	No
Is a visual model presented that illustrates the research?	Yes	No
Is the proper notation used in presenting the visual model?	Yes	No
Are the procedures for data collection and analysis mentioned as they relate to the model?	Yes	No
Are the sampling strategies for both quantitative and qualitative data collection mentioned? Do they relate to the strategy?	Yes	No
Are specific data analysis procedures indicated? Do they relate to the strategy?	Yes	No
Are the procedures for validating both the quantitative and qualitative data discussed?	Yes	No
Is the narrative structure mentioned, and does it relate to the type of mixed methods strategy being used?	Yes	No

Source: From *Research Design*, by J. W. Creswell, 2009, Thousand Oaks, CA: Sage Publications. Copyright 2003 Sage Publications. Reprinted with permission.

This design involves two phases. The first implements quantitative methods in order to inform the second phase of qualitative methods. For example, a survey might be given to explore a specific topic to get quantitative data on the characteristics of a given population. Then, qualitative interviews could be designed specifically for that population (Creswell, 2014).

The two phases of research in explanatory sequential designs must be planned carefully (Creswell, 2014). The quantitative phase must be rigorous and specifically designed to identify the factors most relevant for study by the later occurring qualitative methods. One of the main ideas of this design is that the qualitative phase builds directly on the quantitative phase (Creswell, 2014). Data analysis involves analyzing the results of both phases separately. The results of the quantitative phase are used to plan the qualitative phase (Creswell, 2014).

Banyard and Williams (2007) conducted a mixed method design that was explanatory in nature to study issues surrounding the recovery process of childhood sexual abuse in women. They formed a questionnaire to acquire quantitative data regarding the nature of resilience and the correlates of resilience. They used the data from these interviews to build interviews for a smaller set of participants to investigate their life history, recovery, resilience, and coping abilities.

The final design we discuss is the exploratory sequential mixed method design. This design is a reverse of the explanatory sequential approach to research. The researcher begins the study by researching a specific topic thoroughly utilizing qualitative methods (Creswell, 2014). Then, the researcher initiates the second phase of the project using quantitative methods that are built on the results of the qualitative phase (Creswell, 2014).

In an exploratory sequential mixed method design, qualitative data can be coded to acquire a set of themes that can then be used to group items on a psychometric test, for example. This method can be used to develop scales for assessment (Creswell, 2014). If the qualitative data are thorough and sound, the construct validity of a measurement scale for assessment will be much stronger (Creswell, 2014).

An example of exploratory sequential mixed method design can be found in the 2011 study by Betancourt et al. This study sought to understand how to adapt and evaluate a specific intervention for mental health problems in HIV-affected children living in Rwanda. The investigators chose to begin with an exploration of personal issues of the children and their caregivers via in-depth interviews. They analyzed this qualitative data and utilized these themes to develop survey instruments to be used as pretest and posttest measures for the intervention program they would later implement. This study used qualitative measures to develop an instrument that was later used to acquire quantitative data.

Examples of Multimethod Designs

Multimethod research is used in a variety of health-related fields of study. As can be seen in the examples given so far, it can be a useful tool to accomplish a wide variety of different objectives in research. The following are examples of how mixed method research has been used in communication sciences research studies.

The first example is a pilot study that investigated the perceptions of speech-language pathology student clinicians regarding individuals who stutter (Koutsodimitropoulos et al., 2016). These researchers used a convergent parallel design to administer the Public Opinion Survey of Human Attributes–Stuttering (POSHA-S) as the quantitative component of their study as well as semistructured interviews as the qualitative component. Through the POSHA-S results, they were able to quantify their students' attitudes and compare them to a national average. They also were able to describe more in-depth themes that emerged from the interviews of these students about their attitudes and beliefs about stuttering.

The second example is a study conducted to investigate the difficulties encountered by Hispanic students who struggle with developing adequate writing skills (Perry, 2017). This is a complex issue that is often related to cultural and linguistic differences. Perry conducted a variation of exploratory sequential methods design, which was more embedded. Perry implemented a qualitative analysis of expository essays in order to develop an understanding of the overall structural issues that occur in this type of writing. Then, an intervention was implemented to address these issues and see if they improved after intervention—this was the quantitative portion of the study.

Evaluating Multimethod Research

Questions for evaluating multimethod research were described by Creswell and Clark (2007). These questions reflect relatively general standards, such as basic knowledge of multimethod research, rigor of the research, and advanced knowledge of specific designs. The questions are as follows: (a) Is the study a multimethod study?; (b) Does the study show rigorous multimethod research?; (c) Does the study include advanced multimethod features consistent with multimethod design?; and (d) Does the study show sensitivity of some of the challenges of using the design?

The questions in Table 10–3 may be used to analyze methods research. These questions refer to issues related to quality, which would be referred to as credibility or trustworthiness in qualitative terms or validity in quantitative research.

Table 10–3. Questions for Analyzing Mixed Methods Research

- What are the purposes and questions that justify the use of a mixed-methods design?
- Has the researcher matched the purposes and questions to appropriate methods?
- To what extent has the researcher adhered to the criteria that define quality for the quantitative portion of the study?
- To what extent has the researcher adhered to the criteria that define quality for the qualitative portion of the study?
- How has the researcher addressed the tension between potentially conflicting demands of paradigms in the design and implementation of the study?
- Has the researcher appropriately acknowledged the limitation associated with data that were collected to supplement the main data collection of the study?
- How has the researcher integrated the results from the mixed methods? If necessary, how has the researcher explained conflicting findings that resulted from different methods?
- What evidence is there that the researcher developed the design to be responsive to the practical and cultural needs of specific subgroups on the basis of such dimensions as disability, culture, language reading levels, gender, class, and race or ethnicity?

Source: From *Research and Evaluation in Education and Psychology*, by D. M. Mertens, 2005, Thousand Oaks, CA: Sage Publications. Copyright 2005 by Sage Publications, Inc. Reprinted by permission of Sage Publications, Inc.

Mertens (2005) also described questions for analyzing mixed methods research that are in Table 10–3. The questions require narrative answers.

Summary

Multimethod research is an approach to research that combines quantitative and qualitative methods to answer complex questions. It is a valuable tool in speech-language pathology and is gaining momentum in our field. It is important to remember that multimethod studies follow a specific sequence depending on the problem under investigation. Convergent parallel, explanatory sequential, and exploratory sequential designs can be used to best address issues under investigation. It is true that combining qualitative and quantitative data collection and analysis has several barriers. However, reducing these barriers is worth the time and effort. The truth is that most clinical activities combine quantitative and qualitative research; that is, they are multimethod research. Therefore, using this method to study issues in the fields of speech-language pathology and audiology could be the answer to barriers we face in bridging the gap between research and practice.

DISCUSSION QUESTIONS

1. What is multimethod research?
2. What are characteristics of multimethod research?
3. Why should speech-language pathologists and audiologists understand multimethod research?
4. Describe the major categories of multimethod research.
5. What are the advantages and disadvantages of multimethod research?
6. Identify and describe the different types of component designs.
7. What are the different types of mixed methods designs?
8. Why should a mixed method design be used?
9. How can multimethod research be evaluated?

References

Abusabha, R., & Welfel, M. (2003). Qualitative vs. quantitative methods: Two opposites that make a perfect model. *Journal of the American Dietetic Association, 103*(5), 566–569.

Adamson, J., Gooberman-Hill, R., Woolhead, G., & Donovan, J. (2004). Questerviews: Using questionnaires in qualitative interviews as a method of integrating qualitative and quantitative health services research. *Journal of Health Services Research Policy, 9*(3), 139–145.

Alta Maria Press. (1988). *Field notes.*

Banyard, V. L., & Williams, L. M. (2007). Women's voices on recovery: A multimethod study of the complexity of recovery from child sexual abuse. *Child Abuse and Neglect, 31*(3), 275–290.

Belgrave, L. L., Zablotsky, D., & Guadagno, M. A. (1998). How do we talk to each other? Writing qualitative research for quantitative readers. *Qualitative Health Research, 12*(10), 1427–1439.

Betancourt, T. S., Meyers-Ohki, S., Stulac, S. N., Barrera, A. E., Mushashi, C., & Beardslee, W. R. (2011). Nothing can defeat combined hands (Abashize hamwe ntakibananira): Protective processes and resilience in Rwandan children and families affected by HIV/AIDS. *Social Science and Medicine, 73*(5), 693–701.

Classen, S., Lopez, E., Winter, S., Awadzi, K., Ferree, N., & Garvan, C. (2008). Population-based health promotion perspective for older driver safety: Conceptual framework to intervention plan. *Clinical Interventions in Aging, 2,* 667–693.

Creswell, J. W. (2009). *Research design: Qualitative, quantitative and mixed methods approaches* (3rd ed.). Sage.

Creswell, J. W. (2014). *Research design: Qualitative, quantitative and mixed methods approaches* (4th ed.). Sage.

Creswell, J. W., & Clark, V. L. R. (2007). *Designing and conducting mixed methods research.* Sage.

Depoy, E., & Gitlin, L. N. (2011). *Introduction to research.* Elsevier.

Koutsodimitropoulos, E., Buultjens, M., Louis, K. O., & Monfries, M. (2016). Speech pathology student clinician attitudes and beliefs towards people who stutter: A mixed-method pilot study. *Journal of Fluency Disorders, 47,* 38–55.

McMillan, J. H. (2004). *Educational research.* Pearson.

McMillan, J. H. (2012). *Educational research* (6th ed.). Pearson

McMillan, J. H., & Schumacher, S. (2010). *Research in education.* Pearson.

Meline, T. (2006). *Research in communication science and disorders.* Pearson.

Mertens, D. M. (2005). *Research and evaluation in education and psychology.* Sage.

Mertens, D. M. (2014). *Research and evaluation in education and psychology.* Sage.

Morgan, D. I. (1998). Practical strategies for combining qualitative and quantitative methods: Applications to health research. *Qualitative Health Research, 8*(3), 362–376.

Perry, V. (2017). A mixed methods study of expository paragraph writing in English-proficient Hispanic, middle school students with writing weaknesses. *Perspectives of the ASHA Special Interest Groups, 2*(1), 151–167

Polit, D. F., & Beck, C. J. (2010). *Nursing research: Principles and methods.* Lippincott Williams & Wilkins.

Tashakkori, A., & Teddlie, C. (2003). *Handbook of mixed methods in social and behavioral research.* Sage.

Tashakkori, A., & Teddlie, C. (2010). *Handbook of mixed methods in social and behavioral research* (2nd ed.). Sage.

11

Reporting and Disseminating Research

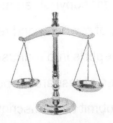

LEARNING OBJECTIVES

Upon completion of this chapter, the reader will be able to:

- Identify reasons for reporting research
- Identify misconceptions about research reporting
- Discuss how to avoid misconceptions about research reports
- Effectively manage time for reporting research and maintain a research log
- Request permission for copyrighted materials
- Discuss the process of rewriting and revision
- Translate research reports into manuscript
- Identify different types of research reports
- Select a journal to submit a manuscript
- Evaluate and review reports

Reporting and disseminating research studies are essential to the advancement of science in speech-language pathology and audiology. Students and practicing professionals are often not prepared to write and publish research reports. What distinguishes the unpublished from the published is a matter of attitude, training, and perseverance. First is a positive attitude of confidence and determination that suggests, "I can and I will publish." Second is the probability that those who do not publish do not know how to publish. Throughout schooling, students have had to write and have been graded on writing, but they have not been taught how to write for publication. Irwin et al. (1992) suggest that "university faculty should instruct students about the process of publishing in a journal" (p. 122). Third, an unpublished paper is often one that someone gave up on. Fourth, many people think they have good writing skills but few do; good writers edit and rewrite, again, and again (Henson, 1993).

The purpose of this chapter is to (a) describe common myths about research reports, (b) identify reasons for reporting the results of research, (c) discuss managing time to report research, (d) describe the organization and style of research reports, (e) explain research reports at professional meetings, (f) classify and describe visual supplements, and (g) explain submission and review of research reports.

Reasons for Reporting Research

There are numerous reasons for reporting research, including ethical responsibility, improving clinical service, aca-demic survival, and personal and group recognition. Hegde (2003) believes "dissemination or research findings are an ethical responsibility" (p. 560). In *A History of the American Speech and Hearing Association 1925–1958*, Paden (1970) stated, "one of the chief reasons for the existence of a profession or learned society is the sharing of knowledge on the field among its members" (p. 21). The American Speech-Language-Hearing Association (ASHA) provides many opportunities for disseminating research, including its scholarly journals, teleseminars, and annual meetings.

Reporting research is fundamental to the advancement of diagnosis and treatment of speech, language, and hearing problems. Silverman (1998) pointed out that if clinical speech-language pathologists and audiologists do not formally disseminate clinical outcome research, the potential to help persons with speech-language-hearing problems is restricted to their caseload and those of colleagues with whom they communicate.

Academic survival is related to understanding "publish or perish." Publication has a significant impact on academic survival and promotion, tenure, and merit salary raises (Anderson, 1992; Boyes et al., 1984; Holcomb & Roush, 1988; Schilling, 2005; Sininger et al., 2003). Publishing makes a difference to speech-language pathologists and audiologists employed in colleges or universities. Those who are promoted have published more than those who have not been promoted. For these reasons, there is tremendous pressure to publish among academicians (Luey, 1987). Academic survival (graduation) of students is also related to completing a thesis or dissertation requirement (Cone & Foster, 2006; Davis & Parker, 1979; Rudestam

& Newton, 2001). There are also several other reasons for reporting, which are listed in Table 11–1. These reasons are institutional as well as individual.

Table 11–1. Reasons for Reporting Research

Ethical responsibility

Advancement of clinical practice

Academic survival; promotion, tenure

Graduation requirement (theses or dissertation)

Stimulate further research

Peer approval

Personal sense of achievement

Evidence of intellectual effort

Entry to professional networks

Quality indicator of group/program/institution

Reasons for not reporting research also warrant consideration. Two of the most frequently cited reasons are lack of time and negative attitudes (Bennett & Taylor, 2003; Meline, 2006). Time management for reporting research is discussed in the next section. Some speech-language pathologists and audiologists do not report research because of the fear of rejection, revisions, or self-censorship (Meline, 2006). In recent years, ASHA journals accepted 52% of the manuscripts that were submitted (Table 11–2). Moreover, one or more revisions were usually required before any manuscript was accepted for publication. Avoiding peer review may also be seen as a related response. Reports based on opinion and testimonials lack significant credibility and are not accepted for publication in peer-reviewed journals. Therefore, peer review is avoided, and such reports are presently directed toward the public and others (Finn et al., 2005).

Table 11–2. Quick Facts About ASHA Sponsored Journals: *AJA, AJSLP, JSHLR, LSHSS, Perspectives*

Number of Journals:	5
Editors-in-Chief:	10
Editors:	59
Editorial Board Members (EBMs):	352
Time from Submission to Decision:	Approximately 4 months
Average Acceptance Rate:	52%
Growth in Amount Published Since 2010:	58%

Source: 2022 (in review). https://academy.pubs.asha.org/asha-journals-author-resource-center/what-to-expect-in-peer-review/

Myths and Facts About Research Reports

Despite attempts to debunk the myths surrounding research reports, there continue to be several common misconceptions, which Sternberg (1993) identified in his book *The Psychologist's Companion: A Guide to Scientific Writing for Students and Researchers*. These myths are described in Table 11–3. Identification and understanding of these myths should facilitate more accurate and realistic concepts about reporting research.

Time Management for Reporting Research

Most productive researchers have no more free time or no fewer commitments than those who do not do research. Instead, those who do research simply make the time to do it. It is a matter of prioritizing and managing time. Like anything else, with practice comes efficiency. The traditional approach to writing requires time for warm-up and reflection, large blocks of time, and uninterrupted working conditions. Another approach preferred by many involves writing in brief spurts (i.e., writing in brief daily sessions; Boice, 1989).

There is a relationship between unproductive researchers and maladaptive delays of "busyness" and binging (Boice, 1989). Busyness involves keeping busy with less important tasks to avoid high-priority tasks. Binging is spending the most time on a less important activity. Those who are too busy cannot get everything done, whereas bingers are likely to overprepare for classes.

According to Leedy and Ormrod (2010), the first step is the development of a reasonable writing schedule and sticking to it. Additionally, suggestions are identification of small accomplishable goals within the project, setting reasonable dates for completing each goal, rewarding yourself each time you meet a goal, seeking regular feedback, and building time into the schedule for at least two or three rewrites.

From the beginning, a target date should be set for completion of the research report. A personal deadline should preempt some time before the actual deadline. The research report should be organized so that it can be completed. If delayed by unavoidable influences, it is necessary to work twice as hard the next day or week or to work over the weekend to stay on schedule. Robertson (2004) described strategies for managing time that may be helpful, such as setting personal goals, using a master list, organizing work space, and being proactive. It is helpful to develop a timetable of activities required to plan, write, and submit a research report (DePoy & Gitlin, 2011; Polit & Beck, 2010). Table 11–4 provides a list of activities and a schedule for completing a research report. Several activities overlap, and some involve little time; others are more time consuming. The identification and scheduling of tasks to complete the report should facilitate completion of the report within a reasonable period of time. In developing a schedule, several factors should be considered: available resources such as technology support and personnel will influence the amount of time required. Other activities that will take time include securing necessary permissions and holding meetings or communicating with coauthors.

Table 11–3. Research Reports: Myths and Facts

Myth:	Clinicians are not researchers.
Facts:	Clinicians should be researchers.
Myth:	Writing the research report is the most routine, least creative aspect of research, requiring much time but little creativity.
Facts:	Writing the research report requires both time and creativity.
Myth:	The important consideration is what is said rather than how it is said.
Facts:	How it is said (professional writing style) is an important consideration.
Myth:	Longer papers are better, more papers also better.
Facts:	Concise papers are better, quality of papers is more important that quantitative of papers.
Myth:	The main purpose of a research paper is presentation of facts, whether newly established (experimental research) or established (literature review, tutorials).
Facts:	Research papers have several purposes: analysis/synthesis of past and current research, drawing conclusions, and providing suggestions for future research.
Myth:	The difference between scientific writing and advertising is that the purpose of the former is to inform and the latter is to persuade.
Facts:	Scientific writing and advertising may both inform and persuade.
Myth:	An acceptable way to gain acceptance of a theory is to refute another theory.
Facts:	An acceptable way to gain acceptance of a theory is to provide credible evidence.
Myth:	Negative results which fail to support a hypothesis are as valuable as positive results that do not support the hypothesis.
Facts:	Both negative and positive results can improve knowledge and understanding.
Myth:	Logical development of ideas in a research paper reflects historical development of ideas.
Facts:	Logical development of ideas in a research paper may not reflect the historical background.

Table 11–4. Steps and Schedule for Writing a Research Report

Steps	Schedule
Prewriting/planning stage	

Review requirement for submitting report
    Obtain permission(s) to use previously published material(s)
    Decide on authorship and order of authors
    Determine level of evidence relevant to topic
    Assemble materials needed to write report	

Writing first draft
    Title page
    Abstract
    Key words
    Introduction (background)
    Statement of problem (purpose)
    Method
    Results
    Discussion
    Conclusions
    Author contributions
    Contact information
    References (all references cited both in text and list)
    Tables and figures
    Documentation of informed consent
    Documentation of IRB approval
    Resources and environment	

Review and revision
    Revise first draft and subsequent revisions
    Editing
    Review and revise the last complete draft
    Final editing and proofreading
    Prepare final report	

Submit manuscript and cover letter Assemble report copies and accompanying materials	

Source: Reprinted from *Writing and Publishing in Medicine*, by E. J. Huth, 1999, Baltimore, MD: Lippincott Williams & Wilkins. Copyright 1999, with permission from Elsevier.

Efficient use of computer technology can increase productivity because of its speed and accuracy. Computers are used for a variety of research tasks: searching the literature, sampling, recording observations, and qualitative and quantitative data analysis (Maxwell & Satake, 2006; McMillan, 2004; Polit & Beck, 2010).

In addition, some types of research are less time consuming than others (Hegde, 2003; Maxwell & Satake, 2006; Meline 2006). Single-subject research designs require less time because clinical service can be integrated with experimental evaluation. Use of single-subject designs can provide answers to many clinically relevant questions. As Connell and McReynolds (1988) concluded, "individual contact with a client over an extended time interval is the basic requirement for implementation of single-subject experimental designs" (p. 1062). This also helps dispel the myth that there is a division between clinical and research activities.

Procrastination

Related to time management is procrastination or needless delay in beginning or completing a research project. Procrasti-

nation may include discomfort, anxiety, busyness, or binging (Boice, 1989). It may reflect a fear of failure or success or it may reflect a need to rebel. Carter-Scott (1989) refers to procrastination as the mañana syndrome and describes it as "the precise behavior which keeps you from meeting deadlines, doing what you say you will do, and reinforcing the fact that you're not up to the challenges" (p. 21). Several strategies have been described to reduce procrastination, such as cognitive behavioral orientation, reprogramming negative attitudes, prioritization, contingency management, procrastination support groups, and time slots. Roth (1989) suggested maintaining a research log or journal from the beginning to the end of a research project, including the completed research report and submission of the report for presentation and/or publication (Table 11–5). This information can also be used to determine authorship contributions.

Some Simple Rules for Dissemination of Research

Ross-Hellaure et al. (2020) defined research dissemination "as a planned

Table 11–5. Research Log Example

Date	Time	Entry
Date of entry	Record time; stop and start	Specify what was done.
3/18/06	10:00–11:45 AM	Computer references search; located articles of interest; requested interlibrary loan for journal articles not available.
3/19/06	1:00–2:30 PM	Reviewed articles.
3/21/06	9:30–11:00 AM	Drafted outline and working title.

process that involves consideration of target audiences, consideration of the setting in which research findings are to be received, and communication and interaction with wider audiences in ways that will facilitate research uptake and understanding" (p. 2). Social networks in academia such as ResearchGate and Academia.edu have millions of users. In the digital age, dissemination of research findings has changed dramatically in the last two decades.

Ross-Hellaure et al. (2020) provide guidance for the dissemination of research with the use of ten simple rules. Summarizing these ten simple rules includes the following:

Rule 1: Get the Basics Right: Researchers should define the objectives about what to achieve through dissemination. Mapping audiences and specifying exactly who one wants to reach. Create a dissemination plan to save time. If working in groups, distribute tasks and efforts to ensure regular updates from your colleagues.

Rule 2: Keep the Right Profile: Use personal websites and social media (e.g., Twitter, LinkedIn, Facebook) accounts to keep research visible. ORCID (http://www.orcid.org) provides a persistent digital identifier that a researcher can own and control and that distinguishes one from every other researcher. ORCID can connect a researcher's professional information with affiliation, grants, publications, peer review, and more.

Rule 3: Encourage participation: This rule involves the engagement of colleagues, consumers of research, and various other organizations.

Zooniverse (https:///www.zooniverse.org) can allow anyone to freely participate in cutting-edge "people-powered research."

Rule 4: Open Science for Impact: Vincente-Saez et. al (2018) stated, "open science is transparent and accessible knowledge that is shared and developed through collaborative research networks" (p. 428). Open science is an innovative method for dissemination. This might involve publishing of datasets, software, and peer reviews that can increase the number of citable research outputs.

Rule 5: Remix Traditional Outputs: Boosting impact of traditional research outputs like research articles or books can be complemented with innovative dissemination. Most universities have an office of public affairs or communication that are interested in science-related stories. Writing a one- to two-page summary of the research for nonspecialists, press releases, and blog posts can increase dissemination. Conference presentations or posters can be uploaded to a general-purpose repository such as Figshare (Figshare.com) or Zenodo (zenodo.org) and a digital object identifier (DOI) can be added.

Rule 6: Go Live: Presentations at formal conferences do not have to be the only method of presenting to a live audience. Science slams are "short talks in which researchers explain a scientific topic to a typically nonexpert audience" (Ross-Hellaure et al., 2020, p. 7). Research presentations can be also be done via YouTube, TEDx talks, and science festivals.

Rule 7: Think Visual: Be creative and find an interesting and easily understandable display of data. There are online tools to upload a sample of research data and develop smart graphs and infographics (e.g., Infogr.am, Datawrapper, Ease.ly, or Venngage).

Rule 8: Respect Diversity: Include diverse groups in research teams as often as possible. Writing and implementing plans in research studies and groups should reflect the principles of diversity, equity, and inclusion (DEI). For scientific communication, messages should be framed to respect all audiences.

Rule 9: Find the Right Tools: The use of innovative dissemination should utilize more tools. For example, OpenUP Hub (http://www.openuphub.eu) is an "open, dynamic and collaborative knowledge environment that systematically captures, organizes and categorizes research outcome, best practices, tools and designs." Similar projects include 101 Innovations in Scholarly Communication (https://101innovations.wordpress.com/).

Rule 10: Evaluate, Evaluate, Evaluate: It is important to know what worked and what did not. The use of quantitative and qualitative indicators should be done in the dissemination plan (Rule 1). Qualitative indicators may include questionnaires, interviews, and observations. Quantitative indicators may include the citation of publications, media coverage, visibility in social media, and feedback from target groups.

Format of Research Reports

Research reports contain most, if not all, of the sections listed in Table 11–6. Further description of selected parts of research reports follows this section: abstracts, key words, author contributions, and tables and figures. Sometimes the results and discussion sections are combined. The format of research is consistent across different types of reports, such as theses, dissertations, journal articles, and papers for professional meetings (Polit & Beck, 2010). Extensive discussions of the format for written reports can be found in the *Publication Manual of the American Psychological Association* (APA, 2020), the *American Medical Association Manual of Style* (AMA, 2020), Orlikoff et al. (2022), and Silverman (1998).

Abstracts

An abstract is a brief comprehensive summary of a report (APA, 2020). The **abstract** may be the most important part of a report because it may be the only part that many people read. Most professional journals use structured abstracts because they provide more detailed and consistent information. In addition, structured abstracts make literature searches easier.

There are two types of structured abstracts. The first is for original reports, and the second is for review or tutorial reports. The primary information for these abstracts is summarized in Table 11–7. No information should be reported in the abstract that does not appear in the text of the paper (AMA, 2020).

Table 11–6. Format for Research Report

Title page	Title, name of authors, and institutional affiliation
Abstract	Summary including methods, results, implications
Key words	Short list of words for indexing
Introduction	Untitled; begins body of paper; review of relevant literature, theoretical foundations and rationale, purpose/research questions or hypothesis
Method	Design of study, subjects, sampling techniques, controls, equipment or test materials, experimental procedures, rationale for choice of statistics
Results	Summary and evaluation of relevant data, tables, and figures
Discussion	Comparison of findings to previous research, limitations, implications for clinical practice, and future research
Author information	Contains information
Author contributions	Disclosure of contributions to report
Acknowledgments	Recognition of support from individuals and/or organizations
References	All cited sources of information
Tables and figures	Visual presentation of information
Appendix	Contains information that cannot be integrated in text; usually contains unpublished information

ASHA journals use a modified abstract, which includes the following sections: purpose, method, results, and conclusions. The *Annals of Internal Medicine* (http://www.acponline.org) added a section on Limitations located immediately before Conclusions. The Limitation section reduced the risk of overgeneralization, overinterpretation, or overexplaining of the evidence. It also helps readers understand how one report differs from another on the same topic.

Key Words (Indexing Terms)

Most journals include a list of key words or indexing terms that represent content of the report, including words in the title or abstract. They are placed on the abstract page following the abstract. These words assist in locating research reports in computer databases such as Medline (http://www.nlm.nih.gov) and the Cumulative Index to Nursing and Allied Health Literature (CINAHL;

Table 11–7. Information Required for Structured Abstract

Original Reporting
1. Objective: exact question(s) addressed by the report
2. Design: the basic design of the study
3. Setting: the location and level of clinical care
4. Patients or participants: the manner of selection and number of patients or participants who entered and completed the study
5. Interventions: the exact treatment or intervention, if any
6. Main outcome measures: the primary study outcome measure as planned before data collection began
7. Results: the key findings
8. Conclusions: key conclusions including direct clinical applications
Review
1. Purpose: the primary objective of the review paper
2. Data sources: a succinct summary of data sources
3. Study selection: the number of studies selected for review and how they were selected
4. Data extraction: rules for abstracting data and how they were applied
5. Results of data synthesis: the method of data synthesis and key results
6. Conclusions: key conclusions, including potential applications and research needs

Source: Adapted from "More Informative Abstracts Revisited," by R. B. Haynes, C. D. Mulrow, E. J. Huth, D. G. Altman, and M. J. Gardner, 1996, *Cleft Palate Craniofacial Journal, 33*(1), pp. 1–9.

http://www.ebsco.com). Medline is the database most used in health care and is one of the largest in the world. CINAHL focuses on publications from the allied health professions.

Author Contributions

Several professional journals require that authors disclose their contributions to a report. Each author specifies their contributions, which are published before the acknowledgement section. Some examples are as follows:

Study concept and design

Acquisition of data

Analysis and interpretation of data

Drafting of the manuscript

Critical revision of the manuscript for important intellectual content

Statistical analysis

Obtaining funding

Administrative, technical, or material support

Study supervision

All authors of a group should have full access to all the data in the report and be responsible for the integrity and accuracy of the report.

Tables and Figures

A wide variety of tables and figures have been described that are used to present complex information in a concise, visual format. Tables generally present exact numerical values, and the data are arranged in an orderly display of columns and rows (APA, 2020). A figure is any kind of graphic illustration other than a table.

Harris (1999) defined and illustrated more than 400 tables and figures. Among the most frequently used figures are pie charts, bar graphs, scatter plots, and curves (DePoy & Gitlin, 2011). Less frequently used figures are concept maps and V-diagrams. Curves refer to any line on a figure used to represent a set or series of data (Harris, 1999).

The Agency for Healthcare Research and Quality (AHRQ; http://www.ahrq.gov) provides guidelines for making charts and graphs to make publications and research findings more easily understood.

Tables and figures should be clear enough to stand alone without explanation in the text (Blessing & Forister, 2011). General guidelines for tables and figures are listed in Tables 11–8 and 11–9.

Diagrams and Maps

There are several reasons for using diagrams and maps to display research data. Among the reasons are to (a) simplify complex information, (b) summarize or enhance certain findings, (c) illustrate complicated results, and (d) demonstrate trends or redundancies in research (Nichol & Pexman, 2003).

According to the APA (2020) manual, both diagrams and maps are types of figures. The main types of diagrams are

Table 11–8. Guidelines for Preparing Tables

- Select a clear and specific table
- Number tables consecutively
- Use subheadings for columns and rows
- Only include information related to the title
- Do not explain table in text it should stand alone
- Use consistent format that conforms to publisher's guidelines. Refer to instructions to authors.
- Avoid excessive lines. Usually vertical lines are not needed
- Use appropriate units of measure

Source: From *Research and Medical Literature*, by J. D. Blessing and J. G. Forister, 2012, Burlington, MA: Jones and Bartlett.

Table 11–9. Guidelines for Preparing Figures

- Labeling table as a figure not a table
- Select appropriate type of figure based on data, statistical analysis and readability
- Title should be self-explanatory
- Refer to figure in text; number consecutively
- Check spelling and plotting of data
- Review publisher's guidelines for overall size, resolution and specification: See instruction for authors
- Include legends if necessary, define abbreviations
- Update permission from copyright holder

Source: From *Research and Medical Literature*, by J. D. Blessing and J. G. Forister, 2012, Burlington, MA: Jones and Bartlett.

graphs and charts. The former is described as displaying the relationship between two quantitative indices or between a continuous quantitative variable. The latter are usually displays of quantitative information such as the flow of subjects through a process (APA, 2020).

Diagrams and maps are often created by using available computer programs, such as Microsoft Word and Microsoft Excel. There are a variety of diagrams and maps for displaying information. A V-diagram consists of 12 elements and is provided in Figure 11–1. Yau (2001) has step-by-step guidelines for graphics from start to finish. These guidelines are for visualizing patterns over time, proportions, relationship differences, and spatial relationships.

The following guidelines for diagrams and maps have been described by Nichol and Pexman (2003):

■ They must be referred to in the text.

■ Information should be as simple as possible.
■ Only relevant information should be included.
■ Labels should be consistent.
■ Use of color should be avoided because most print information is black and white.

General guidelines for evaluating diagrams and maps have been described by Nichol and Pexman (2003). These criteria are as follows: text diagrams and maps use a simple format, font sizes in diagrams and maps do not vary by more than four fonts, captions are typed double spaced on a separate page, lines are thick enough to be clear after reduction, similar diagrams or maps within the same manuscript should have a similar appearance, and diagrams and maps are referred to in the text using the same number(s) as in the caption(s). Detailed strategies for evaluating V-diagrams and concept maps have been developed by Gowin and Alvarez (2005).

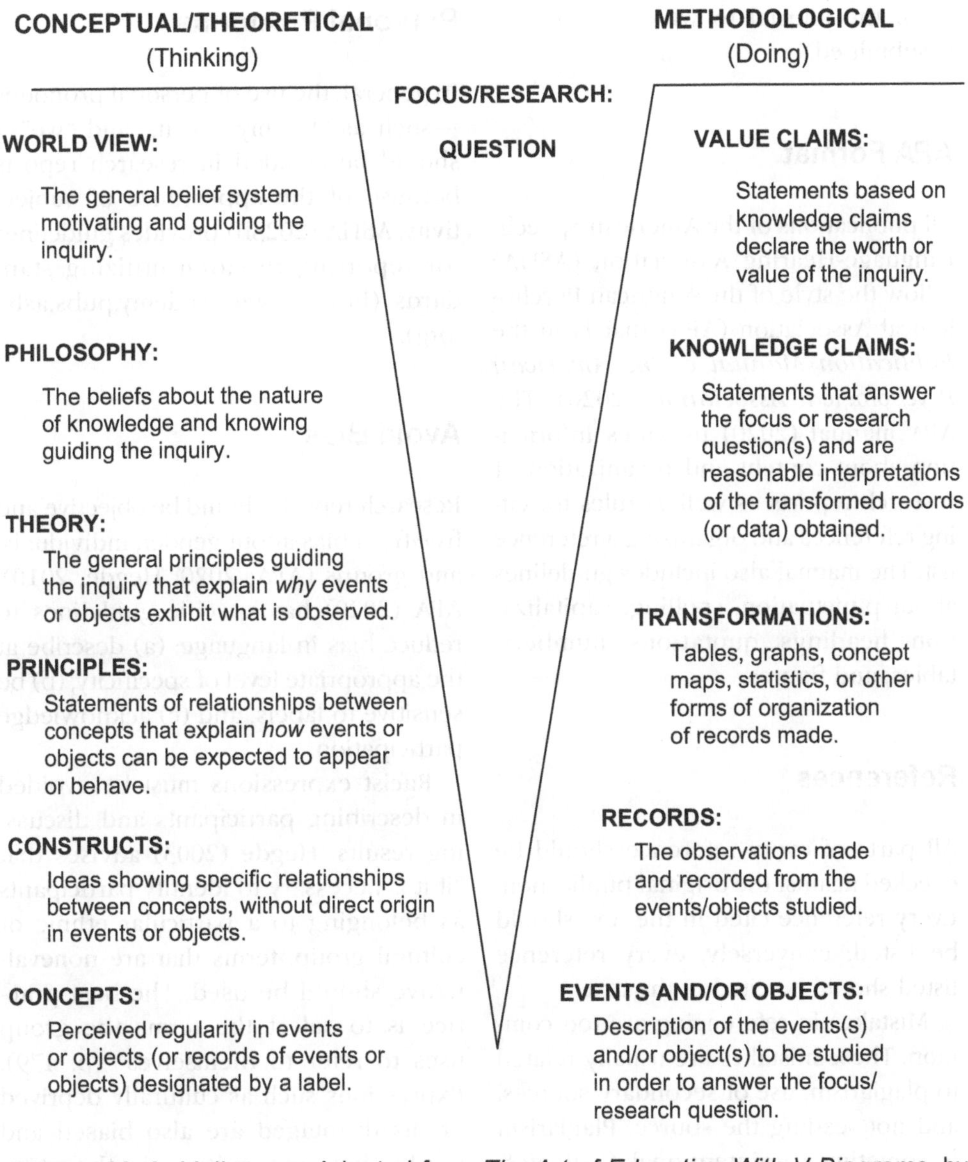

CONCEPTUAL/THEORETICAL
(Thinking)

METHODOLOGICAL
(Doing)

FOCUS/RESEARCH:

QUESTION

WORLD VIEW:

The general belief system
motivating and guiding the
inquiry.

VALUE CLAIMS:

Statements based on
knowledge claims
declare the worth or
value of the inquiry.

PHILOSOPHY:

The beliefs about the nature
of knowledge and knowing
guiding the inquiry.

KNOWLEDGE CLAIMS:

Statements that answer
the focus or research
question(s) and are
reasonable interpretations
of the transformed records
(or data) obtained.

THEORY:

The general principles guiding
the inquiry that explain *why* events
or objects exhibit what is observed.

TRANSFORMATIONS:

Tables, graphs, concept
maps, statistics, or other
forms of organization
of records made.

PRINCIPLES:

Statements of relationships between
concepts that explain *how* events or
objects can be expected to appear
or behave.

RECORDS:

The observations made
and recorded from the
events/objects studied.

CONSTRUCTS:

Ideas showing specific relationships
between concepts, without direct origin
in events or objects.

CONCEPTS:

Perceived regularity in events
or objects (or records of events or
objects) designated by a label.

EVENTS AND/OR OBJECTS:

Description of the events(s)
and/or object(s) to be studied
in order to answer the focus/
research question.

Figure 11–1. V-diagram. Adapted from *The Art of Educating With V Diagrams*, by D. B. Gowin and M. C. Alvarez, 2005, Cambridge.

Writing Styles

Although there are different types of research reports, the style should be similar, that is, as simple and clear as possible. Clear writing is concise, not wordy or redundant. Research reports are of limited value if they are not understandable. Several guides for writing style are available (American Medical Association Manual of Style, 2020; APA, 2020; Hegde, 2010; Strunk & White, 1979; Turabian, 1995). The style should be consistent with the requirements of the university for theses or dissertations or of the journal to which the report is submitted.

APA Format

All publications of the American Speech-Language-Hearing Association (ASHA) follow the style of the American Psychological Association (APA) that is in the *Publication Manual of the American Psychological Association* (2020). The APA manual (2020) provides information about content and organization of research reports as well as rules for citing references and organizing a reference list. The manual also includes guidelines about punctuation, spelling, capitalization, headings, quotations, numbers, tables, and figures.

References

All parts of every reference should be checked against the original publication. Every reference cited in the text should be listed; conversely, every reference listed should be cited in the text.

Mistakes in referencing are too common. These mistakes are usually related to plagiarism, use of secondary sources, and not reading the source. Plagiarism is sometimes unintentional (DePoy & Gitlin, 2011). To avoid this potentially devastating mistake, one should be aware of the standards for referencing. All work written by another person, even if not directly quoted, must be cited. The use of secondary sources is not acceptable; that is, only primary sources should be cited. Another common error is the use of citations that have not been read.

Personal Pronouns

In general, the use of personal pronouns —such as "I," "my," "you," and "we"— should be avoided in research reports because of the appearance of subjectivity. ASHA (2023b) provides guidelines for reporting research utilizing standards (http://www.academy.pubs.asha.org).

Avoid Bias

Research reports should be objective and free from bias about gender, individuals, and groups (APA, 2020; Hegde, 2010). APA (2020) has specific guidelines to reduce bias in language: (a) describe at the appropriate level of specificity, (b) be sensitive to labels, and (c) acknowledge participation.

Racist expressions must be avoided in describing participants and discussing results. Hegde (2003) advises that "if it is necessary to identify participants as belonging to a particular ethnic or cultural group, terms that are nonevaluative should be used. The best practice is to select the terms the group uses to refer to themselves" (p. 479). Expressions such as culturally deprived or disadvantaged are also biased and imply that one culture is the standard against which other cultures are evaluated.

Sexism in language has a long history and may not be easily recognized. It is inherently discriminatory and suggests an unjustified bias against an individual or a group, usually women but sometimes men (Schneider & Soto, 1989). Sexist language should be avoided in speaking and writing. One of the most misused personal pronouns is *he*, which is frequently used to refer to someone of unidentified gender, such as a child, client, customer, or student (Hegde, 2003). Indiscriminate use of personal pronouns may suggest that all authors, bankers, deans, department heads, doctors, editors, executives, firefighters, lawyers, police officers, presidents, or professors are male. The noun *man* is often inappropriately used in ways that also imply sexism. For example, *chairman* of a department or organization. Chair*person* or simply *chair* is appropriate. Apparently, there is some truth in Barzun's (1986) statement that "sex is a source of chaos in language generally, as it is in life" (p. 37).

The ASHA Committee on Equality of Sexes adopted the American Psychological Association Guidelines for Unbiased Language. These guidelines provide specific suggestions and examples for gender-free writing. ASHA (1993) also provided guidelines for gender equality in language usage, which includes "being specific about gender when inclusion of this information is relevant and avoids

generalization which may lead to stereotyping" (p. 42). Other useful references are *The Handbook of Nonsexist Writing* by Miller and Swift (1988), *The Nonsexist Communicator* by Sorrels (1983), and *The Elements of Nonsexist Language Usage* by Drummond (1990).

"Person-first" language should be used to describe individuals with disabilities; that is, put the person first, not the disability. Table 11–10 provides a list of person-first phrases and those that should be avoided. Folkins (1992) described five principles for determining language used to describe individuals with disabilities. These principles are (a) use person-first language, (b) determine disability versus handicap, (c) remember that everyone likes to think of themselves as normal, (d) avoid terms that project unnecessary negative connotations, and (e) do not overdo it.

There are other words that are misused. Huth and Sheen (1984) described some words as dehumanizing; for example, *case* and *patient* or *client*. Case is an episode or example of illness, injury, or disease. Patient or client is the person

Table 11–10. Person First Language

Preferred	Avoid
Children with cleft palate	Cleft palate children
Persons who stutter	Stutterers
Adults with aphasia	Aphasic adults
The lawyer who has dyslexia	The dyslexic lawyer
The client with hearing impairment	The hearing-impaired client

Source: Adapted from *The Language Used to Describe Individuals with Disabilities,* by J. Folkins. Available from http://www.asha.org/about/publications/journal-abstracts/submission/person_first.htm#one. Copyright 1992 by the American Speech-Language-Hearing Association. All rights reserved.

cared for by the speech-language pathologist or audiologist. Patients or clients are cared for, not cases. Another misused word is *subject* or *participant*. The term participants should be used because it acknowledges that participants have an active role in research studies (APA, 2020; ASHA, 2023a).

Permissions

The legal reason for seeking appropriate permission when using previously published materials is related to copyright law (APA, 2020; Huth, 1999). Most publications are copyrighted; legal ownership is vested to the copyright holder. Permission for reproduction of published material must be obtained from the copyright holder, or the writer and publisher are at risk for legal action because of copyright infringement for unauthorized use of published materials. When in doubt about the need for permission, it is probably better to request it. Permission should be sought well in advance. Figure 11–2 provides an example of a letter requesting permission to use copyrighted material. Most publishers have form letters or online forms for requesting permission to use copyrighted material. Additional information about permission is available elsewhere (APA, 2020; Huth, 1999).

Rewriting and Revising

Rewriting and revision are an important part of writing because authors are usu-
ally asked to make revisions (Portney & Watkins, 2009). For most, even those who are experienced writers, writing is hard work. The first or rough draft should not be the final draft. Even experienced writers revise manuscripts several times. Often, the final draft is much different from the first or original draft (Hegde, 2003). Editing and rewriting are the steps to good writing. These steps are listed in Table 11–11.

Rewriting is not easy for several reasons. Self-editing is difficult because it requires critical evaluation of one's own writing (Hegde, 2003). Rewriting requires much focused attention to details and usually reorganization of the paper (Meline, 2006). Lack of time may also prevent revision of a paper. Another problem is related to coauthors who may not be able to respond with suggestions for revision(s) (Huth, 1999). Rewriting and revising increases the likelihood of acceptance, although it is no guarantee. Some writers revise content, structure, and style of a paper at the same time; others revise content and structure first and then style. The content of a paper is more likely to determine whether it is accepted for publications than style. Writing style includes paragraph length and structure, paragraph linkage, sentence variety, and word choices. Further detailed information about writing style is available in Huth's (1999) *Writing and Publishing in Medicine* and the *Publication Manual of the American Psychological Association* (APA, 2020). Strategies for improving writing styles are writing from an outline, putting the first draft aside for a week or two before revising, and having colleagues critically review the draft (APA, 2020; Huth, 1999).

_____

_____

_____

_____

I am preparing a manuscript:

_____
(title of book)

_____
(author/editor of book)

to be published in _____(approx. date) by

_____
(publisher's name and address)

I would like to include in it the material specified below:

Author:
Title:
Date:
Figure or table number(s):

I request permission to reprint the specified material in this book and in future revisions and editions thereof, for possible licensing and distribution throughout the world in all languages. If you do not control these rights in their entirety, would you please let me know where else to write. Proper acknowledgment of title, author, publisher, city, and copyright date (for journals; author, article title, journal name, volume, first page of article, and year) will be given. If the permission of the author is also required, please supply a current address. For your convenience, you may simply sign the release form below. A copy of this request is enclosed for your files.

Thank you,
Author_____   My return address is (please print)
                    (please print)   _____
Date_____   _____
                                                          _____

PERMISSION GRANTED:

_____   _____
Signature   Date

Figure 11–2. Request for permission. From _Singular Manual of Textbook Preparation_, by M. N. Hegde, 1991, Singular Publishing group. Reproduced with permission from copyright holder M. N. Hegde.

Table 11–11. Steps in Writing and Revising Reports

Write first draft
Hold first draft 1–2 weeks, then revise
Second draft
Distribute copies to co-authors and to colleagues willing to critically review
Read draft, make notes on needed revisions
Get written recommendations for revisions from co-authors and colleagues
Third draft same sequences as second
Later drafts
Continue reading to co-authors
Concentrate on content and structure
When satisfied with content, revise style
Review and revise large elements first
Paragraph lengths
External and internal sequence of paragraphs
Consider sentences: length; variety
Elements of sentences: clarify and phrasing; modifying word choices
Read the revised text to identify and correct "overlooked flaws"

Source: Reprinted from *Writing and Publishing in Medicine,* by E. J. Huth, 1999, Baltimore, MD: Lippincott Williams & Wilkins. Copyright 1999, with permission from Elsevier.

Translating Research Reports to Published Papers

Most research presented at professional meetings (platform presentations and poster presentations) is not subsequently published in peer-reviewed journals. There are two reasons for this failure to complete a full manuscript and submit it to a peer-reviewed journal. First, research accepted for presentation at a professional meeting might not stand up under peer review because it is flawed. Second, preparing a manuscript can be overwhelming, especially for beginning presenters.

Many of the reasons for manuscript rejection can be avoided. Therefore, it is useful to be aware of the reasons for rejecting manuscripts. Among the reasons are inappropriate or incomplete statistics, overgeneralization of results, inappropriate or substandard instrumentation, sample too small or biased, writing style flaws, insufficient problem statement, inaccurate or inconsistent data, and inadequate tables or figures (Pierson, 2004).

Types of Research Reports

The organization and style of research reports are consistent across different types of reports, although there is some variation. This section describes the major types of research reports: journal articles, theses and dissertations, textbooks, and presentations at professional meetings. Other types of research reports, systematic reviews, and reports to funding agencies are described in Chapter 13.

Journal Articles

Publication in a journal ensures wide circulation of research findings. Research reports are often submitted for publication after presentation at a professional meeting or they may be reduced reports of research findings from theses and dissertations. Many manuscripts are now submitted online. When submitting a manuscript, it may include a cover letter requesting that the manuscript be considered for publication. The following information should be included in the cover letter:

■ Request that the manuscript be considered for publication
■ Verification that all authors have made contributions that justify authorship
■ Affirmation of compliance with ethical considerations for protection

of human and animal subjects in research
■ Copy of permission granted to reproduce or adapt any copyright material
■ Verification that the manuscript has not been previously published in the same, or essentially the same, form
■ Notice that the manuscript is not currently under review elsewhere
■ Disclosure of any real or potential conflicts of interest
■ Author's professional address, telephone numbers and e-mail address

An example of a cover letter is shown in Figure 11–3.

Manuscripts submitted for publication in peer-review journals are reviewed and evaluated by peers who are experts in the subject area. Non-peer-reviewed journals do not require a critical review of manuscripts by peers with relevant expertise. There is a greater likelihood that the former contributes to the scientific knowledge base in speech-language pathology and audiology and has clinical relevance and credibility.

Selecting a Journal

Selecting a journal to submit a manuscript to is important and should be an early step in planning a paper. Steps in publishing a paper and possible outcomes are shown in Figure 11–4. In addition to ASHA journals, there are several other journals that publish information about speech-language pathology and audiology. Maxwell and Satake (2006) suggested the following questions be considered in selecting a journal:

1. Is the topic of the proposed paper within the scope of the journal?

John Jones, PhD

Editor, Language and Speech Journal

9120 Miracle Road

Greenville, LA 54681

Dear Dr. Jones:

I am submitting this manuscript, "Happy days in Speech and Language," for publication consideration in the Language and speech Journal. The manuscript complies with ethical and authorship guidelines:

— Each authors' contributions are appropriate for authorship

— All of the authors have agreed to the order of authorship

— No copyrighted material is to be reproduced in the material

— The manuscript is not currently under review elsewhere

— Disclosure about previous public presentations elsewhere: the paper was presented in part as a poster session at the annual meeting of the American Speech Language Hearing Association

— There is no real or potential conflict of interest

I have assumed responsibility for keeping the co-authors informed about the status of the manuscript through the editorial review process, the content of the reviews, and any revisions.

Thank you for your time and effort on our behalf. I look forward to hearing from you.

Sincerely,

J. B. Smith

Senior Speech-Language Pathologist

Figure 11–3. Sample letter for submitting a manuscript.

2. Is the topic reported in the journal frequently or only rarely?
3. Would the journal be the best match of readers with that topic?
4. What formats does the journal accept?

5. Does the journal publish an "information for authors" page or issue similar information online?

Information relevant to these questions can usually be found on a journal's

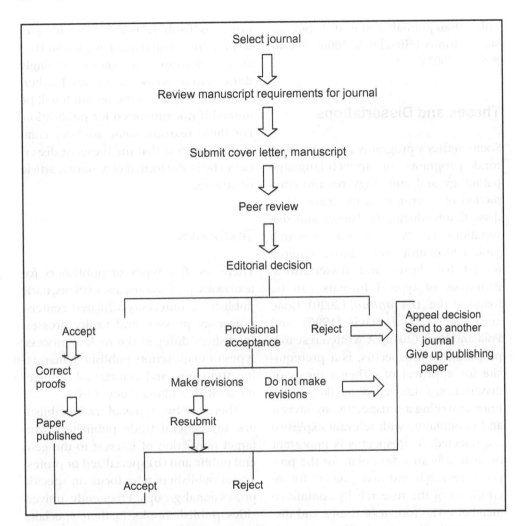

Figure 11–4. Steps in publishing a paper.

information for authors page in the journal or at its website. Huth (1999) suggests if one is uncertain about selecting the right journal, "then write or call the journal's editor" (p. 16). However, this should probably be avoided because many editors of journals do not encourage such questions because the information is usually available elsewhere, that is, in the instructions for authors page.

It also may be helpful to consider the quality of the journals. This can be based on citation analysis, which is an examination of the frequency and patterns of citations of print materials. Citation analysis reflects the quality of journals in print. The impact factor is also used as an indicator of quality. This is the number of times a report is cited each year divided by the total number of reports published. Higher values suggest increased citations and potentially higher impact. There has been criticism about the impact factor relative to its use to evaluate individuals rather than journals and to distribute research funds (Hirschtick 2006; Schutte & Svec, 2007).

Theses and Dissertations

Some master's programs and most doctoral programs in speech-language pathology and audiology require completion of a written thesis (masters) or dissertation (doctoral). Theses and dissertations usually document a research project. Most universities have a required format for theses and dissertations. Examples of typical formats can be found in the *APA Manual* (2020), Cone and Foster (2006), Davis (1997), and Polit and Beck (2010). A written research proposal, or prospectus, is a prerequisite for approval of either a thesis or dissertation (Maxwell & Satake, 2006). Prior to writing a prospectus, an advisor and a committee with relevant expertise are selected. A prospectus is important because it is an action plan for the proposed research and may prevent future criticisms of the research by committee members. The format of theses and dissertations is like a book. The content is very detailed and more comprehensive than required for publication. In other words, the length must be reduced for publication. Some suggestions for reducing length are to narrow the focus to a specific topic, be specific in reporting the results, avoid problems common to beginning authors, omit information that is not appropriate for journal articles, and be selective in the use of references. The only requirement for publication is that enough information is provided to replicate the study.

The best time to publish data from a thesis or dissertation is when the information is "fresh" (Davis, 1997). It is easier to prepare a manuscript while the data are new because it becomes increasingly difficult to do so as time passes. Furthermore, the impact of the research will be limited if not submitted for publication. For these reasons, some advisory committees suggest that the thesis or dissertation be in the format of a journal article or articles.

Textbooks

There are five types of publishers for textbooks: professional associations, trade publishers, university-affiliated centers, university presses, and vanity presses. Publishers differ in the review process, types of manuscripts published, marketing strategies, and contractual arrangements with authors (Luey, 1987).

There are two types of trade publishers: (a) general trade publishers who target nonfiction of interest to the general public and (b) specialized or professional publishers who focus on specific professional groups. Frequently, universities publish books in their specialty areas, although these publications are sometimes limited to research sponsored by the university. University presses are the primary outlet for book-length scholarly reports. They vary greatly in size; some publish hundreds of books a year, others publish less than one a year. Some university presses publish on a variety of subjects; others focus on a few areas. Vanity or subsidy publishers charge money to publish; in other words, if the author pays, the vanity press publishes the book. Obviously, there is no peer review. Therefore, publications by a vanity press carry no prestige and no merit for academic promotion or tenure.

The primary issue in selecting a publisher is whether they publish information about issues related to speech-language pathology and audiology. A book proposal or manuscript submitted to a publisher should be in proper form for the publisher. The author should obtain guidelines for preparing proposals and manuscripts from the publisher to which they plan to submit their manuscript.

University presses and trade houses usually base their publishing decisions on the opinions of reviewers. When a publisher receives a manuscript, it is read by an editor to determine if it is appropriate for the publisher and to assess the quality of the writing. A manuscript may be rejected based on the editor's reading, or it may be sent out to reviewers or referees. Publishers often request that reviewers complete questionnaires like the forms used for evaluating research reports. A manuscript may be accepted with revisions or rejected.

Presentations at Professional Meetings

ASHA, the American Academy of Audiology (AAA), state speech-language-hearing associations, and other professional organizations have meetings at which research is presented, either through oral reports or poster presentations. Presentation at a professional meeting is often linked with publication of similar information in a journal article. That is, oral reports or poster presentations may precede development of a manuscript for publication. Organizing and planning a presentation for a professional meeting and preparing a manuscript are similar up to a point. Presentations of research at professional meetings have

several advantages: (a) there is usually less time between completion of the research and dissemination of the findings; (b) one receives immediate feedback; (c) it is interactive, that is, there is interaction between the author and audience; and (d) it allows networking with others who have similar interests for possible future research (Maxwell & Satake, 2006; Polit & Beck, 2010). Presentations at professional meetings are less valued as scholarly products. Table 11–12 provides a comparison about oral reports and poster presentations. Submitting a presentation for a meeting is somewhat simpler than submitting a manuscript to a journal. ASHA requires electronic submissions through the ASHA website. Some state organizations also require electronic submission.

Usually, the professional organization announces a "Call for Papers" on its website or via written materials (newsletter, journals) about 6 to 9 months before the meeting. The announcement includes instructions/requirements and deadlines for submission. If the submission is accepted, the author is required to appear at the meeting to make the presentation. Regardless of the type of proposed presentation, it must meet certain criteria to be accepted. ASHA's program committee selects proposals based on the following criteria: strength of theoretical rationale, originality of research, strength of research design, credibility of data, integration of findings, and overall clarity.

Oral Reports

Oral reports usually last between 10 and 15 min and are followed by a question and answer period. These presentations frequently use slides and occasionally

Table 11–12. Comparison of Oral Reports and Poster Presentations

Characteristic	Oral Reports	Poster Presentations
Materials	Slides, computer, notes	Poster, Velcro
Subject	Justify objectives; refer to literature, support methods, and results	Justify objectives; refer to literature, support methods, and results
Preparation	Formal speech to adhere to time limits	Answers to expected questions
	Prepare early; practice, review, revise	Prepare early; construct posters, review, revise
Style	More formal; contact one to many	Relatively informal; contact one to one or one to a few
	Speaker standing, audience seated	Both speaker and audience standing
Moderator	Moderator introduces, buffers audience, keeps time	No moderator, direct control, no buffer
Time	Limited	Flexible
Audience	Captive, not likely to leave	Free, only interested stay
Discussion	Declamation from speaker with short questions	Chiefly questions and answer or conversational discussion
Handouts	Possible	Helpful

Source: Adapted from *Scientific Papers and Presentations,* by M. Davis, 1997, New York, NY: Academic Press.

handouts. Organization of oral reports is like that of a journal article (Silverman, 1998). However, there are differences related to length, detail (less detail because of limited time), style, formality (less formal and more redundant), and language (less formal and more conversational).

General characteristics of an oral report are presented in Table 11–12. Additional guidelines include do not "wing it" or read the paper and, whenever possible, use appropriate visual supplements to present complex information (APA, 2020). In addition, the skilled presenter

(a) captures the audience's attention at the very beginning; (b) clearly states the objectives of the presentation; (c) concentrates on concepts, not confusing details; (d) presents important concepts in different ways; (e) uses slides of less complexity than published tables and figures; and (f) prepares for a question-and-answer period.

A first-time presenter is usually more anxious than an experienced presenter. Also, to be considered is the size of the audience—typically the larger the audience, the greater the anxiety. Presenters should also be aware of other factors that affect oral presentations. These factors include the

■ quality of the presenter's speech and manner;
■ physical or nonverbal aspects of the presenter (appearance, eye contact, facial expression, gesture enthusiasm, dress, grooming);
■ confidence and poise; and
■ knowledge of information related to effective presentations. (Goldfarb & Serpanos, 2009)

Poster Presentations

Poster sessions have become a major format for presenting research at a professional meeting. A poster session at a professional conference consists of several simultaneous visual displays of research studies. Attendees circulate around the posters during the session (Polit & Beck, 2010). Poster presentation may be formal or open. In formal poster presentations, the author presents an overview of the poster with a moderator who guides discussion about each poster in a symposium format. The author is present at an open session to answer attendees' questions. Most organizations have specific instructions for poster presentations. Generally, the title is at the top followed by author(s) and affiliation. The introduction is in the upper left corner and the conclusions in the right lower corner. Traditional posters have the advantage of permitting simultaneous sessions within the same time period. Poster presentations allow participants to select information of interest, receive substantial information within a short period of time, and avoid posters dealing with topics of less interest to them. For some presentations, poster presentations are less threatening

(Maxwell & Satake, 2006). Traditional poster presentations also have disadvantages. First, preparing posters requires more effort and expense than preparing for an oral report. Second, posters, like wedding dresses, are often not used subsequently. Third, a presentation can be seriously disadvantaged if placed in an awkward, crowded location or in poor lighting conditions (Simmonds, 1984). It might be best, if possible, to check the room in advance when doing a poster presentation (Deep & Sussman, 1990). Problems identified early may be resolved. An example involves placing posters on a crowded stage that was inaccessible to participants in wheelchairs or on crutches. Fourth, posters at times can be difficult to transport (Bordens & Abbott, 1988).

In recent years, more poster presentations have been electronic. The primary differences between traditional and electronic poster presentations are related to the presence of an author and attendees. These and other differences are compared in Table 11–13.

General guidelines for posters according to Blessing and Forister (2011) are as follows:

■ Keep the poster simple.
■ Include only enough information to support the conclusions.
■ Use tables and figures; less text is better.

Templates are available for preparing posters as well as computer-generated programs, such as PowerPoint, Microsoft Excel, and Statistical Programs for the Social Sciences (SPSS). Leedy and Ormrod (2010) provided detailed descriptions of Microsoft Excel and SPSS. Nichol and Pexman (2003) provided guidelines

Table 11–13. Characteristics of Traditional and Electronic Poster Presentations

	Traditional	Electronic
Access	Live	Remote
Audience	Restricted	Widespread
Schedule	Fixed	Flexible
Frequency	Nonrepeatable	Repeatable
CEUs	Inconsistent	Consistent
Duplication	Impossible	Possible
Author and audience	Present	Not present
Access	Direct	Indirect or direct

for the content and style of posters. Considerations related to content were to consider the main point, key points of information for attendees, crucial details, methodology, the most important results, and realistic conclusions. Style was related to available space: one large poster or a poster consisting of small panels.

Visual Supplements

Visual supplements are essential to oral presentations and posters. A visual supplement is any illustration used to clarify and analyze information in written reports and oral presentations. The most common visual supplements are tables and figures, which were discussed earlier in the chapter under the section on Format of Research Reports. Handouts may be used to supplement oral reports and poster presentations. They should include the title of the report, the authors' names and affiliation, and

where and when presented. PowerPoint slides or a mini poster are frequently used as handouts. It is recommended that handouts for oral reports be distributed prior to the presentation, not while the presentation is occurring. Instead of, or in addition to handouts, some presenters distribute diskettes containing information about the presentation (Nichol & Pexman, 2003). However, this can be expensive.

Guidelines for visual supplements are listed in Table 11–14. Criteria for visuals are simplicity, legibility, unity, quality, and feasibility. Visuals should be cohesive and uniform with other visual supplements and with the written or spoken words. Production and presentation of visual supplements should be possible with available materials, facilities, and time (Davis, 1997). The *Publication Manual of the American Psychological Association* (2020) provides extensive guidelines about traditional tables and figures.

Table 11–14. Guidelines for Visual Supplements

• Make them simple
• Make the images or letters large enough to be seen clearly
• Make a trial run long enough before the presentation to permit you to revise the visual aids if needed
• Coordinate the visual aids with the oral report or written text so that the audience is not distracted and the visual aid is relevant to the oral report or text
• Prior to a presentation that uses visual aids, be sure that any needed equipment is available and operational

Source: Adapted from *Scientific Papers and Presentations*, by M. Davis, 1997, San Diego, CA: Academic Press.

Evaluating and Reviewing Research Reports

Research reports should be read critically; just because a report has been published does not ensure its quality. Another consideration is the impact factor, which indicates how many times a journal's paper is cited in other journals (Huth, 1999). Some journals provide this information at the end of reports.

Readers are responsible for critically reviewing research reports and deciding their value. Critically evaluating and reviewing research reports is a skill that requires knowledge and experience. The most important considerations are scientific relevance, soundness of methodology, and the author(s). Several guidelines for evaluating research reports are available (APA, 2020; Hegde, 2010; Polit & Beck, 2010; Orlikoff et al., 2022; Silverman, 1998). These guidelines can also be used to evaluate oral reports and poster presentations.

Evidence-based practice uses specific criteria to evaluate the quality of evidence. The criteria differ according to whether the evidence is related to decisions about diagnosis or treatment (ASHA, 2023b).

These guidelines can also be used to evaluate oral presentation and posters. There are also guidelines with specific focus, such as the type of research, qualitative or quantitative (Leedy & Ormrod, 2010; McMillan, 2004), clinical services, diagnosis, or treatment (ASHA, 2005), and level of evidence (Haynes & Johnson, 2009; Jewell, 2011).

Dollaghan (2007) developed brief summaries of evidence for a variety of topics:

■ CATE—Critical Appraisal of Treatment Evidence
■ CADE—Critical Appraisal of Diagnostic Evidence

- CASM—Critical Appraisal of Systemic Review or Meta-Analysis
- CAPE—Checklist for Appraising Patient/Practice Evidence
- CAPP—Checklist for Appraising Patient Preferences

Answers to questions can be used for evaluating reports (Blessing & Forister, 2011). These questions are listed in Table 11–15.

CATs

Two methods have been suggested for brief critical reevaluations of the literature. Critically Appraised Topics (CATs) and Evidence-Based Communication Assessment and Intervention (EBCAI) structure appraisal abstracts.

A CAT is a brief summary of clinical quality and appraisal of the evidence that typically begins with a clinical bottom line that is a recommendation about use and application (Polit & Beck, 2010). Al-Jundi and Sakka (2017) provided guidance regarding the components of the Critical Appraisal of Clinical Research.

There are several templates for CATs available online. CATS have two distinguishing characteristics: (a) they are based on specific clinical questions and developed by using the Problem/Population, Intervention, Comparison, Outcome (PICO) format; and (b) they include the bottom line or conclusions about the value of the findings. The major advantage of CATs is the potential to improve patient care. Other advantages include a standard format, specific/focused questions, and brevity as well as possibly reducing the amount of time for critical

Table 11–15. Questions to Ask and Answer About Research

- What is the source of the report?
- Was the publication peer-reviewed?
- Who are the authors and their affiliations?
- What was the main subject of the study?
- What was the problem(s) investigated?
- What was the purpose or rationale for the study?
- Who or what constituted the sample or populations?
- What was the design?
- What statistical analyses were used?
- Are the results clear?
- Did the results answer the identified question(s)?
- Are the conclusions consistent with the design and analysis?
- Are the results consistent or contradictory with the results of similar studies?
- What do the results mean relative to clinical practice, and patients?
- Can the results be applied to your research or clinical practice?

Source: From *Research and Medical Literature*, by J. D. Blessing and J. G. Forister, 2012, Burlington, MA: Jones and Bartlett.

review. Disadvantages are short-term use as new evidence becomes available, limited access to the literature, based on only one or two studies, and variable skills and methods of analysis. Structured appraisal abstracts can be used to evaluate evidence (Lackey & Ogletree, 2012). These abstracts are published in the peer-review journal *Evidence-Based Communication Assessment and Intervention* (EBCAI). EBCAI abstracts can be used to evaluate credibility and determine the potential for application to clinical practice.

Summary

There are several reasons for reporting research. Among these reasons are ethical responsibility to contribute and disseminate professional information as an indicator of institutional quality as well as recognition and academic survival.

It is difficult to report research without effective time management. Research is frequently not reported because of failure to make time to write and revise reports. There are, however, several strategies that can facilitate managing time for reporting research.

Research might be considered incomplete until the reports have been disseminated at a professional meeting, as a written report, or both. The form and content of oral and written research reports are similar, although there are differences primarily in manner of presentation and length. Written reports are usually longer. There are different types of written reports: journal articles, theses and dissertations, and textbooks. Evaluating and reviewing research reports is an important professional responsibility. Critical review and evaluation of research reports are an integral part of evidence-based practice, which emphasizes the application and use of research evidence to make clinical decisions.

DISCUSSION QUESTIONS

1. What distinguishes the unpublished from the published writer?
2. What are the reasons for reporting research?
3. Define "publish or perish."
4. Why is research not reported?
5. Explain the myths about research reports.
6. Why and how can these myths be eliminated?
7. How can time management facilitate research productivity?
8. What is the difference between "busyness" and binging?

9. Why should a timetable be developed and implemented for reporting research?
10. How can computer technology be used to increase productivity?
11. Why do single-subject research designs require less time?
12. Describe procrastination.
13. How can procrastination affect research?
14. How can procrastination be avoided or reduced?
15. How can a research log be used to determine order of authorship?

16. List and briefly describe the major sections of research reports.
17. What is a structured abstract?
18. Compare structured abstracts for original and review of tutorial reports.
19. Why are key words important?
20. Why do professional journals require the authors to disclose their contributions to a report?
21. What is the difference between tables and figures?
22. Why are tables and figures valuable to research reports?
23. What is meant by writing style?
24. How is writing style developed?
25. What is APA format?
26. Why are mistakes in referencing so common?
27. How can mistakes in referencing be eliminated or reduced?
28. What is biased language? How can it be avoided?
29. What is person-first language?
30. When and why should one request permission to use previously published materials?
31. What are the steps in rewriting and revising a report?
32. Why are rewriting and revising challenging?
33. List and briefly describe the types of research reports.
34. What is a cover letter? What information is included in a cover letter?
35. Define peer review. Why is peer review important?
36. How does one select an appropriate journal to submit a manuscript?
37. What types of articles are published in ASHA journals?
38. Briefly describe the different types of textbook publishers.
39. What is a vanity press? What are the limitations?
40. What are the advantages and disadvantages of presenting research at professional meetings?
41. What is a "call for papers"?
42. What are the advantages and disadvantages of poster presentations?
43. What are the differences between traditional and evidence-based poster presentations?
44. How can visual supplements be used in written reports and oral presentations?
45. Why should published research reports be evaluated and reviewed?
46. How can research reports be reviewed?
47. What percentage of papers submitted for publication to ASHA journals, within the last few years, are accepted for publication? What are the implications?
48. What are the guidelines for tables and figures? Why is it important to be familiar with these guidelines?
49. What are the advantages and disadvantages of presenting research findings at professional meetings?
50. What are the major components of a V-diagram?

51. What information should be included in a cover letter when submitting a manuscript?
52. What factors can affect presentation of research findings at professional meetings?
53. What are CATs? What are the different types of CATs?
54. How can research be evaluated?
55. Why should research be evaluated?
56. What factors influence poster presentation?
57. Compare traditional and electronic poster presentations. Which would have the most advantages? Why?

References

Al-Jundi, A., & Sakka, S. (2017). Critical appraisal of clinical research. *Clinical of Diagnostic Research, 11*(5), JE01–JE05. https://www.doi.org/10.7860/JCDR/2017/26047/9942

American Medical Association. (2020). Instructions for authors. *Journal of the American Medical Association*. https://doi.org/10.1093/jama/9780190246556.001.0001

American Psychological Association. (2020). *Publication manual of the American Psychological Association* (7th ed.).

American Speech-Language-Hearing Association. (1993). Guide for gender equality: Language usage. *ASHA, 35*(10), 42–46.

American Speech-Language-Hearing Association. (2005, June 1). Examples of levels-of evidence hierarchies. *ASHA Leader.*

American Speech-Language-Hearing Association. (2023a). *Code of ethics.* http://www.asha.org

American Speech-Language-Hearing Association. (2023b). *Guidelines for reporting your research.* http://www.academy.pubs.asha.org

Anderson, M. (1992). *Imposters in the temple.* Simon & Schuster.

Barzun, J. (1986). *Writing, editing, and publishing.* University of Chicago Press.

Bennett, D. M., & Taylor, D. M. (2003). Unethical practices in authorship of scientific papers. *Emergency Medicine, 15*(3), 263–270.

Blessing, J. D., & Forister, J. G. (2011). *Introduction to research and medical literature for health professionals* (3rd ed.). James and Bartlett Learning

Boice, R. (1989). Procrastination, busyness, and binging. *Behavioral Research Therapy, 27*(6), 605–611.

Bordens, K. S., & Abbott, B. B. (1988). *Research designs and methods.* Mayfield.

Boyes, W., Happel, J., & Hogen, T. (1984). Publish or perish: Fact or fiction. *Journal of Economics Education, 15*(2), 136–141.

Carter-Scott, C. (1989). *Negaholics.* Fawcett Crest.

Cone, J. D., & Foster, S. L. (2006). *Dissertations and theses from start to finish.* American Psychological Association.

Connell, P., & McReynolds, L. (1988). A clinical science approach to treatment. In N. J. Lass, L. McReynolds, J. Northern, & D. Yoder (Eds.), *Handbook of speech-language pathology and audiology* (pp. 1058–1073). B. C. Decker.

Davis, G. B., & Parker, C. A. (1979). *Writing the doctoral dissertation.* Barron's Educational Services.

Davis, M. (1997). *Scientific papers and presentations.* Academic Press.

Deep, S., & Sussman, L. (1990). *Smart moves.* Addison-Wesley.

DePoy, E., & Gitlin, L. N. (2011). *Introduction to research.* C. V. Mosby.

Dollagham, C. A. (2007). *The handbook of evidence-based practice in communication disorders.* Brookes.

Drummond, V. (1990). *The elements of nonsexist language usage.* Prentice Hall.

Finn, P., Bothe, A. K., & Bramlett, R. E. (2005) Science and pseudoscience in communication disorders: Criteria and application. *American Journal of Speech-Language Pathology, 14*(3), 172–186.

Folkins, J. (1992). *The language used to describe individuals with disabilities.* http://www.asha.org/publication/

Goldfarb, R., & Serpanos, Y. C. (2009). *Professional writing in speech-language pathology and audiology.* Plural Publishing.

Gowin, D. B., & Alvarez, M. C. (2005). *The art of educating with V diagrams.* Cambridge University Press.

Harris, R. L. (1999). *Informative graphics.* Oxford University Press.

Haynes, R. B., Mulrow, C. D., Huth, E. J., Altman, D. G., & Gardner, M. J. (1996). More informative abstracts revisited. *Cleft Palate Craniofacial Journal, 33*(1), 1–9.

Haynes, W. O., & Johnson, C. E. (2009). *Understanding research and evidence-based practice in communication disorders.* Pearson.

Hegde, M. N. (2003). *Clinical research in communicative disorders.* Pro-Ed.

Hegde, M. N. (2010). *Coursebook on scientific and professional writing for speech language pathology.* Singular Publishing.

Henson, K. T. (1993, June). Writing for successful publication. *Phi Delta Kappan,* 799–802.

Hirschtick, R. E. (2006). A piece of my mind. Copy-and-paste. *JAMA: The Journal of the American Medical Association, 295*(20), 2335–2336. https://doi.org/10.1001/jama.295.20.2335

Holcomb, J., & Roush, R. (1988). A study of the scholarly activities of allied health facilities in southern academic health science center. *Journal of Allied Health, 17*(11), 227–293.

Huth, E. J. (1999). *Writing and publishing in medicine.* Williams & Wilkins.

Huth, E. J., & Sheen, A. (1984). How to write and publish papers in the medical sciences. *Plastic and Reconstructive Surgery, 73*(1), 153–154.

Irwin, D. L., Pannbacker, M. D., & Kallail, K. (1992). Writing for communication disorders and related journals. *Journal of the National Student Speech-Language Hearing Association, 19,* 119–122.

Iverson, C., Flanagin, A., Fontanarosa, P. B., Glass, R. M., Glitman, P., & Lantz, J. C., . . . American Medical Association. (1993). *American Medical Association manual of style.* Lippincott, Williams, & Wilkins.

Jewell, D. V. (2011). *Guidelines to evidence based physical therapist practice.* Jones and Bartlett.

Lackey, K. C., & Ogletree, R. T. (2012). EBCAI structured abstracts. *Evidence-Based Communication Intervention and Treatment, 10,* 177–165. doi:10.1080/17489539.2011.649891

Leedy, P. D., & Ormrod, J. E. (2010). *Practical research.* Pearson.

Luey, B. (1987). *Handbook for academic authors.* Cambridge University Press.

Maxwell, D. L., & Satake, E. (2006). *Research and statistical methods in communication sciences and disorders.* Thomson-Delmar Learning.

McMillan, J. H. (2004). *Educational research.* Pearson.

Meline, T. (2006). *Research in communication science and disorders.* Pearson.

Miller, C., & Swift, K. (1988). *The handbook of nonsexist language.* Harper and Row.

Nichol, A. A., & Pexman, P. M. (2003). *Displaying your findings.* American Psychological Association.

Orlikoff, R. F., Schiavetti, N., & Metz, D. A. (2022) *Evaluating research in communication disorders.* Pearson Education.

Paden, E. P. (1970). *A history of the American Speech and Hearing Association, 1925–1958.* American Speech-Language-Hearing Association.

Pierson, D. J. (2004). The top ten reasons why manuscripts are not accepted for publication. *Respiratory Care, 49,* 1246–1252.

Polit, P. F., & Beck, C. T. (2010). *Nursing research: Principles and methods.* Lippincott Williams & Wilkins.

Portney, L. G., & Watkins, M. P. (2009). *Foundations of clinical research: Applications to practice* (3rd ed.). Prentice Hall.

Robertson, S. (2004, September 24). I used to have a handle on life, but it broke! *ASHA Leader, 9,* 13, 37.

Ross-Hellauer, T., Tennant, J. P., Banelytė, V., Gorogh, E., Luzi, D., Kraker, P., . . . Vignoli, M. (2020). Ten simple rules for innovative dissemination of research. *PLoS Computational Biology, 16*(4), e1007704. https://doi.org/10.1371/journal.pcbi.1007704

Roth, A. J. (1989). *The research paper.* Wadsworth.

Rudestam, K. E., & Newman, R. R. (2001). *Surviving your dissertation.* Sage.

Schilling, L. S. (2005). Publish or perish: Writing under pressure. *Pediatric Nursing, 31*(3), 234–236.

Schneider, S., & Soto, A. M. (1989). Sexist language: Should we be concerned? *Journal of the American Women's Medical Association, 44*(3), 79–83.

Schutte, H. K., & Svec, J. G. (2007). Reaction of Folia Phoniatrica et Logopaedica on the current trend of impact factor measures. *Folia Phoniatrica, 59,* 281–285.

Silverman, F. H. (1998). *Research design and evaluation in speech-language pathology and audiology.* Allyn & Bacon.

Simmonds, D. (1984). How to produce good posters. *Medical Teacher, 6*(1), 10–13.

Sininger, T., March, R., Walden, B., & Wilber, L. A. (2003). Guidelines for ethical practice in research for audiologists. *Audiology Today, 15*(6), 14–17.

Sorrels, B. D. (1983). *How to complete and survive a doctoral dissertation.* St. Martin's Press.

Sternberg, R. J. (1993). *The psychologist's companion: A guide to scientific writing for students and researchers.* Cambridge University Press.

Strunk, W., & White, E. B. (1979). *The elements of style.* MacMillan.

Turabian, K. L. (1995). *A manual for writers of term papers, theses, dissertations.* University of Chicago Press.

University of Chicago Press. (2017). *The Chicago manual of style* (17th ed.). https://doi.org/10.7208/cmos17

Vincente-Saez, R., & Martinez-Fuentes, C. (2018) Open science now: A systematic literature review for an integrated definition. *Journal of Business Research, 88*(July), 428–436.

Yau, N. (2001). *Visualize this.* Wiley.

12

Evaluating Tests and Treatments

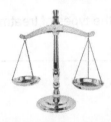

LEARNING OBJECTIVES

Upon completion of this chapter, the reader will be able to:

- Discuss reasons for evaluating tests and treatments
- Distinguish between decisions based on evidence and opinions
- Apply specific criteria to evaluation of tests and treatments
- Define terms related to testing: true/false negative, true/false positive, specificity, and sensitivity
- Distinguish between the types of treatment outcome research

The evaluation of tests and treatments involves both qualitative and quantitative research—that is, multimethod research. In speech-language pathology and audiology, data are collected about individuals for diagnosis and treatment. Options for data collection include tests, checklists, quality-of-life measuring, observation, and various documents (case history, medical charts, and educational records). Evaluating diagnostic tests and treatment outcomes is a type of research relevant to the clinical practice of speech-language pathology and audiology. This type of research involves

- being skeptical;
- considering the source of the information;
- distinguishing between cause and effect;
- differentiating observation from inference;
- ensuring that describing a product is not only to sell it; and
- recognizing that an example is not evidence for what is claimed. (Lum, 2002)

Evidence-based practice and ethics are important in evaluating tests and treatments. It is a method of using the highest available level of evidence to make clinical decisions.

Evidence-based tests and treatments are an ethical responsibility. The present Code of Ethics of the American Speech-Language-Hearing Association (ASHA, 2023) contains several related references to ethical research. Moreover, selection of tests and treatments is significant in terms of cost and benefit. Speech-language pathologists and audiologists should be discerning consumers

of diagnostic and treatment resources. A test or treatment should be selected on the best available evidence. Obsolete and outdated evaluation and treatment methods should be discarded. New diagnostic and treatment products constitute a growing market that may be heavily promoted because of high profit margins (Lum, 2002).

Evaluation Issues

Speech-language pathologists and audiologists should assume responsibility for critical review of diagnostic tests and treatment materials to avoid products without evidence being used because there is great variability in the quality of tests and treatments. With any test or treatment, speech-language pathologists and audiologists should always ask, "What is the evidence?"

An evaluation of diagnostic tests and treatment methods based on opinion is incompatible with evidence-based practice. All sources of evidence are not equal—that is, bad to poor evidence that is low (weak) to high (strong) level. Opinion is considered to be weak evidence (Reilly, 2004). Unfortunately, many speech-language pathologists and audiologists more frequently use clinical experience and opinion than research or clinical practice guidelines to make clinical decisions (Zipoli & Kennedy, 2005). Several trends have decreased the emphasis on general psychometric checklists for evidence about sensitivity and specificity of tests (Pena et al., 2006). Opinion and blind acceptance should not be the basis for making clinical decisions. Speech-language pathologists and audiologists should be skeptical and admit to not knowing unless there is sufficient evidence (Lum, 2002).

Tests

Tests are used by speech-language pathologists and audiologists for a variety of reasons. They may be used to establish whether or not someone has a speech, language, or hearing problem; to monitor response to treatment; to make informed treatment decisions; to assess progress; or to assess the risk of developing a speech, language, or hearing problem (Mart, 1999).

The primary purpose of any test is to determine whether or not someone has a speech, language, or hearing problem. A good test is one that can correctly detect that a problem is truly present (true positive) or that someone does not have a problem (true negative). Test results can be misleading if there is a high false-negative or false-positive result (Mart, 1999). In other words, low false-positive and false-negative results are desired.

Haynes and Pindzola (1998) believe uncritical acceptance of tests is "probably the rule rather than the exception" (p. 83). Test accuracy is based on sensitivity and specificity. The *sensitivity* of a test is the proportion of people who actually have the problem who had a true positive test—that is, accuracy of the test in identifying people with the problem. It is further defined as the probability of a diagnostic test finding a problem among those who have the problem or the proportion of people with the problem who have a positive test result (true positive; Melynk & Fin-

eout-Overholt, 2005). The specificity of a test is the equal and opposite of sensitivity. It is the proportion without the problem with a true negative test result (Lum, 2002; Maxwell & Satake, 2006). Specificity is further defined as the probability of a diagnostic test finding no problem among those who do not have the problem or the proportion of people free of a problem who have a negative test (true negative; Melynk & Fineout-Overholt, 2005). An accurate test will have a high positive likelihood ratio and a low negative likelihood ratio, indicating that the test correctly identified people who have the problem and those people who do not (Dollaghan, 2004). Sensitivity and specificity can be calculated as follows:

$$\text{Sensitivity} = \frac{\text{true positives}}{\text{true positives} + \text{false negatives}}$$

$$\text{Specificity} = \frac{\text{true negatives}}{\text{true negatives} + \text{false positives}}$$

The composition of normative groups should be considered in interpreting test scores and making diagnostic decisions. Pena et al. (2006) reviewed descriptions of the normative groups for 32 child language tests. If the normative group includes a mixed sample of normal and language-impaired children, measurement precision decreases for absolute score interpretation but may increase for relative interpretations. Thus, clinicians should be aware of two principles: (a) determine if test characteristics are appropriate for interpretation and (b) a single test may not support multiple diagnostic purposes.

Another consideration in evaluating tests is the *predictive value*. The predictive value of a test has practical implications for predicting actual clinical outcomes based on test results (Maxwell & Satake, 2006). There are two major components or predictive values of a diagnostic test: (a) *predictive value positive* and (b) *predictive value negative*. Predictive value positive (PV+) is the probability that a person has a problem given the test result is positive. Predictive value negative (PV–) is the probability that a person does not have a problem given that the test result is negative. These values are calculated as follows:

$$PV+ = \frac{\text{true positives}}{\text{true positives} + \text{false positives}}$$

$$PV- = \frac{\text{true negatives}}{\text{true negatives} + \text{false negatives}}$$

Many tests have tables for converting raw scores into age and/or grade equivalent scores. These scores, according to Haynes and Pindzola (1998), "are the least useful and most dangerous scores to be obtained from standardized tests because they lead to gross misinterpretation of a client's performance" (p. 72). Age and grade-equivalent scores are the least useful types of scores because they tend to distort performance and lead to misinterpretations by both consumers and professionals. Nonetheless, these scores are often used to interpret test performance and make diagnostic decisions. Furthermore, many state departments of education mandate the use of age-equivalent scores for making decisions about eligibility for services (Haynes & Pindzola, 2012).

There are two basic types of review for evaluating diagnostic tests and treatment methods: traditional and evidence based. There are major differences between traditional and evidence-based reviews. The former tends to be subjective and use vague criteria. The latter involve application of specific criteria for evaluation, diagnosis, and treatment. This reduces the risk for bias. ASHA (2018) has provided examples of levels of evidence hierarchies for both diagnosis and treatment as presented in Tables 12–1 and 12–2.

Some evaluation strategies have multiple purposes. For example, ASHA has a series of questions for evaluation, treatment procedures, purchasing a product, or attending an educational program. These questions can also be used for evaluating tests. Table 12–3 lists ASHA's questions.

Another method of evaluation is to differentiate between science and pseudoscience characteristics of a test or treatment. These criteria are shown in Table 12–4. Several authors have described criteria for evaluating tests (Haynes & Pindzola, 2012; Hutchinson, 1996; Lum, 2002; Mertens, 2005; Shipley & McAfee, 2009; Stein & Cutler, 1996). These criteria are related to the test manual, descriptive statistics, and normative sample.

Haynes and Pindzola (1998) suggested obtaining a test for evaluation because test brochures and catalogs may not provide adequate information. Furthermore, "if possible, order a test for appraisal, and pay for it only if you are satisfied with its psychometric adequacy and what it will actually tell you about a client" (p. 77). Therefore, psychometric adequacy should be evaluated on the basis of identifiable criteria.

Table 12–1. Examples of Levels-of-Evidence Hierarchies for Diagnostic Studies

Level	Type of Diagnostic Study
1a	Systematic review or meta-analysis of 1c studies (high-quality trials)
1b	Independent replication of a 1c study
1c	A diagnostic study having a representative and consecutive sample and appropriate reference standard (e.g., gold-standard test) in an independent blind comparison demonstrating validated specificity and sensitivity that are almost absolute
2a	Systematic review or meta-analysis 2b diagnostic studies
2b	A cohort study with a good reference standard
3a	Systematic review or meta-analysis 3b studies
3b	A diagnostic study having a nonconsecutive sample or a consistently applied reference standard
4	One or more case-control study Expert opinion without explicit critical appraisal

Note: Levels 1 through 3b could be further fractioned by experimental precision. For example, level 2a could become 2a(+) and 2a(−) for grouping high- and low-precision experiments respectively.

Source: From "Examples of Levels-of-Evidence Hierarchy," by American Speech-Language-Hearing Association, 2005. Retrieved from http://www.asha.org/About/publications/leader-online/archives/2005/f050524a3.htm

Table 12–2. Examples of Levels-of-Evidence Hierarchies for Treatment Studies

Level	Type of Treatment Study
1a	Systematic reviews or meta-analyses of high-quality randomized controlled trials
1b	High-quality randomized controlled trials
2a	Systematic reviews or meta-analyses of high-quality nonrandomized controlled trials
2b	High-quality nonrandomized controlled trials
3a	Systematic reviews of cohort studies
3b	Individual cohort study or low quality randomized controlled trials
4	Clinical outcome studies
5a	Systematic review of case-control studies
5b	Individual case-control studies
6	Case-series
7a	Expert opinion without explicit critical appraisal

Source: From "Examples of Levels-of-Evidence Hierarchies," by American Speech-Language-Hearing Association, 2005. Retrieved from http://www.asha.org/about/Publications/leader-online/archives/2005/f05024a3.htm

Table 12–3. ASHA's Questions for Evaluating Treatments, Procedures, Products, or Programs

Stated uses:	What are the stated uses of the procedure, product, or program?
Population:	To which client/patient population does it apply? Is there documented evidence that it is valid for use with a specific population?
Generalization:	To which other populations does it claim to generalize?
Outcomes:	Are outcomes clearly stated?
Publications:	Are there publications about this procedure, product, or program? Is the information published in a peer-reviewed journal? Is promotional material the only published source of information?
Peer-reviewed:	Is there peer-reviewed research that supports or contradicts research: the stated outcomes or benefits?
Developers:	What is the professional background of the developers of the procedure/product/program?
Availability:	Are there similar procedures, products, or programs currently: available? How do they compare in performance and cost?
Experience:	Have you talked with others who have experience with this product, procedure, or program? What was their expertise? Have you considered posting a query on ASHA's interactive member forum on its website?
Scope of Practice:	Is it within my profession's Scope of Practice? Is it within my personal scope of practice (i.e., personal training, competence, experience) to use this procedure, product, or program?
Information/ Policies:	Have you checked to see if there are any ASHA statements or guidelines on this topic?
Cost:	Based on the factors above, is the cost reasonable and justifiable?

Source: From "When Evaluating Any Treatment, Procedure, Product, or Program Ask Yourself the Following Questions," by American Speech-Language-Hearing Association, n.d. Retrieved from http://www.asha.org/members/evaluate.htm

Table 12–4. Ten Criteria for Distinguishing Between Science and Pseudoscience

Yes	No	
☐	☐	1. Untestable: Is the treatment unable to be tested or disproved?
☐	☐	2. Unchanged: Does the treatment approach remain unchanged even in the face of contradictory evidence?
☐	☐	3. Confirming evidence: Is the rationale for the treatment approach based only on confirming evidence with disconfirming evidence ignored or minimized?
☐	☐	4. Anecdotal evidence: Does the evidence in support of the treatment rely on personal experience and anecdotal accounts?
☐	☐	5. Inadequate evidence: Are the treatment claims incommensurate with the level of evidence needed to support those claims?
☐	☐	6. Avoiding peer-review: Are treatment claims unsupported by evidence that has undergone critical scrutiny?
☐	☐	7. Disconnected: Is the treatment approach disconnected from well-established scientific models or paradigms?
☐	☐	8. New terms: Is the treatment described by terms that appear to be scientific but upon further examination are found not to be scientific at all?
☐	☐	9. Grandiose outcome: Is the treatment approach based on grandiose claims or poorly specified outcomes?
☐	☐	10. Holistic: Is the treatment claimed to make sense only within a vaguely described holistic framework?

Source: From "Science and Pseudoscience in Communication Disorders: Criteria and Applications," by P. Finn, A. K. Bothe, and R. E. Bramlett, 2005, *American Journal of Speech-Language Pathology, 14*(3), pp. 172–186.

Dollaghan (2004) described criteria from the evidence-based practice literature to use in evaluating diagnostic tests, which are presented in Table 12–5. Three evidence-based propositions were considered:

■ The opinions of expert authorities, singly or in groups, such as consensus panels, should be viewed with skepticism and discounted entirely when they contradict evidence from rigorous scientific studies.

■ Not all research is relevant to decisions about clinical practice.

■ Being judgmental about evidence is a goal, not a character flaw.

Another consideration is reporting diagnostic findings that involve both quantitative and qualitative data, namely,

Table 12–5. Checklist of Questions for Evaluating Evidence of a Diagnostic Measure

Yes	No	
☐	☐	Was the measure compared to a gold standard (GS)?
☐	☐	Was the gold standard valid, reliable, and reasonable?
☐	☐	Were both measures administered to all participants?
☐	☐	Were both measures administered to all participants?
☐	☐	Were participants identified prospectively?
☐	☐	Were participants described clearly?
☐	☐	Did participants include individuals with and without the disorder of interest?
☐	☐	Did participants exhibit a range of severity levels?
☐	☐	Did participants include some with confusable symptoms?
☐	☐	Were the two measures administered independently, by different examiners?
☐	☐	Were examiners blinded to performance on the other test?
☐	☐	Were examiners blinded to other patient information?
☐	☐	Was the positive likelihood ratio in at least the intermediate range (≥4.0)?
☐	☐	Was the negative likelihood ratio in at least the intermediate range (≥0.4)?
☐	☐	Was the confidence interval reasonably narrow?
☐	☐	Is the new measure feasible in usual clinical practice?
☐	☐	Does the new measure offer a significant advantage over the gold stand?

Source: From "Evidence-Based Practice in Communication Disorders: What Do We Know and When Do We Know It?" by C. A. Dollaghan, 2004, *Journal of Communication Disorders, 37*(5), pp. 391–400.

multimethod research. A worksheet for organizing and interpreting diagnostic findings is shown in Figure 12–1. The worksheet can be used as the final report or as the prerequisite to a narra- tive report. The worksheet serves as a reminder that diagnosis of communication disorders is a type of research that combines both quantitative and qualitative data.

Diagnostic Worksheet

Date of Evaluation: _____ _____ _____

Date of Birth: _____ _____ _____

Chronological Age: _____ _____ _____

		Qualitative	Quantitative
Language	**Oral Language (general)**		
	· Receptive Language Content/Semantics (vocabulary) Form/Syntax, Morph. (grammar) Use/Pragmatics		
	· Expressive Language Content/Semantics (vocabulary) Form/Syntax, Morph. (grammar) Use/Pragmatics		
Speech	**Articulation/Phonology** Inventory, distribution, sequences Phonological rules, intelligibility, consistency, stimulability, prosody		
	Voice		
	Fluency		
	Oral Mechanism		*Fail* / *Pass*
H	**Hearing**		*Fail* / *Pass*
Other	**Cognitive**		
	Adaptive Behavior		
	Achievement Reading Math Other		

Key: ■ - Lower Extreme;   - (Well) Below Average; ▦ - Average: ▨ - (Well) Above Average: ■ - Upper Extreme

O - Observed Score; R - Reported Score; ? - Estimated Level. (68% confidence bands should be indicated if possible)

Figure 12–1. Diagnostic worksheet (Powell, 2006).

Treatment

Treatment outcome is a broadly defined term that refers to change, or the lack of it, that may occur as a result of time, treatment, or both (Golper et al., 2001). Moreover, treatment outcomes are generalized, maintained, indirect, and clinically valid results of treatment (Hegde, 2003). A distinction is frequently made between efficacy, effectiveness, and efficiency of treatment. The following questions can be used to make this distinction:

■ Has the treatment been shown to be beneficial in controlled research, that is, ideal conditions (efficacy)?

■ Is treatment useful in applied clinical settings (average conditions) and, if so, with what patients and under what circumstances (effectiveness)?

■ Is treatment efficient (minimal waste, expense, and unnecessary effort) in the sense of being cost effective relative to other alternative interventions (efficiency; Golper et al., 2001; Maxwell & Satake, 2006)?

There are major differences between various types of treatment research. Uncontrolled or nonexperimental research is designed to document improvement such as case studies (Hegde, 2003). Controlled treatment research, or experimentation, is designed to establish a cause-and-effect relationship between treatment (independent variable) and positive changes (dependent variable). Controlled treatment research is used to determine effectiveness. It requires either a single subject or group experimental design. Directly replicated research or experimentation is designed to determine if results (improvement or effects) in an uncontrolled or controlled study can be replicated when there is no change in treatment, setting, or clinicians; the only change is new clients.

Two other variations of treatment studies warrant consideration: retrospective (past) and prospective (current; Lum, 2002). *Retrospective studies* involve examination of existing case records, which has limitations if the records are incorrect or inaccurate. Retrospective studies can be completed quickly and economically because they are based on existing data (Maxwell & Satake, 2006). *Prospective* means the data needed for study are determined before they are collected. In prospective studies, current information is used to predict future status.

Silverman (1998) provided a series of questions for evaluating treatment that focused on space and time. These questions are listed in Table 12–6. To assess treatment outcomes with a single client,

Table 12–6. Questions for Evaluating Treatment

— What are the impacts of the treatment on specific behaviors that contribute to a client's speech-language problem at given points in time?
— What are the effects of the treatment on other aspects of a client's speech-language at given points in space-time?
— What are the effects of the treatment on a client other than those directly related to speech-language at given points in space-time?
— What are the client's attitudes about the treatment and its impact on his or her speech-language and other behaviors at given points in space-time?
— What are the attitudes of a client's clinician, family, friends, and others toward the treatment and toward its effect on the client's speech-language and other attributes of behavior in space-time?
— What investment is required of client and clinician at given points in space-time?
— What is the probability of relapse following termination of treatment?

Source: From *Research Design and Evaluation in Speech-Language Pathology and Audiology,* by F. H. Silverman, 1998, Boston, MA: Allyn & Bacon.

Lum (2002) described a number of factors to consider in evaluating treatments, as presented in Table 12–7. These factors utilize elements related to single-subject research design. Robey and Schulz (1998) and Robey (1998, 2004) described a five-phase outcome model for clinical outcome research that involves developing a treatment; testing its efficacy; testing its effectiveness; examining its efficacy; and determining its cost effectiveness, cost benefit, and cost utility. The model is presented in Figure 12–2.

Additional measures of treatment outcome include traditional instrumental and behavioral data, cost-benefit analysis, and quality-of-life scales. Integrated data systems linking these data produce comprehensive reports that provide better information about treatment outcomes. Further information related to treatment outcome research is available in books edited by Frattali (1998), Law (2002), and Schlosser (2003).

Table 12–7. Factors to Consider in Evaluating Treatment

— Specify the nature of the client's problem

— Deciding on the time frame for evaluation

— Selecting the behaviors to be changed

— Deciding on control and treatment behaviors and tasks

— Deciding on the format of the treatment tasks

— Deciding on the content of the treatment task items

— Deciding on the staging of treatment

— Deciding on the strategy for changing behavior

— Deciding which tasks to use to measure performance

— Deciding on the length of the baseline phase

— Deciding on the number of data measurements

— Deciding whether to use probes or continuous measurement

— Defining time intervals for reassessment and maintenance

— Stating predictions about generalization effects

— Developing treatment tasks

— Documenting decisions in treatment and obtaining the client's response

Source: From *Scientific Thinking in Speech and Language Therapy*, by C. Lum, 2002, Mahwah, NJ: Lawrence Erlbaum Associates.

Phase V
- study of efficiency, cost-effectiveness, cost-benefit; cost utility
- patient and family satisfaction; quality of life
- large samples

Phase IV
- test treatment effectiveness
- average conditions
- day to day practice
- typical conditions (patients, clinicians, intensity, and duration)
- large samples
- external control (no-treatment) not required
- a analysis of efficacy studies
- single subject studies with multiple replication; large single group designs
- examine variations in populations, intensity, and duration of treatment, level of clinician training

Phase III
- efficacy of treatment under ideal conditions (ideal patients, ideal clinicians, ideal treatment, ideal intensity and duration, ideal outcome measures)
- typically randomized control trial; (random assigned treatment or no treatment)
- large samples
- multiple sites
- parallel group designs; single subject studies

Phase II
- refine primary research hypothesis
- develop explanation for efficaciously and effectiveness
- specify treatment protocol
- determine discharge criteria
- demonstrate validity and reliability of outcome measures
- case studies, single-subject studies, small, single group studies

⇧

Phase I
- develop hypothesis to be tested in later phases
- establish safety of treatment
- demonstrate if treatment active (patients improve)
- brief, small sample size
- does not require external controls
- case studies, single subject studies
- small group pre-post studies, retrospective studies

Figure 12–2. Five-phase model for communication sciences and disorders from highest to lowest level. From "A Five-Phase Model for Clinical Outcome Research," by R. R. Robey, 2004, *Journal of Communication Disorders*, 37(5), pp. 401–411; and "A Model for Conducting Clinical Outcome Research: An Adaptation of the Standard Protocol for Use in Aphasiology," by R. R. Robey and M. C. Schultz, 1998, *Aphasiology*, 12, pp. 787–810.

Summary

Careful evaluation of tests and treatments is a fundamental responsibility for justifying clinical services. There are a variety of methods for evaluating tests and treatments, either individually or collectively. Clinical decisions are often made on the basis of opinion rather than critical review and the best available research evidence. Clinical services are enhanced by evidence-based decisions as opposed to beliefs and opinions.

? DISCUSSION QUESTIONS

1. What type(s) of research is(are) involved in evaluating tests and treatments?
2. Why should speech-language pathologists and audiologists be discerning consumers of tests and treatments?
3. Why are clinical decisions based on opinion(s) incompatible with evidence-based practice?
4. How can false-negative and false-positive results affect clinical decisions?
5. Explain the importance of specificity and sensitivity to test accuracy.
6. What is the difference between positive and negative predictive values?
7. Differentiate between traditional and evidence-based review for evaluating tests and treatments.
8. How do science and pseudoscience differ?
9. What are the criteria for pseudoscience?
10. What are the primary criteria for evaluating tests?
11. What are the evidence-based criteria for evaluating tests?
12. Differentiate between efficiency, effectiveness, and efficacy of treatment.
13. Describe the major differences between various types of treatment research.
14. What is the difference between retrospective and prospective studies?
15. What factors should be considered in evaluating treatment with a single client?
16. Describe a five-phase model for clinical outcome research.

References

American Speech-Language-Hearing Association. (2018). *Levels of evidence in communication sciences and disorders.* https://www.asha.org/research/ebp/assessing-the-evidence/

American Speech-Language-Hearing Association. (2023). *Code of ethics.* http://www.asha.org/policy

Dollaghan, C. (2004). Evidence-based practice in communication disorders: What do we know, and when do we know it? *Journal of Communication Disorders, 37*(5), 391–400.

Finn, P., Bothe, A. K., & Bramlett, R. E. (2005). Science and pseudoscience in communication disorders: Criteria and application. *American Journal of Speech Language Pathology, 14*(3), 172–186.

Frattali, C. M. (1998). *Measuring outcomes in speech-language pathology.* Thieme.

Golper, L., Wertz, R. T., Frattali, C., Yorkston, K., Myers, P., Katz, R., . . . Wambaugh, J. (2001). Evidence-based practice guidelines for the management of communication disorders in neurologically impaired individuals. *ANCDS, Practice Guidelines Project*, 1–12.

Haynes, W. O., & Pindzola, R. H. (1998). *Diagnosis and evaluation in speech pathology.* Allyn & Bacon.

Haynes, W. O., & Pindzola, R. H. (2012). *Diagnosis and evaluation in speech-language pathology.* Pearson.

Hegde, M. N. (2003). *Clinical research in communication disorders.* Pro-Ed.

Hutchinson, T. A. (1996). What to look for in the technical manual: Twenty questions for test users. *Language, Speech and Hearing Services in Schools, 27*, 109–121.

Law, M. (2002). *Evidence-based rehabilitation.* Slack.

Lum, C. (2002). *Scientific thinking in speech and language therapy.* Lawrence Erlbaum.

Mart, J. (1999). Is this test effective? In M. Dawes, P. Davies, A. Gray, J. Marx, K. Seers, & R. Snowball (Eds.), *Evidence-based practice.* Churchill Livingstone.

Maxwell, D. L., & Satake, E. (2006). *Research and statistical methods in communication sciences and disorders.* Thomson-Delmar Learning.

Melynk, B. M., & Fineout-Overholt, E. (2005). *Evidence-based practice in nursing and healthcare.* Lippincott Williams & Wilkins.

Mertens, D. M. (2005). *Research and evaluation in education and psychology.* Sage.

Pena, E. D., Spaulding, T. J., & Plante, E. (2006). The composition of normatic groups and diagnostic decision-making: Shooting ourselves in the foot. *American Journal of Speech, Language Pathologists, 15*, 247–254.

Powell, T. W. (2006). *Diagnostic worksheet* [Unpublished data].

Reilly, S. (2004). What constitutes evidence? In S. Reilly, J. Douglas, & J. Oates (Eds.), *Evidence-based practice in speech pathology* (pp. 18–34). Whurr.

Robey, R. R. (1998). A meta-analysis of clinical outcomes in the treatment of aphasia. *Journal of Speech, Language, and Hearing Research, 41*, 172–187.

Robey, R. R. (2004). A five-phase model for clinical-outcome research. *Journal of Communication Disorders, 37*(5), 401–411.

Robey, R. R., & Schultz, M. C. (1998). A model for conducting clinical-outcome research. An adaptation of the standard protocol for use in aphasiology. *Aphasiology, 12*, 782–810.

Schlosser, R. W. (2003). *The efficacy of augmentative and alternative communication.* Academic Press.

Shipley, K. G., & McAfee, J. G. (2009). *Assessment in speech-language pathology.* Singular Publishing.

Silverman, F. H. (1998). *Research design and evaluation in speech-language pathology and audiology.* Allyn & Bacon.

Stein, F., & Cutler, S. K. (1996). *Clinical research.* Singular Publishing.

Zipoli, R. P., & Kennedy, M. (2005). Evidence-based practice among speech-language pathologists: Attitudes, utilization, and barriers. *American Journal of Speech Language Pathology, 14*(3), 208–220.

13

Evidence-Based Practice: Application of Research to Clinical Practice

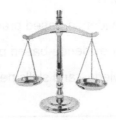

LEARNING OBJECTIVES

Upon completion of this chapter, the reader will be able to:

■ Define evidence-based practice, research utilization, and information literacy

■ Discuss myths surrounding evidence-based practice

■ Evaluate quality and credibility of communicative evidence to patients and other professionals

■ Describe the clinical issues related to evidence-based practice

■ Describe clinical traits

■ Identify barriers to evidence-based practice

■ Locate resources for evidence-based practice

■ Recognize the knowledge and skills needed for evidence-based practice

Evidence-based practice (EBP) is the application of research data to clinical decisions. Speech-language pathologists and audiologists who base their practice on the best available evidence use a systematic approach to selecting assessment and treatment procedures (Cornett, 2001). The most compelling reason for speech-language pathologists and audiologists to be evidence-based practitioners is to ensure that clients receive the best possible services (Johnson, 2006).

Speech-language pathologists and audiologists in all work settings should be aware of the advantages of evidence-based practice or research-based practice. Meline (2006) believes evaluating research for its application to clinical practice is one of the most important resources available for ensuring best clinical practice in speech-language pathology and audiology. There is growing interest in developing an evidence-based practice through research used in making clinical decisions.

Over the previous 20 years, changes in education and research have led to an awareness of the need for a better evidence base for the clinical practice of speech-language pathology and audiology. Most training programs have modified their curricula to include evidence-based practice and critical analysis of the research literature. There has also been an increased focus on research related to clinical practice. Both students and practicing professionals need hands-on, interactive, practical experience in translating research into clinical practice (Gallagher, 2001).

There are other factors that may account for the increasing use of evidence-based practice. Among these factors are the development of strategies for efficiently finding evidence, systematic clinical practice guidelines, electronic databases, and continuing education (Sackett et al., 2001). In spite of these developments, there have not been major changes in research utilization among clinicians; underutilization of research continues to be a problem. Research evidence is not routinely used in making clinical decisions about assessment and treatment. Unfortunately, many clinicians continue to make clinical decisions in the absence of evidence and on the basis of opinion, testimony, and/or advertisements. Opinions, singly or in groups, even from respected authorities, should be viewed with skepticism (Dollaghan, 2004). In this chapter, various aspects of evidence-based practice are discussed.

Defining Evidence-Based Practice

Evidence-based practice utilizes the best available research to make clinical decisions about patient care. It is based on critical appraisal of research findings and applying what is known to clinical practice (Frattali & Worrall, 2001). Research utilization is the application of some aspect of research to clinical practice. Polit and Beck (2010) described research utilization as a continuum ranging from direct application of research findings to clinical practice (instrumental utilization) to situations in which research findings are ignored or not used. Research utilization is a matter of degree; clinicians even with limited effort can accomplish some degree of evidence-based practice (Schlosser, 2004). In essence, evidence-based practice is the utilization of research findings to make decisions about patient care.

The major steps for using evidence-based practice are as follows:

- Selecting a topic or problem (Schlosser & O'Neil-Pirozzi, 2006)
- Assembling and evaluating evidence (Law & Plunkett, 2000; Meline, 2006)
- Assessing for potential implementation (Nye & Harvey, 2006)
- Developing or identifying evidence-based practice guidelines or protocols (Law & Plunkett, 2000)
- Implementing the treatment
- Evaluating outcomes (Bernstein-Ratner, 2006; Herder et al., 2006)
- Deciding to adopt or modify the treatment or revert to prior practice (Konnerup & Schwartz, 2006)

Evidence-Based Practice: Terms and Definitions

Evidence-based practice is utilization of the best available research to make clinical decisions about patient care. It is based on critical appraisal of research findings and applying what is known to clinical practice (Frattali & Worrall, 2001). Other terms related to evidence-based practice are as follows:

- Clinical expertise: proficiency of clinical skills and abilities, informed by continually expanding knowledge that individual clinicians develop through experience learning and reflection about their professional practice.
- Cost-effectiveness, Cost benefit, Cost utility: terms that compare cost of service to outcome.
- Effectiveness: extent to which an intervention or service produces

a desired outcome under usual conditions.

- Efficacy: extent to which an intervention or service produces a desired outcome under ideal conditions.
- Efficiency: extent to which an intervention produces an outcome with a minimum of waste, expense, or unnecessary effort.
- Evidence: any empirical observation about apparent relations between events constitutes potential evidence.
- Evidence-based designs: emphasizes the importance of using credible evidence.
- Evidence-based management: evaluation of best evidence for making decisions.
- Fidelity: truthfulness; degree to which administration of a test or treatment corresponds to the prototype.
- Intent to treat: analysis based on initial treatment intent.
- Outcome: result.
- Randomized controlled trial (RCT): experimental study in which patients meeting specific criteria are randomly assigned to treatment and nontreatment groups. (Golper et al., 2001; Jewell, 2011; Kaderavek & Justice, 2010).

Research Utilization

Research utilization is the application of research to clinical practice. Polit and Beck (2010) described research utilization as a continuum ranging from direct application of research to clinical practice (instrumental utilization) to situations in which research is ignored or not used. Therefore, research utilization is a matter of degree; clinicians even with minimal effort can use research to some degree to make clinical decisions that are based on evidence. Audiologists and speech-language pathologists' use of research to make clinical decisions is limited (Kloda & Bartlett, 2009). Zipoli and Kennedy (2005) reported that speech-language pathologists most often consult colleagues and do not use scholarly journals for clinical information. Although, the use of EBP appears to be on the rise among speech and language pathologists (Greenwell & Walsh, 2021).

Information Literacy

Information literacy is the ability to recognize when information is needed and the ability to locate, critically review, and effectively use information (Cobus, 2008). Many audiologists and speech-language pathologists have inadequate information-seeking abilities (McCurtin & Roddam, 2012; Moodle et al., 2011; Nail-Chiwetalu & Ratner, 2006). There is a need for information literacy instruction in the university curriculum, and this instruction should continue for practicing audiologists and speech-language pathologists in the form of continuing education (Nail-Chiwetalu & Ratner, 2007). It was suggested that librarians work with audiology and speech-pathology training programs to integrate a high level of information into the curriculum and that librarians provide continuing education activities focusing on information literacy for practicing professionals.

Information literacy is essential for evidence-based practice (Nail-Chiwetalu & Ratner, 2006). Five standards for information literacy have been identified (Nail-Chiwetalu & Rattner, 2006):

1. Determine the nature and extent of information needed

2. Access needed information effectively and efficiently
3. Evaluate information and sources critically, and incorporate selected information into a knowledge-based and values system
4. Individually, or as a member of a group, use information effectively to accomplish a specific purpose
5. Understand the economic, legal, and social issues about the use of information, and access and use of information ethically and legally

Clinical Trials

Clinical trials are typically associated with evidence-based practice. Sometimes referred to as clinical research trials or outcome measures, clinical trials are research designed to study the safety, efficacy, effectiveness, efficiency, and cost-benefit of an assessment or treatment (DePoy & Gitlin, 2011; Polit & Beck, 2010).

Clinical trials are classified according to purpose (Portney & Watkins, 2009). The six purposes are (a) prevention, (b) screening, (c) diagnostic, (d) treatment, (e) quality of life, and (f) compassionate use.

There are six hierarchical phases of clinical trials ranging from the pre-clinical phase to the lowest or highest phase that involves cost-effectiveness and cost-benefit. These phases are listed and described in Table 13–1. Each phase provides information about assessment or treatment.

A major limitation of phase III is related to RCTs. According to Polit and Beck (2009), RCTs are not relevant to real-life situations. Moreover, there is the ethical dilemma of having a treatment

Table 13–1. Phases of Clinical Trials

Phase	Description
Pre-clinical	Exploratory to determine safety under laboratory conditions.
I	Develop questions to be considered in later phases.
II	Refine primary hypothesis and develop plan for evaluating efficacy and effectiveness of assessment or treatment.
III	Efficacy under ideal conditions: typically a randomized controlled trial.
IV	Efficacy under average conditions
V	Study of efficiency, cost effectiveness, cost benefit, or cost utility.

Source: From "Evidence-Based Practice Guidelines for the Management of Communication Disorders in Neurologically Impaired Individuals," by L. A. Golper et al., 2001, *ANCDS Practice Guidelines.*

and nontreatment group and blinding or masking, which are typically needed for a control group—that is, withholding treatment. Therefore, the focus is on practical information that can be used in routine clinical practice. Another problem related to the professions is that most studies in audiology and speech-language pathology do not adequately address assessment and treatment relative to setting or condition. Other problems are related to extremely limited information from phase IV treatment in audiology and speech-language pathology.

Advantages and Disadvantages of Evidence-Based Practice

Evidence-based practice has the potential to improve assessment and treatment of children and adults with communication disorders, increase resources for clinical services, and enhance the perception of the professionals of speech-language pathology and audiology (Mullen, 2007).

Disadvantages include limited or no evidence about some clinical practices, evidence unrelated to routine clinical practice, conflicting evidence, increased cost bias, conflict of interest, erroneous concepts, and overemphasis on randomized controlled trials (Mullen, 2007). There is also the possibility the evidence is wrong (Dodd, 2007). There are other issues as well: one is the limited discussion of settings and conditions in many research reports and the other is the limited information about the rule of instituting in evidence-based practice (Dodd, 2007).

Myths About Evidence-Based Practice

Several myths surrounding evidence-based practice exist and should be considered. Table 13–2 lists those myths

Table 13–2. Evidence-Based Practice: Myths and Facts

Myth:	Evidence-based practice already exists.
Fact:	Many clinicians use opinions not evidence to make clinical decisions.
Myth:	Evidence-based practice is impossible to initiate.
Fact:	It is impossible to initiate with minimal time.
Myth:	Clinical experience is not relevant to evidence-based practice.
Fact:	Clinical experience is relevant to evidence-based practice.
Myth:	Cost is not an important consideration.
Fact:	Cost-benefit is an important consideration.
Myth:	Expert opinion is the highest level of evidence.
Fact:	Expert opinion is not considered credible evidence.
Myth:	All research is related to clinical decisions.
Fact:	Basic research is not related to clinical decisions, but applied research is related to clinical decisions.
Myth:	Evidence based on opinion is best.
Fact:	Evidence based on empirical research is best.
Myth:	Textbooks contain high levels of evidence.
Fact:	Textbooks contain low levels of evidence copying.
Myth:	Clinical practice guidelines are not detailed
Fact:	Some clinical practice guidelines are detailed.

Source: From "Introduction to Evidence-Based Practice," by M. Law, 2002. In M. Law (Ed.), *Evidence-Based Rehabilitation* (pp. 2–12), Thorofare, NJ: Slack; "Evidence-Based Medicine: What It Is and What It Isn't," by D. L. Sackett, E. M Rosenberg, J. Gray, R. B. Haynes, and W. S. Richardson, 1996, *British Medical Journal, 312*(7023), pp. 71–72; and "Evidence-Based Practice: Myths and Misconceptions," by C. Dollagham, 2004, *ASHA Leader.*

that contribute to misunderstanding evidence-based practice and may make it difficult, if not impossible, to implement evidence-based practice. Eliminating or reducing these misconceptions increases the likelihood of using evidence-based practice to support clinical decision-making.

Barriers to Evidence-Based Practice

A major disadvantage of evidence-based practice is related to barriers that prohibit or impede its implementation. Barriers should be considered so that strategies can be developed to reduce or eliminate these barriers, thereby facilitating research use and evidence-based practice. A major barrier to evidence-based practice is failure to integrate research and clinical activities. There have also been delays between the completion of a research study and the time the results were reported, which might make the results no longer applicable to clinical practice.

The evidence base itself is frequently cited as a barrier (Mullen, 2005a, 2005b). Barriers to evidence-based practice were also identified by Worrell and Bennett (2001). These barriers were:

- limited access and ability to use databases;
- all related literature not listed;
- frequently a lack of evidence about the topic;
- level of evidence not high;
- evidence not matching the reality of clinical services; and
- no database of published clinically appraised topics (CATs).

Nonexistent, conflicting, or irrelevant evidence is considered to be a formidable problem. Overreliance on RCTs is also a source of controversy (Elman, 2006). Sackett et al. (1996) believe that evidence-based practice is not restricted to RCTs and meta-analysis, and it should involve finding the best available evidence to answer clinical questions.

Other barriers to EBP are related to bias about funding, publication, consumer-research mismatch, and reduced clinical applicability (Elman, 2006). There are limited research funds and a trend to allocate funds on the basis of evidence. There is a tendency for positive

trials to be published more than once and the possibility of subjective publication decisions. Also, there may be a mismatch between the treatments that are researched and those that are desired or prioritized by consumers. Reduced clinical applicability results from a trade-off between subject selection criteria and clinical applicability. Clients with severe problems or comorbidities may be underrepresented in clinical trials that have a homogeneous subject selection. The type of evidence also warrants consideration. The RCT is considered the gold standard or highest level of evidence, although the information needed to understand human problems is not necessarily amenable to RCT (DePoy & Gitlin, 2011). A related limitation is that RCTs are not the only valid design. RCTs may not be appropriate for evaluating treatment provided to heterogeneous populations that have a wide range of differences, such as, aphasia, dysphagia, and developmental language disorders. For many types of speech and language disorders, RCTs cannot be conducted (Dodd, 2007).

Additional barriers to EBP include research utilization and information literacy, negative attitudes about research, resistance to change, and limited collaboration and communication between researchers and clinicians. Some speech-language pathologists and audiologists do not read research journals or do not critically review published research findings (information and examples of this process are provided in Chapter 14). Lack of knowledge about how to access and critically review research evidence has also been identified as a barrier to using research evidence in clinical practice. Research is sometimes reported in a way that makes findings inaccessible for clinicians. Complex statistical information and dense research jargon may pose barriers to acquiring knowledge about evidence-based practice (Polit & Beck, 2010). Some speech-language pathologists and audiologists do not attend professional conferences where research is reported. Another consideration is that researchers sometimes ignore the research needs of clinicians.

Other barriers are related to time and change. Sometimes, clinicians are overwhelmed or overstretched because they believe they do not have enough professional time for evidence-based practice (Frattali & Worrall, 2001; Meline & Paradiso, 2003; Mullen, 2005a, 2005b; Zipoli & Kennedy, 2005). Sometimes, clinicians are resistant to change because it requires retraining and reorganization. Some clinicians may lack administrative support to implement evidence-based practice (Rose & Baldac, 2004). Both time and cost are reported as barriers to EBP by some speech-language pathologists (Mullen, 2005). Critical appraisal of research is fundamental to evidence-based practice, yet it may be difficult for some speech-language pathologists and audiologists (hopefully not after reading Chapter 14!).

Other barriers to evidence-based practice are related to the shortage of PhD-level researchers in speech-language pathology and audiology (American Speech-Language-Hearing Association [ASHA], 2002; Justice & Fey, 2004). There are problems associated with the PhD shortage: (a) almost half of new PhD graduates choose nonacademic positions, which are probably nonresearch positions; and (b) an aging faculty is facing imminent retirement (Meline & Paradiso, 2003).

Last, there are barriers related to organizations and the professions. Professional organizations may be reluctant to expend resources for teaching and/or using evidence-based practice. The professionals may also have barriers related to a shortage of role models for evidence-based practice or may carry historical baggage that causes them to perceive themselves as not being capable of doing research or recommending changes based on research results (Polit & Beck, 2010).

Quality of Evidence: Levels and Grades of Evidence

Assessment of the quality of evidence is essential to evidence-based practice. Levels of evidence refer to a hierarchy for evaluating the quality and credibility of evidence. There are several methods for determining levels of evidence.

ASHA modified the levels of evidence from the Scottish Intercollegiate Guidance Network (Table 13–3). The levels of evidence hierarchical model is based on research design and ranges from highest/most credible or strongest to lowest/least credible or weakest. Randomizing and controlling are considered within research design. Tickle-Degnen and Bedell (2003) criticized this model because "it is wrong when applied in a manner that excludes the use of all relevant valid, and available research evidence for clinical decision making" (p. 234). Other limitations noted were lack of information about patients and causality.

ASHA's Advisory Committee on Evidence-Based Practice and the National

Table 13–3. ASHA's (2005a) Levels of Evidence

Level	Creditability Description
Ia	Well-designed meta-analysis of >1 randomized controlled trial
Ib	Well-designed randomized controlled study
IIa	Well-designed controlled study without randomization
IIb	Well-designed *quasi-experimental* study survey
III	Well-designed nonexperimental studies, i.e., correlational and case studies
IV	Expert committee report, consensus conference, clinical experience of respected authorities

Source: From *Evidence-based practice in communication disorders: An introduction* by ASHA, 2004. Available at http://www.asha.org

Center for Evidence-Based Practice developed a system for levels of evidence (Mullen, 2007). This system is shown in Table 13–4. The system involves four processes: (a) appraising the quality of studies, (b) identifying the research stage of each study, (c) assessing the quality relative to the stage of the research, and (d) synthesizing the information into a single table. Eight factors were identified for evaluation.

The type of clinical study, diagnostic or treatment oriented, can be used to determine the level of evidence. ASHA (2005) described hierarchies of evidence for diagnosis and treatment. In addition to these levels of evidence, studies are graded with recommendations about use for making clinical decisions (Figure 13–1). The grades range from A (highly recommended) to E (not recommended).

Regardless of the criteria used for evaluation of the quality of evidence, five common themes were identified by ASHA (2005a). These themes are (a) independent confirmation and converging evidence, (b) experimental control, (c) avoidance of subjectivity and bias, (d) effect sizes and confidence intervals, and (e) relevance and feasibility.

Knowledge and Skills Needed for Evidence-Based Practice

Audiologists and speech-language pathologists should understand that evidence-based practice utilizes the best available evidence in research and clinical practice. Research utilization and information literacy are basic perquisites to evidence-based practice. ASHA's (2005b) position statement about evidence-based practice outlines the skills needed for evidence-based practice. Audiologists and speech-language pathologists should

■ recognize the needs, abilities, values, preferences, and interests of

Table 13–4. ASHA's (2007) Levels of Evidence

Study Design
- Controlled Trial
- Cohort Study
- Single-Subject Design or Case Control Study
- Cross-Sectional Study or Case Series
- Case Study

Blinding
- Assessors blinded
- Assessors not blinded or not stated

Sampling
- Random sample adequately described
- Random sample inadequately described
- Convenience sample/hand-picked sample or not stated

Subjects
- Groups comparable at baseline on important factors (between subject design) or subject(s) adequately described (within subject design)
- Groups/subjects not comparable at baseline or comparability not reported or subject(s) not adequately described

Outcomes
- At least one primary outcome measure is valid and reliable
- Validity unknown, but appears reasonable; reliable
- Invalid and/or unreliable

Significance
- p value reported or calculable
- p value neither reported nor calculable

Precision
- Effect size and confidence interval reported or calculable
- Effect size or confidence interval, but not both reported or calculable
- Neither effect size nor confidence interval reported or calculable

Intention to Treat (controlled trials only)
- Analyzed by intention to treat
- Not analyzed by intention to treat or not stated

Source: From "The State of the Evidence," by R. Mullen, 2007, *ASHA Leader.*

A

Good evidence for inclusion
Peer-review evidence
Supporting use for treatment

B

Fair evidence for inclusion
Peer-review evidence supports
Consideration of use for treatment

C

Insufficient evidence
Lack of peer-review evidence: however
recommendation(s) for use possible
on other grounds

D

Fair evidence for exclusion
Peer-review evidence supports treatment
should be excluded

E

Good evidence for exclusion
Peer-review supports treatment
should be excluded

Figure 13–1. Outcomes from systematic review. Reprinted with permission from "Evidence-Based Practice in Schools: Integrating Craft and Theory With Science and Data," by L. M. Justice and M. E. Fey, 2004, *ASHA Leader, 9*(4–5), pp. 30–32. Copyright by American Speech-Language-Hearing Association. All rights reserved.

patients and families and combine this information with best current research evidence and clinical expertise;

■ acquire and maintain knowledge and skills necessary to provide high-quality professional service, including knowledge about evidence-based practice;

■ evaluate clinical services and procedures for cost-effectiveness using recognized appraisal criteria described in the evidence-based literature;

■ evaluate efficacy, effectiveness, and efficiency of clinical and research protocols using criteria described in the evidence-based literature;

■ evaluate the quality of evidence in journal reports, textbooks, continuing education newsletters, advertisements, and web-based products; and

■ monitor and apply new and high-quality evidence.

Haynes and Johnson (2009) provided a detailed discussion for each of these skills. The discussion was related to skills for both students and practicing professionals. In addition, audiologists and speech-language pathologists should

■ use scientific criteria for making decisions about research and clinical practice (Finn et al., 2005);

■ effectively communicate about evidence to patients, families, and other professions;

■ determine level of evidence for clinical and research studies (Mullen, 2007);

■ educate students and other professionals about the use and application of evidence-based practice;

- evaluate effectiveness and outcomes of education and training about evidence-based practice;
- develop and implement strategies to reduce barriers to evidence-based practice;
- dispel the myths and misconceptions about evidence-based practice;
- create an evidence-based environment; and
- document fidelity.

Developing and Implementing Evidence-Based Practice

To utilize EBP, speech-language pathologists and audiologists must (a) discount the opinions of authorities when there is counterevidence; (b) focus on research relevant to clinical practice; and (c) use rigorous criteria to evaluate the quality of evidence, including validity, importance, and precision (Dollaghan, 2004).

Education and training are the foundation for developing and implementing evidence-based practice. The December 2009 issue of *Evidence-Based Communication Assessment and Intervention* focused on teaching evidence-based practice to speech-language pathologists. Table 13–5 is a list of the authors and titles of these reports.

The decision-making process can be used to implement and develop evidence-based practice. Boswell (2005) and Kully and Langeven (2005) described similar procedures for evidence-based decision-making. The steps were (a) asking a clear, focused question; (b) finding the best evidence; (c) critically appraising the evidence; (d) integrating the evidence with clinical judgment and clinical values; and (e) evaluating the decision-making process. According to Schlosser et al. (2007), the first step in EBP is asking well-built questions. However, this is often difficult for clinicians. To facilitate well-built questions, the PESICO template was proposed. PESICO stands

Table 13–5. Teaching Evidence-Based Practice from December 2009 *Evidence-Based Communication Assessment and Intervention*

Author	Title
Klee and Stringer	Teaching evidence-based practice to speech and language therapy students in the United Kingdom
McCabe, Purcell, Baker, Madill, and Trembath	Case-based learning: One route to evidence-based practice
Proxy and Murza	Building speech-language pathologists capacity for evidence-based practice: A unique graduate course approach
Raghavendra	Teaching evidence-based practice in a problem-based course in speech-language pathology
Schlosser and Sigafoos	Teaching evidence-based practice: An impetus for further curricular innovation and research

for person (problem), environments, stakeholders, intervention, comparison, and outcome. Johnson (2006) provided specific examples for making evidence-based decisions about childhood speech-language disorders.

Threats (2002) suggested the World Health Organization's International Classification of Disorders for developing evidence-based practice that could bridge the gap between research and clinical practice by providing a common framework and language. The purposes were to (a) collect statistical data about functioning and disability, such as in population studies; (b) conduct clinical research, such as measurement of outcomes, quality of life, or impact of environmental factors on disability; (c) use for clinical needs assessment, matching treatments with specific conditions, program outcome evaluation, and rehabilitation documentation; and (d) use for social policy, such as social security planning, governmental oversight of disability programs, and policy decision-making.

There are several strategies for implementing and developing evidence-based practice. Some of these strategies include the following:

- Create a culture for evidence-based practice
- Provide evidence-based practice training and experience for both students and practicing professions
- Develop critical thinking skills (Finn, 2011)
- Integrate evidence-based practice into speech-language pathology and audiology curriculum (Forrest & Miller, 2001)
- Eliminate dichotomy between research and clinical practice

- Develop awareness of misconceptions about evidence-based practice
- Provide high levels of research evidence
- Encourage collaboration of researchers and clinicians
- Use systematic reviews to introduce evidence-based practice (McCauley & Hargrove, 2004; Mullen, 2005b)
- Communicate research results widely and clearly
- Specify clinical implications of research
- Expect evidence that a diagnosis or treatment procedure is effective
- Practice in a journal group
- Form collaborative work groups (Johnson, 2006)
- Use ASHA's registry of evidence-based practice guidelines and systematic reviews (Evidence-Based Practice Tool Available, 2006)
- Indicate level of evidence in professional presentations and publications and continue education
- Seek professional environment that supports evidence-based practice
- Identify and eliminate sources of bias about EBP (Elman, 2006)
- Volunteer to participate in clinical research trials (Logemann & Gardner, 2005)
- Audit the degree and extent of research utilization
- Form on-site or online journal clubs (Betz et al., 2005)
- Provide multidisciplinary evidence-based practice courses
- Use formats for case presentations and critical reviews such as those suggested by C. Dollaghan (2004), C. A. Dollaghan (2004), Frattali and Worrall (2001), Threats (2002), and Worrall and Bennett (2001)

Evidence-based practice is a process by which the current best evidence is critically appraised, clinical expertise is considered, and a course of action is selected. Several decisions may be made. For example, what is the best and most current research evidence? How can the evidence be integrated with clinical expertise and client preferences?

Because of the relative newness of evidence-based practice in speech-language pathology and audiology, little evidence exists to guide identification of the best strategies for implementing evidence-based practice. Some strategies are successful in some settings and with some professional groups but not with other settings or groups (Cilisla et al., 2005).

Organizational Support for Evidence-Based Practice

Professional organizations have supported evidence-based practice. Among these organizations are the Academy of Neurological Communication Disorders and Sciences, American Academy of Audiology, American Speech-Language-Hearing Association, Australian Speech and Hearing Association, and the Canadian Speech and Hearing Association.

ASHA has devoted considerable effort to increase research utilization through evidence-based practice. The major activities include a website for evidence-based practice (ASHA, 2005a); a position statement (ASHA, 2005a); levels of evidence (ASHA, 2005b); a technical report (ASHA, 2005b); and evidence maps for amyotrophic lateral sclerosis, aphasia, autism, cerebral palsy, cleft lip and palate, dementia, head and neck cancer, Parkinson's disease, traumatic brain injury-adult, and traumatic brain injury-children (National Center for Evidence-Based Practice in Communication Disorders, 2012). In addition, ASHA has established the National Center for Evidence-Based Practice in Communication Disorders. The center has a registry of clinical practice guidelines and systematic reviews (Mullen, 2007). Only guidelines and reviews with an overall rating of highly recommended or recommended with provisions are included in the registry. ASHA also has several practice guidelines, which provide information to assist clinicians in making decisions based on available research evidence and prevailing expert opinion. The purpose of such guidelines is to improve the quality of service, identify the most cost-effective treatment, prevent unfounded practices, and stimulate research (Golper et al., 2001).

ASHA also established the Communication Sciences and Disorders Clinical Trials Research Group (CSDRG), which is devoted solely to the development and conduct of clinical trials by audiologists; speech-language pathologists; and speech, language, and hearing scientists (Baum et al., 1998; Logemann, 2004; Logemann & Gardner, 2005). CSDRG's clinical trials involve dysarthria, dysphagia, and language stimulation.

ASHA's Research and Scientific Affairs Committee had a series of reports about research concepts and their application to speech-language pathology and audiology (Feeney, 2006). Topics include "Back to the Basics: Reading Research Literature" (Golper et al., 2006), "Developing a Research Question" (Nelson & Goffman, 2006), "Bias and Blinding" (Finn, 2006), and "Interpretation of Correlation" (Oller, 2006).

In addition, two ASHA journals have had issues focusing on EBP. *Communication Issues in Communication Services and Disorders* (CICSD) described the specific task(s) needed to conduct a systematic review and meta-analysis that would facilitate EBP. *Language, Speech, and Hearing Services in Schools* (LSHSS), the other journal, discussed making evidence-based decisions for speech sound disorders, reading problems, and child language intervention.

The American Academy of Audiology emphasized EBP in a special 2005 issue of the Academy's journal, the *Journal of the American Academy of Audiology*. These papers focused on the effectiveness of hearing rehabilitation.

The Academy of Neurologic Communication Disorders and Sciences (ANCDS) applied the principles of evidence-based practice to the development of practice guidelines with support of ASHA's Special Interest Division, Neurophysiologic and Neurogenic Speech and Language Disorders (Golper et al., 2001). "The purpose of such guidelines is to improve and assure the quality of care by reducing unacceptable variation in its provisions" (Golper et al., 2001, p. 2). The practice guidelines were completed when research evidence was available in the literature.

There are three types of clinical practice guidelines based on evidence: traditional or narrative (TPG), systematic reviews (SR), and evidence-based practice (Hargrove & Gruffer, 2008). Differences between these clinical practice guidelines were described in Chapter 5.

There is hierarchy of clinical practice guidelines with tradition-narrative reviews ranking the lowest (meeting the fewest criteria) and evidence-based reviews ranking the highest (meeting the most criteria). Specifically, traditional reviews met only two of seven criteria, systematic reviews met five of seven criteria, and evidence-based reviews met all seven criteria. This information is useful in making decisions about using and recommending clinical practice guidelines.

The National Evidence-Based Center of ASHA uses the Appraisal of Guidelines for Research and Evaluation (AGREE) for evaluating and recommending systematic reviews. These reviews are highly recommended, recommended with reservations, or not recommended. The Academy of Neurologic Communication Disorders and Sciences (ANCDS) has developed evidence-based practice guidelines (EBPG). These EBPGs focus on five areas: aphasia, acquired apraxia, cognitive dysarthria, and communication disorders related to traumatic brain injury and dementia.

Obviously, there is a variation in reporting clinical practice guidelines. Shiffman et al. (2003) developed and standardized a format for reporting clinical practice guidelines which is based on 15 factors and is followed by systematic reviews by writing committees within ANCDS (Golper et al., 2001; Yorkston et al., 2001). These guidelines reflected a moderate degree of clinical certainty and are usually based on Class II evidence or strong consensus from Class III evidence (Golper et al., 2001).

The Canadian Association of Speech-Language Pathologists and Audiologists (CASLPA) has promoted evidence-based practice in classrooms, clinics, and research (Orange, 2004). In 1996, CASLPA affiliated with the Canadian Cochrane Network and Center. Evidence-based practice has been incorporated into the academic coursework, clinical practice, and thesis research at the University of Western Ontario.

The Australian Speech Pathology Association published a series of reports about clinical practice (Baker, 2005). The first in this series of articles was "What Is the Evidence for Oral Motor Therapy" by Bowen (2005). Reports about evidence-based practice have continued to be published in the association's journal.

Resources for Evidence-Based Practice

Finding evidence is a fundamental aspect of evidence-based practice. Electronic searches can be an efficient way to locate evidence (Dollaghan, 2007). There are several electronic databases related to evidence-based practice: PubMed, Cumulative Index of Nursing and Allied Health (CINAHL), and the Cochrane Collection. The American Speech-Language-Hearing Association developed evidence-based maps related to clinical expertise/expert opinion, external scientific evidence, and client/patient/caregiver perspectives. There are evidenced-based maps for amyotrophic lateral sclerosis, autism spectrum disorder, Parkinson's disease, and traumatic brain injury in children and adults.

Several books are available that focus on evidence-based practice in communication disorders:

- *Evidence-Based Practice in Speech Pathology* (Reilly et al., 2004)
- *The Efficacy of Augmentative and Alternative Communication: Toward Evidence-Based Practice* (Schlosser, 2000)

- *The Handbook for Evidence-Based Practice in Communication Disorders* (Dollaghan, 2007)
- *Understanding Research and Evidence-Based Practice in Communication Disorders* (Haynes & Johnson, 2009)
- *Evidence-Based Practice in Audiology: Evaluating Interventions for Children and Adults With Hearing Impairment* (Wong & Hickson, 2012)
- *Evaluating Research in Communication Disorders* (Orlikoff et al., 2021)

In addition, there are two journals exclusive to evidence-based practice:

- *Evidence-Based Communication: Assessment and Intervention* is a peer-reviewed journal published by Psychology Press. This journal brings together professionals from several different disciplines to facilitate evidence-based services for children and adults with communication disorders. These professionals include speech-language pathologists, special educators, regular educators, applied behavior analysts, clinical psychologists, physical therapists, and occupational therapists.
- *Evidence-Based Practice Briefs (EBP Briefs)* is an open-access online journal meant for clinicians who need to search for best evidence in a timely manner. It began publication in 2006 by Pearson Publications.

Evidence-based practice guidelines integrate evidence about a single topic (Polit & Beck, 2010). The evidence is summarized and evaluated from previous studies for use in clinical practice. Systematic reviews, meta-analyses, and clinical practice guidelines are useful resources for evidence-based practice.

Communicating Evidence

Communication is important for implementing and developing evidence-based practice. Communicating evidence to clients and others improves understanding, involvement in decisions, and outcomes (Epstein et al., 2004). Speech-language pathologists and audiologists should discuss possible options, including relevant research evidence, risks, and benefits. The goal is to provide sufficient information to the client and/or family so that an informed decision can be made (Johnson, 2006).

Tickle-Degnen (2002) described four steps for effectively communicating information: (a) identify the relative role or the decision-maker relative to the clinician, (b) identify the decision that the decision-maker will make with the clinician, (c) locate and interpret which evidence is related to the information need of the decision-maker and the clinician, and (d) translate the evidence in a comprehensive communication that facilitates informed delegating with the decision-maker so that decisions can be made and action taken.

Methods for communicating evidence include visual supplements, tables and groups, decision aids, graphic representation, and quantitative translation of clinical evidence. Systematic reviews and clinical practice guidelines can be used to communicate evidence for clinical decision-making among professionals, third-party payees, and policy makers.

Another approach for communicating evidence among professionals is the peer-reviewed journal *Evidence-Based Communication Assessment and Intervention* (EBCAI; Taylor & Francis Group, 2006). The primary aims of EBCAI are (a) promoting EBP in communication assessment and treatment, (b) appraising the latest evidence in communication evaluation and treatment, (c) providing a forum for discussions that advance EBP, and (d) disseminating EBP research.

Ethical Considerations

There are several ethical principles and practices to evidence-based practice: beneficence, nonmaleficence, justice, autonomy, control groups, risks-benefits, and fidelity (Chabon et al., 2011). Beneficence is doing good or kindness, seeking to maximize benefits for study participants and prevent harm (Polit & Beck, 2010). Nonmaleficence means do no harm, in other words, avoiding harm to subjects or patients (Aiken, 2002). Justice is fairness to equitable distribution of risks and benefits (Portney & Watkins, 2009). Autonomy is independence or freedom to make decisions.

Control Groups

The use of control groups in RCTs has been criticized because withholding treatment is wrong; therefore, many studies have only experimental groups and not control groups. These studies are considered to be weaker than those utilizing control groups. RCTs, however, are considered to be the gold standard for evidence (Brown & Golper, 2012).

Double Blinding

Double blinding (when the researcher and subject are both unaware of group assignment—treatment or no treatment) is possible in audiology and speech-language pathology research but is rarely used because of ethical issues related to withholding treatment from a control group (Dodd, 2007).

Risks and Benefits

Risks and benefits are an ethical principle with an element of informed consent in which risks and benefits are compared and related to outcomes. Studies are compared to the benefits of the study outcome (Portney & Watkins, 2009). Essentially, the question is, do the benefits outweigh the risks? The research board at each institution will approve studies, in part, based on the details of risks and benefits provided by the researcher.

Fidelity

Fidelity is the extent to which a clinical procedure is administered according to the author's instructions. It is an important but neglected concept that can affect clinical research findings. Fidelity can be enhanced by using a detailed unified

protocol so that the procedure can be delivered consistently, is producible, and is independent of style; providing training and monitoring through observation or review of audio or video recordings; and providing training compliance (DePoy & Gitlin, 2011).

Summary

There has been progress in implementing evidence-based practice in speech-language pathology and audiology, although this process has been slow. It does not seem that clinicians have increased their recognition of the need for evidence-based practice or research utilization.

Several organizations have undertaken efforts to facilitate implementation and development of evidence-based practice. Among these organizations are ASHA, ANCDS, and CASLPA.

There are barriers to evidence-based practice. The primary barriers are related to the evidence base itself, time, and resistance to change. There are a number of strategies to implement evidence-based practice that may improve the extent to which research is used for making clinical decisions. Information about evidence in audiology and speech-language pathology must be communicated to decision-makers—that is, patients, third-party payees, and other professionals. Several ethical issues are especially related to evidence-based practice: use of control groups, risks-benefits, and blinding.

DISCUSSION QUESTIONS

1. What are evidence-based practice, research utilization, and information literacy?
2. What factors may account for the increased interest in evidence-based practice?
3. How do speech-language pathologists and audiologists make decisions about assessment and treatment?
4. Why is the research underutilized? Why is the poorest evidence overutilized?
5. How can research utilization be improved?
6. What is meant by the statement that "research utilization is on a continuum"?
7. How do speech-language pathologists and audiologists make clinical decisions?
8. Why should levels of evidence be considered in making clinical decisions?
9. What are the myths about evidence-based practice? How do these myths affect clinical decisions?
10. What activities has ASHA undertaken to facilitate imple-

mentation of evidence-based practice?
11. What is CSDRG?
12. Define clinical trials. What are the phases?
13. What is blinding or masking?
14. What are the indications and contradictions for blinding?
15. What are the steps in making evidence-based decisions?
16. What are the barriers to evidence-based practice? How can these barriers be reduced or eliminated?
17. What can be done to develop and implement evidence-based practice?
18. How can evidence be communicated to patients? Other professionals?
19. How have professional organizations supported evidence-based practice?
20. What resources are available for evidence-based practice?
21. What are the major ethical issues related to evidence-based practice?

References

Aiken, T. D. (2002). *Legal and ethical issues in health occupations*. W. B. Saunders.

American Speech-Language-Hearing Association. (2002). *PUD program survey results*. http://www.asha.org/members/pud

facilityresearch/reports/pud_survey_sum.htm

American Speech-Language-Hearing Association. (2005a). *Evidence-based practice in communication disorders: An introduction*. http://www.asha.org/about

American Speech-Language-Hearing Association. (2005b). *Evidence-based practice in communication disorders: Position statement.*

Baker, E. (2005). What's the evidence from? *Acquiring Knowledge in Speech, Language, and Hearing, 8*(3), 144–147.

Baum, H. M., Logemann, J., & Lilenfeld, D. (1998). Clinical trials and their application to communication sciences and disorders. *Journal of Medical Speech-Language Pathology, 6,* 55–64.

Bernstein-Ratner, N. (2006). Evidence-based practice: An examination of its ramifications for the practice of speech-language pathology. *Language, Speech, and Hearing Services in Schools, 37*(4), 257–267.

Betz, C. L., Smith, A., Melnyk, B. M., & Rickey, T. (2005). Disseminating evidence. In B. M. Melynk & E. Fingout-Overholt (Eds.), *Evidence-based practice in nursing and healthcare* (pp. 351–403). Lippincott Williams & Wilkins.

Boswell, S. (2005, September 27). Finding the evidence for school-based clinical decision making. *ASHA Leader,* 26–27, 39.

Bowen, C. (2005). What is the evidence for oral motor therapy? *Acquiring Knowledge in Speech, Language, and Hearing, 7*(3), 144–147.

Brown, K. E., & Golper, L. A. (2012). Applying evidence to clinical practice. In R. Lubinski & M. W. Hudson (Eds.), *Professional issues in speech-language pathology and audiology* (pp. 582–601). Delmar.

Chabon, S., Morris, J., & Lemoncello, S. (2011). Ethical deliberations: A foundation for evidence-based practice. *Seminar in Speech Language, 31,* 298–308.

Cilisla, D., DeCenso, A., Melynk, B. M., & Stelter, C. (2005). Using models and strategies for evidence-based practice. In B. M. Melynk & E. Fingout-Overholt (Eds.), *Evidence-based practice in nursing and healthcare* (pp. 185–219). Lippincott Williams & Wilkins.

Cornett, B. S. (2001). Service delivery issues in health care settings. In R. Lubinski & C. Frattali (Eds.), *Professional issues in speech-language pathology and audiology* (pp. 229–250). Delmar.

DePoy, E., & Gitlin, L. N. (2011). *Introduction to research.* C. V. Mosby.

Dodd, B. (2007). Evidence-based practice and speech-language pathology: Strengths, weaknesses, opportunities, and threats. *Folia Phoniatrica, 9,* 118–119.

Dollaghan, C. (2004). Evidence-based practice myths and realities. *ASHA Leader, 12,* 4–5, 12.

Dollaghan, C. (2007). *The handbook of evidence-based practice in communication disorders.* Brookes.

Dollaghan, C. A. (2004). Evidence-based practice in communications disorders: What do we know, and when do we know it? *Journal of Communication Disorders, 3*(5), 391–400.

Elman, R. J. (2006). Evidence-based practice: What evidence is missing? *Aphasiology, 20,* 103–109.

Epstein, R. M., Alper, B. S., & Quill, T. E. (2004). Communicating evidence for participatory decision-making. *Journal of the American Medical Association, 219*(19), 2359–2386.

Feeney, P. (2006, May 2). Primer on research: An introduction. *ASHA Leader, 11*(6), 14, 26.

Finn, P. (2006, June 13). Bias and blinding. *ASHA Leader, 11*(8), 16–17, 22.

Finn, P. (2011). Critical thinking: Knowledge and skills for evidence-based practice. *Language, Speech, and Hearing Services in Schools, 42,* 69–72.

Finn, P., Bothe, A. K., & Bramlet, R. F. (2005). Science and pseudoscience in communication disorders: Criteria and application. *American Journal of Speech Language Pathology, 14,* 172–185.

Forrest, J. L., & Miller, S. (2001). Integrating evidence-based decision-making into Allied Health curricula. *Journal of Allied Health, 30*(4), 215–222.

Frattali, C., & Worrall, L. E. (2001) Evidence-based practice: Applying science to the art of clinical care. *Journal of Medical Speech-Language Pathology, 9*(1), iv–xiv.

Gallagher, T. M. (2001). Implementation of evidence-based practice in communication disorders coursework and practice. *Proceedings of Academic Programs in Communication Sciences and Disorders, 29–45.*

Greenwall, T., & Walsh, B. Evidence-based practice in speech-language pathology: Where now? *American Journal of Speech and Language Pathology, 30*(1), 186–198.

Golper, L., Wertz, R. T., Frattali, C., Yorkston, K., Myers, P., Katz, R., . . . Wambaugh, J. (2001). Evidence-based practice guidelines for the management of communication disorders in neurologically impaired adults. *Academy of Neurological Communication Disorders and Science Report Practice Guidelines,* 1–12.

Golper, L. C., Wertz, R. T., & Brown, K. E. (2006). Back to basics. Reading research literature. *ASHA Leader, 11*(5), 10–11, 28, 34–35.

Hargrove, P., & Gruffer, M. (2008). Procedures for using clinical practice guidelines. *Language, Speech, and Hearing Services in Schools, 39,* 289–302.

Haynes, W. O., & Johnson, C. E. (2009). *Understanding research and evidence-based practice.* Pearson.

Herder, C., Howard, C., Nye, C., & Vanryckeghem, M. (2006). Effectiveness of behavioral stuttering treatment: A systematic review and meta-analysis. *Contemporary Issues in Communication Sciences and Disorders, 33,* 61–73.

Jewell, D. V. (2011). *Guide to evidence-based physical therapy.* Jones and Bartlett.

Johnson, C. E. (2006). Getting started in evidence-based practice for childhood speech-language disorders. *American Journal of Speech-Language Pathology, 15,* 20–35.

Justice, L. M., & Fey, M. E. (2004, September 21). Evidence-based practice in schools: Integrating craft and theory with science and data. *ASHA Leader,* 30–32, 45.

Kaderavek, J. N., & Justice, L. M. (2010). Fidelity: An essential component of evidence-based practice in speech-language pathology. *American Journal of Speech-Language Pathology, 19,* 269–279.

Kloda, L., & Bartlett, J. C. (2009). Clinical information behavior of rehabilitation therapists: A review of the research or occupational therapists, physical therapists, and speech-language pathologists. *Journal of the Medical Library Association, 97,* 194–202.

Konnerup, M., & Schwartz. J. (2006). Translating systematic reviews into policy and practice. *Contemporary Issues in Communication Sciences and Disorders, 33,* 79–82.

Kully, D., & Langeven, M. (2005, October 18). Evidence-based practice in fluency disorders. *ASHA Leader,* 10–11, 23.

Law, J., & Plunkett, C. (2000). Grading study quality in systematic reviews. *Contemporary Issues in Communication Disorders and Sciences, 33,* 28–36.

Law, M. (2002). Introduction to evidence-based practice. In M. Law (Ed.), *Evidence-based rehabilitation* (pp. 2–12). Slack.

Logemann, J. A. (2004). Clinical trials: CSD-RGG overview. *Journal of Communication Disorders, 37*(5), 419–423.

Logemann, J. A., & Gardner, P. M. (2005, August 16). Help find the evidence clinicians need. *ASHA Leader,* 8–9.

McCauley, R. J., & Hargrove, P. (2004). A clinician's introduction to systematic reviews in communication disorders: The course review paper with muscle. *Issues in Communication Sciences and Disorders, 31,* 173–181.

McCurtin, A., & Roddam, H. (2012). Evidence-based practice: SLT's under siege opportunity for growth: The use and nature of research evidence in the profession. *International Journal of Language and Communication Disorders, 17,* 22–26.

Meline, T. (2006). *Research in communication science and disorders.* Pearson.

Meline, T., & Paradiso, T. (2003). Evidence-based practice in schools. *Language, Speech, and Hearing Services in Schools, 34,* 273–283.

Moodle, S. T., Kothari, A., Bagatto, M. P., Seewald, R., Miller, L. T., & Scollie, S. D.

(2011). Knowledge translation in audiology: Promoting the clinical application of best evidence. *Trends in Amplification, 15,* 5–22.

Mullen, R. (2005a, August 16). Evidence-based practice planning addresses member needs skills. *ASHA Leader, 1,* 21.

Mullen, R. (2005b, November 8). Survey test members' understanding of evidence-based practice. *ASHA Leader, 4,* 14.

Mullen, R. (2007, March 6). The state of the evidence. ASHA develops levels of evidence for communication sciences and disorders. *ASHA Leader,* 8–9, 24–25.

Nail-Chiwetalu, B., & Ratner, N. (2006). Information literacy for speech-language pathologists: A key to evidence-based practice. *Language, Speech, and Hearing Services in Schools, 17*(2), 151–167.

Nail-Chiwetalu, B., & Ratner, N. (2007). Assessment of the information seeking abilities and needs among speech-language pathologists. *Journal of the Medical Library Association, 95*(2), 182–188.

National Center for Evidence-Based Practice in Communication Disorders. (2012). http://www.ncepmap.org

Nelson, P., & Goffman, L. (2006, May 2). Primer on research: Developing research questions. *ASHA Leader, 11*(6), 15, 26.

Nye, C., & Harvey, J. (2006). Interpreting and maintaining the evidence. *Contemporary Issues in Communication Sciences and Disorders, 33,* 56–60.

Oller, D. K. (2006, November 7). Interpretation and correlation. *ASHA Leader,* 24–26.

Orange, J. B. (2004). Evidence-based clinical practice: A Canadian perspective. *American Journal of Speech-Language Pathology, 13*(3), 1264–1265.

Orlikoff, R., Schiavetti, N., & Metz, D. (2021). *Evaluating research in communication disorders* (8th ed.). Pearson.

Polit, P. F., & Beck, C. T. (2010). *Nursing research.* Lippincott.

Portney, L. G., & Watkins, M. P. (2009). *Foundations of clinical research: Applications to practice.* Pearson.

Reilly, S., Oates, J., & Douglas, J. (2004). Evidence-based practice in speech-language pathology: Future directions. In S. Reilly, J. Douglas, & J. Oates (Eds.), *Evidence-based practice in speech-language pathology* (pp. 330–352). Whurr.

Rose, M. I., & Baldac, S. (2004). Translating evidence into practice. In S. Reilly, J. Douglas, & J. Oates (Eds.), *Evidence-based practice in speech pathology* (pp. 317–329). Whurr.

Sackett, D. L., Rosenberg, W. M., Gray, J., Haynes, R. B., & Richardson, W. S. (1996). Evidence-based medicine: What it is and what it isn't. *British Medical Journal, 312*(7023), 71–72.

Sackett, D. L., Strauss, S. E., Richardson, W. S., Rosenberg, W. M., & Haynes, R. B. (2001). *Evidence-based medicine.* Churchill Livingstone.

Schlosser, R. W. (2000). *The efficacy of augmentative and alternate communication: Evidence-based practice.* Elsevier.

Schlosser, R. W. (2004). Evidence-based practice in ACC: 10 points to consider. *ASHA Leader,* 6–7, 10–11.

Schlosser, R. W., Koul, K., & Costello, J. (2007). Asking well-built questions for evidence-based practice in augmentative and alternative communication. *Journal of Communication Disorders, 40,* 225–238.

Schlosser, R. W., & O'Neil-Pirozzi, T. M. (2006). Problem formulation in evidence-based practice and systematic reviews. *Contemporary Issues in Communication Sciences and Disorders, 33,* 5–10.

Shiffman, R. M., Shekelle, P., Overhage, M., Slutsky, K., & Grimshaw, J. (2003). Standardized reporting of clinical practice guidelines. *Annals of Internal Medicine, 139,* 493–498.

Taylor & Francis Group. (2006). *Evidence-based communication and intervention.* http://www.tandfico/journals/titles/17489539.asp

Threats, T. T. (2002). Evidence-based practice research using a WHO framework. *Journal of Medical Speech-Language Pathology, 10*(3), xvii–xxiv.

Tickle-Degnen, N. (2002). Communicative evidence to clients, managers, and funders. In M. Law (Ed.), *Evidence-based rehabilitation* (pp. 221–254) Slack.

Wong, L., & Hickson, L. (2012). *Evidence-based practice in audiology: Evaluating interventions for children and adults with hearing impairment.* Plural Publishing.

Worrall, L. E., & Bennett, S. (2001). Evidence-based practice: Barriers and facilitators for speech-language pathologists. *Journal of Medical Speech-Language Pathology, 9*(2), xi–xvi.

Yorkston, K. M., Spencer. K. A., Duffy, J., Beukelman, D., Golper, L. A., & Miller, R. (2001). Evidence-based medicine and practice guidelines: Application to the field of speech-language pathology. *Journal of Medical Speech-Language Pathology, 9*(4), 243–256.

Zipoli, R. P., & Kennedy, M. (2005). Evidence-based practice among speech-language pathologists: Attitudes, utilization, and barriers. *American Journal of Speech-Language Pathology, 14*, 208–220.

14

Critical Review of Quantitative and Qualitative Research Articles

Tobias A. Kroll and Jeremy J. Donai

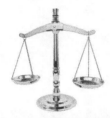

LEARNING OBJECTIVES

Upon completion of this chapter, the reader will be able to:

■ Describe what is meant by the term consumer of research and why being an effective consumer of research is important for clinicians.

■ Discuss the process of critically analyzing quantitative peer-reviewed research articles

■ Discuss the process of critically analyzing qualitative peer-reviewed research articles

Consumers of Research

Following graduation, most students from speech-language pathology and audiology graduate programs pursue careers in clinical practice rather than careers conducting research. However, it is vital for clinicians to be able to read, understand, and apply research findings to inform clinical decision-making, all skills involved in being an effective **consumer of research** (someone who can effectively utilize research to guide clinical decision-making based on available evidence). This chapter summarizes information from previous chapters regarding how to critically evaluate, interpret, and apply findings from both quantitative and qualitative research articles.

General Critical Review Strategies: Quantitative Articles

This section discusses considerations related to critically analyzing sections of quantitative research articles including the Introduction, Methods, Results, and Discussion/Conclusion. A description of the process along with some questions the reader should ask while reading each section are provided.

Introduction

The primary goal of the Introduction section is to provide an overview of the rationale for conducting the study. Included in this section should be references to and interpretation of previous and current literature; discussion of

any gaps in the literature; review of any relevant theory, conceptual framework, or clinical application regarding the topic; and motivation for conducting the study. This section is where the authors should "sell" the importance or need for the study, including clinical and/or theoretical implications. Some common questions to ask when critically analyzing the Introduction section include the following:

1. What is the underlying problem or question, and is it a clinical or theoretical problem or issue?
2. Has the relevant literature (past and present) been reviewed, and does it support the research question(s) being posed?
3. What are the aims and objectives of the study, and are they clearly stated and sufficiently motivated?
4. What are the hypotheses and expected outcomes of the study, and are they clearly stated?

Methods

The Methods section should provide a detailed description of the technical details of the study. From a research perspective, it is critical that this section provide sufficient detail to allow for replication of the study by other researchers. Common questions to consider when critically analyzing the Methods section include the following:

1. How did the researcher attempt to answer the research question (i.e., what specific methods or techniques were used), and were those attempts appropriate for the research question?

2. What were the specific inclusion and exclusion criteria for subject selection?
3. What were the specific independent and dependent variables?
4. Did the authors provide sufficient detail about the technical aspects of the study to allow for replication?

Results

The primary purpose of the Results section is to present the data obtained during the study. In this section, the author should avoid making claims or drawing conclusions based on the study outcomes but rather simply present the data in a straightforward, efficient, and easy to interpret manner. Some questions to consider include the following:

1. Are the data easy to view and organized for maximum understanding?
2. Are the visuals (tables and figures) displaying the data easy to read and understand?
3. What analytic methods were used, and were they appropriate in answering the research question?
4. Were the results of the study clinically and statistically significant, and if so, were effect size measures reported (and what does all this mean)?

Discussion/Conclusion

The last section of quantitative research articles is the Discussion/Conclusion section. This section is where questions from the study are answered and the implications (clinical or theoretical) of

these findings are discussed. The results are often compared to other, similar, studies considering the similarities and differences. Limitations of the study and directions for future research are often provided in this section. New information related to the study should not be presented in this section. Some questions to consider for this section include the following:

1. Do the results answer the proposed research question(s)?
2. Did the author(s) sufficiently interpret the data with regards to the research question(s)?
3. Were the results similar to or different from other similar studies?
4. What were the strengths, weaknesses, and limitations of the study?
5. What are the practical implications of the study (related to theory development or clinical service provision)?

General Critical Review Strategies: Qualitative Articles

Given the emergent and interpretive nature of qualitative research (see Chapter 9), critical review of qualitative studies proceeds in a more "organic" manner than that of quantitative studies. Rather than evaluating, for example, sampling procedures, sample size, and data analysis according to relatively stringent criteria, consumers of qualitative research have more flexibility and, at the same time, more responsibility when it comes to gauging the appropriateness of the study in front of them. They can be more flexible because qualitative research itself is more flexible than quantitative and experimental approaches. The process may resemble a "**bricolage**" more than a stepwise procedure (Denzin & Lincoln, 1994) and has been likened to a dance (Janesick, 1994). Hence, researchers have more leeway in approaching their work and so do reviewers.

By the same token, this flexibility makes for a higher potential of researcher biases creeping into findings or of methodological sloppiness. And since the criteria for detecting either are not as straightforward, a comparably larger burden is placed on the consumer. An important aspect of handling this burden is to know one's epistemology. Our (the authors of this text) stance is a pragmatist one (Creswell & Creswell, 2023, pp. 11–12; Patton, 2015, pp. 152–157): we contend that it is *our* best reading of a study that determines if it is of use *to us*, and we should not be surprised if our evaluation of it differs considerably from that of others.

That said, criteria and guidelines for evaluating qualitative studies do exist; Chapter 9 lists a variety of them that will be taken up in this chapter to illustrate their use. Table 14–1 lists the criteria for validity and reliability in the left column and evaluative questions in the right column.

When checking the study in question against the criteria presented in the left-hand column of Table 14–1, we may make a distinction between *procedural* and *interpretive* criteria. **Procedural criteria** pertain to the more material, formal aspects of the qualitative process; these can be gauged by their presence or absence and may involve quantification. *Triangulation, member checking, disclosure of bias, presentation of con-* *tradictory evidence, time spent in the field, peer debriefing, external audition,* and *cross-checking of transcripts as well as codes* all fall under this rubric. For example, authors may state (or not) that they performed a member check (or not); they may or may not disclose their biases; they may report the time spent in the field; and so forth. Note, however, that simply using the criteria previously described as a checklist and "score" the study in question on it would be to miss the point of qualitative inquiry. A study may be deemed flawed because too many of these criteria are absent or insufficiently addressed; it may also be deemed adequate or at least informative because it has other redeeming qualities not listed here, notable interpretive strengths or the like. As mentioned previously, reviewer and consumer have more flexibility when evaluating qualitative research but also more responsibility.

Interpretive criteria are those that pertain to the less tangible dynamics of the process; this would include *rich/thick description* and *constant comparison*. An amount of these is needed in any qualitative study, but it is rather difficult to gauge directly whether they were utilized sufficiently and appropriately; the reader must come to their own conclusion as to the quality and the richness of the writing. Note that *quality* is used as a technical term in this chapter: it refers to the intangible aspects of a piece of writing that are neither readily quantifiable nor explicable, but nonetheless obvious to most readers (Pirsig, 1974).

The evaluation questions in the right-hand column of Table 14–1 offer a window in the complexity of assessing quality in this sense; they rely on terms that are either open to interpretation (*appropriate, clear, accepted,* and *adequate*), or

Table 14–1. Criteria and Questions for Evaluating Qualitative Research

Criteria for Validity and Reliability	Evaluation Questions
Do researchers report use of (any, some, all of) the following: 1. Triangulation 2. Member checking 3. Rich, thick description 4. Disclosure of author bias 5. Present contradicting evidence 6. Spending a significant amount of time in the field 7. Peer debriefing 8. External auditor 9. Cross-checking of transcripts 10. Constant comparison 11. Regular exchange between researchers 12. Cross-checking of codes	1. Are the methods of research appropriate to the nature of the question being asked? 2. Is the connection to an existing body of knowledge or theory clear? 3. Are there clear accounts of the criteria used for the selection of cases for study and of the data collection and analysis? 4. Does the sensitivity of the methods match the needs of the research question? Were the data collection and record keeping systematic? 5. Is reference made to accepted procedures of analysis? 6. How systematic is the analysis? 7. Is there adequate discussion of how themes, concepts, and categories were derived from the data? 8. Is there adequate discussion of the evidence for and against the researcher's arguments? 9. Is a clear distinction made between the data and their interpretation?

borrowed from the quantitative sciences, where they have a specific meaning that is not transferable to the qualitative realm (*sensitivity, systematic, analysis*). Nonetheless, they provide valuable guidance, once the reader has accepted that she cannot use them in a step-by-step way or expect to exhaustively answer them.

We will use the criteria and questions listed in Table 14–1 as guideposts for walking the reader through the review process for qualitative study. To reiterate, though, neither the criteria nor the

questions apply to every study in equal measure, nor are they of equal relevance. In our view, the ultimate arbiter for the quality of any given study is the reader, and the reader's verdict is intimately wedded to the usefulness of the study to the reader's specific purpose. The challenge, whether as a producer or consumer of qualitative research, is the same: to transcend one's subjectivity while steering clear of rigid notions of objectivity.

When evaluating a study, it is helpful to consider the differences between the various qualitative methodologies, including the ones outlined in Chapter 9. While the cautionary notes described previously do apply to all of them, they do not apply to all of them in equal measure. Ethnographic and phenomenological studies can be much more varied and "liberal" in the ways they approach their subject matter (Damico & Simmons-Mackie, 2003; Rehorick & Bentz, 2008); consequently, the criteria and questions in Table 14–1 are meant to be applied rather loosely to them. Grounded theory, by contrast, was explicitly developed as a rigorous qualitative alternative to quantitative methodologies (Charmaz, 2006), hence a reader may apply criteria and questions much more stringently to it. The same is true for Conversation Analysis (CA), although its descriptive (rather than interpretive) bent (Damico & Simmons-Mackie, 2003) makes it a bit of an outlier among qualitative methods—to the extent that a truly thorough evaluation of a CA study should ideally proceed along CA-internal criteria, rather than general qualitative ones. Case studies, finally, may run the whole gamut of "loose" to "stringent," depending on the field they originate in and the questions they are meant to answer. Readers should pay careful attention to both and decide whether a more or less rigid application of criteria and questions is appropriate for the study in front of them.

Introduction and Literature Review

Similar to quantitative works, an Introduction and Literature Review in a qualitative research article should cover the rationale for the study and any background knowledge and existing research as needed. However, the similarities end there. Sequence and scope of sections are less rigid; they may look more like an ongoing reflection than like the stepwise progression typical for quantitative papers. There may be no clear distinction between Introduction and Literature Review or even between any of the "normal" sections of a research paper.

Depending on the approach, the rationale for the study may be carefully constructed out of existing research, or it may be based on a researcher's hunch or curiosity. Likewise, literature reviews may be comprehensive and exhaustive, or cursory as needed. Generally speaking, ethnographic and grounded theory studies should have a clear rationale, while phenomenological approaches may proceed mainly based on researcher interest. However, researchers are expected to clearly articulate which school of phenomenological analysis they use and why. (See Patton [2015, pp. 85–168] for a concise overview of a variety of qualitative approaches.) Case studies typically share a rationale among them: that they are, to an extent, unique. A similar rationale applies to conversation analytic studies, which tend to focus on specific mechanisms of sequential actions.

Ethnography, conversation analysis, and case studies normally include a more or less comprehensive literature review, while grounded theory studies may proceed with minimal reference to extant literature so as to not obscure researchers' view on the data. It is still expected that researchers complete a comprehensive literature review after the fact, possibly as part of their own interpretive analysis (Charmaz, 2006). Phenomenological studies may be found anywhere on this continuum. No matter the approach, qualitative literature reviews typically allow more room for reflection and for a wider variety of sources than quantitative ones. Their style may be less formal, with interspersion of personal narratives or experiences.

That said, general yardsticks for scholarly writing still apply. Any beginning to a qualitative study must be carefully reasoned, adhere to the basic rules of logic, and, where applicable, precisely define terms. The problem and the reason for investigating it should be clearly stated (but note, as mentioned previously, that the term *clearly* itself is open for interpretation). Often, qualitative authors go well beyond what quantitative researchers offer in terms of higher-order reflection, veering into the philosophical and the personal (cf. Hinckley, 2005; Rehorick & Bentz, 2008). This applies not only to rationale and literature review but also to definitions, methods, and so forth.

With regard to the criteria listed in Table 14–1, number 4 (disclosure of author bias) may be found in this beginning part of an article; as for questions, the reader may most likely find answers to number 1 and number 2 here (appropriateness of methods, connection to existing knowledge). Note that it is perfectly appropriate, in our view, to judge a qualitative study as invalid or less-than-useful based on the authors' stated theoretical background or choice of methods. (The same is true for quantitative studies, of course, but since the criteria for selection of methodology are generally more stringent in the quantitative realm, and researcher bias is—technically—not supposed to play any role, the criteria for rejecting a study are equally more stringent.) Worldviews clash more openly in the qualitative world, and methodological disputes have long become epistemological ones, with some qualitative

researchers questioning the validity of the entire qualitative enterprise (cf. Denzin & Lincoln, 2005). By the same token, the consumer of interpretive research enjoys considerable liberty in judging a theoretical background or choice of methodology as adequate or not.

Methods and Results

What applies to the Introduction and Literature Review is equally true for the Methods and Results sections of a qualitative paper. They may be clearly outlined and distinguished, as in a "hard science" study. Or they may blend into each other, particularly when researchers approach their work more as a "dance" than as a laboratory procedure (Janesick, 1994). In this mode, sometimes called **iterative coding** where explicit coding procedures are involved (Srivastava & Hopwood, 2009), data collection and analysis are not clearly distinguishable. Analysis begins while data is still being collected, codes and even themes that emerge from the analysis may be changed or amended as new data comes in, and subsequent data collection may be informed by prior findings. Presentation of results may proceed using visuals, tables, graphs and figures, or—in a narrative or even poetic fashion—a blend of both. As previously described, the quality of a study must be gauged carefully by the reader's judgment. That said, the reader typically has more helpful pointers in this part of a study, as it is here where most of the criteria and questions listed in Table 14–1 apply.

Evidently, criteria 1 and 2 as well as 5 through 12 should be addressed in the Methods section—*if* they are relevant to the study. The caveat, again, is that there is no rule, algorithm, or checklist that the reader can simply follow. Whether or not a certain criterion is reported is less relevant than whether it should be present based on the authors' chosen method. For an ethnographic study, a researcher should spend a certain amount of time in the field and member checking should be utilized; for a grounded theory study, interpretive depth is more relevant (evidenced for example by triangulation, contradicting evidence, constant comparison, and cross-checking of codes). With regard to Results, rich and thick description is expected in any type of qualitative research, and whether the authors succeeded in this regard will be one of the main criteria by which the reader judges the quality of their work.

Along the way, the questions in Table 14–1 are helpful to the reader, again to different degrees and in different ways. Questions 1 and 4 are of utmost importance, as the quality of any qualitative (or quantitative) study hinges on whether researchers' chosen methods are capable of addressing the questions they are asking. It would be inadequate, for example, to use a first-person narrative from the author's perspective in order to understand the culture of a workplace or a particular problem with which employees are struggling. An ethnographic approach would be much more suitable to capture culture—a grounded theory one to understand employees' grievances. By the same token, an inner shift in a researcher's perspective may be best expressed in narrative or even poetic form, rather than a formalized procedure.

In contrast to this, questions 2 and 3 as well as 5 through 9, need to be tackled keeping in mind the character of the study in its entirety. Similar to our previous discussion of criteria, they are more or less applicable and relevant to a given project, depending on the chosen method, researchers' epistemological background, and so forth.

Discussion/Conclusion

Given the interpretive nature of qualitative research, it is easy to see how the Discussion and Conclusion sections lend themselves most readily to author biases. Of note, however, if the discussion overshoots the study's findings, the ground for that is typically prepared earlier. Sloppy collecting and coding of data makes it easier to come to unwarranted conclusions. Again, much responsibility is placed on the reader: in the end, it is up to us to carefully decide on the *quality* of a given study. That decision should be based on a close comparison of the authors' data and their interpretation, and their fidelity to their self-proclaimed interpretive framework. It will also depend on the study's usefulness for the reader's purposes, as mentioned previously.

Given that the qualitative research enterprise is inherently reflective, the concluding section of a well-written paper should show evidence of further reflectiveness on the authors' part. Thus, after interrogating themselves on their choice of methods and approaches to interpretation, they should now also question their own conclusions and, ideally, provide alternative conclusions as well as arguments for not choosing those. Then again, reflectiveness is not limited to this particular format. Ultimately, it is the reader who must reflect on their own assessment of the authors' reflectiveness. And the reader may well find that the process of interpreting, assessing, and reflecting on one's interpretations and assessments is inherently unending, and any stop to it—for example, the conclusion of an article or the reader's final takeaway—is at least partly arbitrary. Thus, while claims to finality are inappropriate for any type of research (Popper, 1959), they are particularly out of place in the qualitative realm.

Critical Review (Quantitative)

The following article entitled "Audibility-Based Hearing Aid Fitting Criteria for Children With Mild Bilateral Hearing Loss" by McCreery et al. (2020) will be critically reviewed. It is recommended that the reader review the article and consider the questions provided in this chapter for each section of the paper prior to proceeding with the chapter. This correlational study (nonexperimental) examined the issue of audibility needs of children with mild hearing loss where decisions regarding fitting hearing aids are not straightforward (as they are in other instances of more severe hearing loss). Each question from the previous section on quantitative research is provided with examples from the article under review.

Introduction

1. What is the underlying problem or question, and is it a clinical or theoretical problem or issue?
   ■ The first paragraph of the paper discusses the issue at hand which relates to uncertainty regarding the clinical question

of whether to fit amplification to children with milder degrees of hearing loss. The authors cite a literature review by Winiger et al. (2016) suggesting inconsistent amplification recommendation practices for children with mild bilateral hearing loss. The authors also provide definitions of salient audiologic terminology related to the clinical question, which assists the reader in their general understanding of the topic.

2. Has the relevant literature (past and present) been reviewed, and does it support the research question(s) being posed?
   ■ Pages 56–59 contain a review of the relevant literature. Specifically, the article discusses the negative effects of mild bilateral hearing loss on developmental outcomes in children and then provides a review of the literature on current candidacy criteria for children with mild bilateral hearing loss. Figure 1 (p. 58) provides a visual representation of the effects of age-related ear canal acoustics and their effect on audibility for children with similar hearing loss in the mild range. A review of information from the Introduction section supports the study and the research questions posed.

3. What are the aims and objectives of the study, and are they clearly stated and sufficiently motivated?
   ■ A primary objective of the study was to determine the unaided speech intelligibility index (SII) value (a measure of sound audibility without amplification)

where language delays begin to emerge and to explore hearing aid recommendations using the unaided SII as a clinical tool (p. 59). This is a nonexperimental, correlational design as no experimental manipulation is used and relationships between variables of interest are studied. The detailed review of information from the Introduction section sufficiently motivates the study.

4. What are the hypotheses and expected outcomes of the study, and are they clearly stated?
   - The authors suggest that the development of a criterion for amplification based on unaided SII values could have significant value for clinical decision-making for children with mild degrees of hearing loss (p. 59). As such, it is hypothesized that the unaided SII as a tool for determining audibility without the use of amplification may hold value for clinical decision-making.

Methods

1. How did the researcher attempt to answer the research question (i.e., what specific methods or techniques were used), and were those attempts appropriate for the research question?
   - Beginning on page 59, the authors provide methodological information related to the study. To determine the relationship between better ear unaided SII values and language outcomes, the authors recruited 52 subjects with various degrees of hearing

loss and applied a linear regression model with unaided SII as a predictor of language outcome (p. 60) to effectively answer the research question. Additionally, a piecewise regression model was used to determine the unaided SII value where decreases in language outcomes began to occur.

2. What were the specific inclusion and exclusion criteria for subject selection?
   - On page 59 under *Participants*, the authors provide the inclusion criteria related to degree of hearing loss, the absence of developmental conditions or diagnoses, and requirements for spoken English as the primary language used in the home. Additional inclusion criteria were specified for subjects with amplification. Exclusion criteria were participants who did not meet inclusion requirements. The authors also collected data from 52 children with normal hearing matched for age, socioeconomic status (SES), and nonverbal intelligence.

3. What were the specific independent and dependent variables?
   - The independent (predictor) variable for the study is unaided SII. The dependent (outcome) variables for the study are the language function tests (Peabody Picture Vocabulary Test Fourth Edition [PPVT-4], Wechsler Abbreviated Scale of Intelligence [WASI] vocabulary section, and the syntax construction subtest of the Comprehensive Assessment of Spoken Language

[CASL]). These variables are described on page 59.

4. Did the authors provide sufficient detail about the technical aspects of the study to allow for replication?

- Throughout the *Methods* on pages 59–60, the authors describe, in detail, the audiological methods and language measures used in the study. All materials used in the study are commonly accepted in audiological practice (e.g., converting hearing thresholds in dB HL to dB SPL using reference equivalent thresholds for SPL and real ear to coupler differences [RECD] for the transducer used during testing) or are standardized test measures (such as the PPVT-4, WASI vocabulary section, and the syntax subsection of the CASL). Providing these details and the use of standardized measures and accepted procedures will allow for study replication by interested researchers in the future.

Results

1. Are the data easy to view and organized for maximum understanding?

- Figures 2 to 4 (pp. 61 and 62) show performance (interquartile range and 95% confidence interval) on the three language outcome measures for children with normal hearing and children with hearing loss. Figures 5 to 7 (pp. 62 and 63) show results of the piecewise

regression analysis and location where the better ear unaided SII values intersect with the median language outcomes for children with normal hearing as well as the point at which the relationship between the better ear unaided SII and language outcome changes (known as the "knot"). Table 2 provides a summary of the piecewise regression model for each language outcome (PPVT-4 knot = better ear unaided SII of 76, CASL Syntax Construction = better ear unaided SII of 72, WASI Vocabulary = better ear unaided SII of 80).

2. Are the visuals (tables and figures) displaying the data easy to read and understand?

- The tables and figures used in the paper (described in the previous section) succinctly and clearly display the descriptive data (Figures 2–4) and piecewise regression analyses (Figures 5–7).

3. What analytic methods were used, and were they appropriate in answering the research question?

- The authors used a combination of descriptive analyses (Figures 2–4), linear regression (Figures 5–7), and piecewise regression (Table 2) in answering the research questions. Each technique was appropriate and allowed the authors to answer unique portions of the research questions.

4. Were the results of the study clinically and statistically significant, and if so, were effect size measures

reported (and what does all this mean)?

- Significant differences between children with HL and children with NH were found (children with NH performing better) on PPVT-4 (p = .0031) and the syntax construction subsection of CASL (p = .042) but not on the WASI vocabulary score (p = .21).

- Linear regression models using better ear unaided SII (for children with HL) to predict language outcomes provided the following effect sizes (i.e., strength of relationship between SII values and specific language outcomes): R^2 = .25 for PPVT-4; R^2 =.11 for CASL syntax score; and R^2 =.17 WASI vocabulary score. These values are generally considered *medium* (R^2 = .11 and .17) to *large* (R^2 = .25) effect sizes, meaning that better ear unaided SII accounted for 25% of performance on the PPVT-4, 17% of performance on the WASI Vocabulary score, and 11% of performance on the CASL syntax score.

- Piecewise regression was used to determine the point at which the regression function predicting language outcome from better ear unaided SII changed for children with HL (known as the "knot" represented by the solid vertical line in Figures 5–7). These values are provided: PPVT–4 = better ear unaided SII of 76, CASL syntax score = better ear unaided SII of 72, WASI vocabulary score = better

ear unaided SII of 80 (all shown in Table 2).

Discussion/Conclusion

1. Do the results answer the proposed research question(s)?
   - The reported purposes of this study were to determine the unaided SII values associated with risk of negative language outcomes among children with mild bilateral hearing loss and secondarily to evaluate the possibility of using the unaided SII as a tool to inform clinical decision-making regarding the fitting of children with mild bilateral hearing loss (p. 64). Considering the findings of the study, the authors propose unaided SII values to consider when determining whether or not to recommend amplification for children with mild degrees of bilateral hearing loss.

2. Did the author(s) sufficiently interpret the data with regards to the research question(s)?
   - This study utilized descriptive and inferential statistics to answer the research questions. Linear and piecewise regression analyses were used to elucidate the relationship between unaided better ear SII and language outcomes and the unaided SII values associated with the risk of negative language outcomes.

3. Were the results similar to or different from other similar studies?
   - To the knowledge of the authors of this text, this is the first study

to utilize better ear unaided SII values in children with mild bilateral hearing loss to predict language outcomes. As such, this study represents initial support for the use of unaided SII values in this patient population. Future research should be conducted to replicate and extend the findings of this initial study.

4. What were the strengths, weaknesses, and limitations of the study?

   ▪ The authors report one strength of the study was use of the piecewise regression model, which is a statistical method blind to the purpose and hypothesis of the study, for determining criterion levels of audibility (p. 64).

   ▪ The authors report limitations related to a lack of consistent hearing aid use among this clinical population affecting practical benefit and issues related to the homogenous sample (all from homes with English as primary language, free from other developmental comorbidities, and from more economic advantaged homes compared to the general population) used in the study. All of these factors likely reduce the representativeness of study findings (p. 65).

5. What are the practical implications of the study (related to theory development or clinical service provision)?

   ▪ The authors report that the criteria developed in this study were based on levels of unaided audibility equivalent to the median level of performance

for an age-matched group of children with typical hearing and a model that determined the level of unaided audibility where language outcomes began to deviate from median levels of age and SES matched peers with normal hearing (pp. 65–66).

   ▪ As such, the authors advocate for the use of an unaided SII score of 80 (or .80) or lower for recommending amplification for children with mild bilateral hearing loss (pp. 64–66).

Summary

In summary, the McCreery et al. (2020) article represents a correlational (non-experimental) *quantitative* research study. The authors effectively provide information to answer the questions posed in this chapter for each section of the research paper (which were individually discussed in the previous section of the chapter). The Introduction section effectively motivates the study, reviews relevant literature (including any gaps), and provides clear goals. The Methods section clearly describes the procedures, instruments, and inclusion and exclusion criteria used in the study to allow for study replication, which is critical for advancing the knowledge base in research or clinical service provision through the accumulation of evidence (eventually resulting in the use of meta-analytic techniques). Inclusion and exclusion criteria are also clearly stated. The Results section effectively reports and displays study findings using easy to read and interpret figures and tables. The Discussion/Conclusion section reviews how the findings answer the questions posed, highlights strengths and limitations of the study, and describes potential clinical implications for children with mild bilateral hearing loss.

Critical Review (Qualitative)

In this section, we will review two qualitative articles that, we hope, speak to the depth and the breadth of the qualitative paradigm in Communication Sciences and Disorders (CSD) research. It is recommended that the reader familiarize themselves with them before delving into the review. Even a cursory overview will demonstrate how different they are and how a critical review should proceed accordingly.

Reviewing an Autoethnographic Study

The first article is "The Piano Lesson: An Autoethnography About Changing Clinical Paradigms in Aphasia Practice (Hinckley, 2005). The title indicates the kind of study the reader may expect. Autoethnography is an approach located at the intersection of ethnography and phenomenology, where a researcher attempts to understand a concept of interest based on their own experience while living through or with it (Holman Jones, 2005; Patton, 2015, pp. 100–104). (Note also the relative proximity to case studies—in a sense, the researcher investigates themselves as a particular case.) By default, then, data gathering and analysis will be less structured and systematic than in other paradigms—not only because ethnography and phenomenology are less structured and systematic but also

because the object of inquiry is a subjective experience, hence any attempts at distancing the experiencer from it via structured practice would amount to self-deception. In fact, autoethnography may take the opposite route, expressing its findings in such variegated forms as journal entries, evocative narrative, or even poetry (Holman Jones, 2005). Rigor, then, is achieved not via structure but via increased reflectiveness, and this is for what the reader should be looking.

An Overview of Hinckley (2005)

Hinckley begins her paper with a brief rationale, outlining why therapists' emotional experience of therapy should be a legitimate subject of study. Her argument is (a) that therapeutic schools of thought —"ideologies," in her words—for example, about what does and does not constitute therapy, what the clinician's and the patient's roles are, and so forth shape our practice for the better or the worse and (b) that beneficial shifts in therapeutic ideology are usually precipitated or accompanied by an emotion-laden experience. Hence, these experiences are important to understand; her goal is to share an autoethnographic narrative that illustrates this.

After a brief review of autoethnography as a method, Hinckley delves into the narrative itself. It centers on a past therapy session with a stroke survivor who is a highly respected pianist and piano teacher but can no longer move her right hand. Hinckley decides that in order to restore the patient's ability to resume her previous occupation, she— the therapist—will assume the role of a piano student, allowing her patient to take the role of the teacher and practice different ways to compensate for her disability. The narrative details the first session where she adopts this "flipped" paradigm of clinician-as-student, including her own emotional reaction (characterized by insecurity and doubt) and the patient's deft developments of compensatory techniques that allow her to fulfill her teaching role. The story ends on an emotional high note: two years later, the patient gives a concert playing a piece written for the left hand only.

Hinckley ends her article with three separate Discussion sections, only one of which is titled *Discussion*. Recall the flexibility qualitative research affords: "The Piano Lesson" contains neither a Methods or Results section in the traditional sense, and to someone looking for a discussion as typical in the quantitative realm—a sum-up of the findings—the three different sections may appear disjointed. To achieve Hinckley's aim, however, they are quite fitting. The first section—the one titled *Discussion*—reports that the clinician's perceptions, detailed in the narrative, differ substantially from those of the patient in one crucial point of the narrative where Hinckley fears she may have set the patient up for failure. Her fears are found unsubstantiated, and she uses this as a springboard to the second section, where she reiterates the importance of investigating the emotional lives of clinicians, particularly when it comes to beneficial changes in therapeutic ideologies. She then closes her paper by discussing the usefulness of autoethnography to this end (in the third section).

Evaluating Hinckley (2005)

It appears, from this brief review, that Hinckley's paper achieves its stated aim; namely, to advocate for the investigation of clinicians' inner lives and for auto-ethnography as a tool to do so. Before making this conclusion final, however, we will rereview her piece, this time using the criteria and questions laid out in Table 14–1. Beginning with the criteria, we may note that *member checking* and *rich, thick description* are both present, as is evidence that Hinckley spent a *significant amount of time* with the patient, getting to know her well. Due to the nature of the study, *triangulation* was not possible, as there is by necessity only one dataset (the narrative of the session in question, retrieved from memory). The member check, however, fulfilled a similar function.

In addition to the necessarily subjective mode of inquiry, Hinckley stresses the personal and intimate nature of her research; both aspects ensure that the formal criteria pertaining to collaboration with other researchers (peer debriefing, regular exchange) are less relevant to her study than they would be to a more structured and larger-scale inquiry of others' experience. That said, her paper could have benefited from an *external auditor*, if only to raise questions not readily visible from the first-person perspective.

Similarly, transcript checking, **constant comparison**, and cross-checking of codes are not applicable to a study whose aim is simply to use a first-person narrative for illustrating the usefulness of a certain mode of inquiry; by contrast, disclosure of author bias would have been extremely valuable to the reader in order to better understand Hinckley's original impetus for this kind of study, her therapeutic background, her view on communicative encounters, and so forth. Note that **author bias** does not simply refer to preconceptions an author might carry, but to their entire worldview and deeply held beliefs, even if they do not appear directly connected to the study at hand. Not all clinicians are able to intuit that a role reversal may be helpful to their patient, and most clinicians, it may be surmised, are not inclined to subsequently write about their experience. It would be helpful to know, for each of these, whence Hinckley drew her inspiration. All that said, while information about her background is missing, reflectiveness is evident by virtue of her presenting *evidence contradicting her perspective* (as result of the member check).

With regard to the evaluation questions, we note that Hinckley's approach is entirely appropriate in order to achieve her stated aim (our previous and subsequent caveats notwithstanding), as is her case selection. Given the nature of autoethnography, then, questions 4 through 7 are simply not applicable to her study and should not be weighed against it. Questions 8 and 9 (pertaining to reflectiveness) are adequately addressed, as mentioned previously. What is missing, in our view, is a sufficient account of *connection to an existing theory* (question 2), specifically the theoretical backdrop to the author's methodology. The paper would have benefited from a more comprehensive introduction to autoethnography, including the different forms it may take and the ends those forms may serve. While an extensive methodological discussion is not necessary, the paper delves into the narrative *too* quickly in its current form, failing to fully justify its choice of methods, and leaving the reader inadequately prepared for what is to come.

In sum, after gauging it using established criteria and questions, we find that Hinckley's paper does achieve its aim.

The narrative at the center of her piece is evocative and illustrates in depth how trying out new modes of intervention can tax the clinician emotionally and in their professional sense of self. Rigor is ensured by her detailed reflection on the "why" of the paper, on the retrieval of the memory at the heart of the narrative, and on the member check. Aside from the caveats we outlined previously, we find that "The Piano Lesson" is a qualitative paper of high *quality*.

Reviewing a Formal Ethnography

We will now proceed to the second study titled "Communicative Accessibility in Aphasia: An Investigation of the Interactional Context of Long-Term Care Facilities" (Azios et al., 2018). This paper, too, uses ethnography but takes a rather different approach to it. First, it is an "actual" ethnography; namely, the study of someone other than the researcher. Appropriately, it is therefore much more structured than Hinckley (2005), involving distinct methods of data collection (**participant observation, semistructured interviews, artifact analysis**) as well as coding of data to identify patterns (recall that Hinckley relied solely on narrative and reflection). Note also that while formal ethnography is clearly distinct from other qualitative methodologies in terms of data *collection*, it is considerably similar to them in terms of data analysis and reporting. Coding and identifying patterns (or themes) are common to several structured qualitative methodologies, including, for example, grounded theory. Consequently, the reader may expect, from this study and similarly structured ones, a more systematic and explicit approach to reporting, more akin to a quantitative research paper than to Hinckley (2005).

An Overview of Azios et al. (2018)

The authors begin their paper with a formal literature review, providing background information on stroke survivors in long-term care facilities (LTCFs), their communication needs, and the culture of such facilities, which oftentimes impedes person-centered care, including meeting said needs. They close their literature review with two research questions and an aim with two sub-aims. Their questions are as follows: "How does the LTCF environment impact social encounters in PWAs [persons with aphasia]?" and "How do behaviors and attitudes of other people influence communication?" (p. 1475). Consequently, their stated aim is "to unpack the relationship between aphasia and LTCF environments to better understand how context impacts interaction for PWAs in LTCFs" (p. 1475) and includes the sub-aims of "learning about the physical and interactive context, the behaviors of PWA and staff members as they navigated communicative events, and facilitators and barriers to successful communication between PWA and others" (p. 1475). Note that while these look similar to the formal questions, aims, or hypotheses utilized in quantitative research, the relationship between questions/aims on the one hand and findings on the other is not as "algorithmic" in qualitative research. The reader should not expect a format of the type "for question a, we found answer x" or "regarding aim b, we will discuss findings y and z" for the Results or Discussion sections. Rather, themes emerging

from the data will be used to elucidate all questions and aims as applicable, and examples from codes or the raw data will be used to illustrate the phenomenon at hand and support the authors' reasoning.

Azios et al. (2018) then proceed to detailing their methods—including a discussion of ethnographic methodology and its place in the wider qualitative realm, of their participants' characteristics and of recruitment procedures, and of data collection and analysis including ways of establishing trustworthiness (an umbrella term for the qualitative equivalent of validity and reliability; cf. Chapter 9). We will review this section in more detail in the following; for now, the reader may note that the structure of this section bears strong similarity to that of a quantitative study, in all the ways that Hinckley (2005) did not.

The heart of the article is, in many ways, the Results section. Here, Azios et al. (2018) describe their findings in detail. The reader will note that this section is much more extensive than the corresponding section in a quantitative paper; this is due to the nature of qualitative results. Where quantitative (especially experimental) researchers can limit themselves to reporting whether or not a hypothesis was confirmed (including significance, effect size, and such), qualitative authors have to go to great lengths to justify their conclusions, as they must make transparent, to the extent possible, the interpretive process that led them there. Azios et al. do this by providing a glimpse into ethnographic writing at the beginning of the section, by listing their themes and subthemes with extended explanations, and giving ample examples from their data for further illustration. We cannot do the richness of their writing justice here; hence we will confine ourselves to listing their themes and subthemes.

Theme 1 is *lack of support,* that is, a dearth of efforts to meet the communicative needs of the LTCFs' residents with aphasia. The reason for this lack is found in its **subthemes**: *physical layout, shortage of resources, knowledge of aphasia,* and *time and space pressures.* Facilities' lighting was either bright and impersonal or semidark, with poor acoustics throughout. Speech therapy was often not provided, and participants with aphasia lacked access to basic communication devices such as a telephone or the internet. Both staff and residents had little knowledge about aphasia, the importance of communication, or best practices to facilitate it. In addition, staff workload all but guaranteed that staff had little time for communicative interchanges with participants; tight spaces and difficulties with mobility added to the dearth of communication and the frequent breakdowns when it did occur.

Theme 2 is titled *social hierarchy,* indicating that the lack of communication opportunities for residents was partly due to an implicit hierarchy into which LTCF culture sorted them. *Independence* emerged as a *metric* (subtheme 1) by which staff and residents alike "ranked" residents; less independent seniors were quickly aided by more independent ones when struggles arose, but also faced segregation and patronizing. This sometimes worked to the advantage of the PWAs, as they were more mobile than other residents, but it worked to their disadvantage in communication situations, where they were often misinterpreted or spoken for. Also, residents with

aphasia appeared to select communication *partners* from an implicit *taxonomy* (subtheme 2), with staff members and nondisordered residents "ranking high" for desirable interaction and residents with cognitive impairments "ranking lower" than the PWAs.

Theme 3 is *focus on performance,* with subthemes of *task oriented, physical needs,* and *emphasis on group.* This cluster elucidates LTCFs' staff culture and how it influences patient culture. Staff was found to be largely concerned with getting concrete tasks done (e.g., administering medication), which minimized their orientation toward social interaction and led them to disregard PWAs' attempts at conversation. In addition, facilities' culture prioritized physical needs over psychosocial needs, leading even residents to minimize their verbal interactions with one another. Relatedly, residents' individuality was rarely acknowledged, leading to further lack of meaningful interaction opportunities.

Azios et al. (2018) close their paper with a Discussion section including clinical implications, future directions, and limitations. (Note again the formal similarities to a quantitative report format.) Here, they place their findings in a cultural analysis context, noting that LTCFs are necessarily "hybrid" cultures ("home" for residents, workplace for employees) and that the resulting conflict was skewed, in the facilities studied, in favor of workplace culture, resulting in a less than adequate interactional environment for residents. They point out that this is a factor of a traditional, top-down culture of care where procedures are shaped by those who oversee the facilities' functions; they contrast this to a resident-centered approach, where psychosocial needs and quality of life are the primary drivers of procedures; and they call for a culture change in traditionally managed LTCFs. After suggesting similar adjustments (i.e., from an expert- to a patient-centered approach) to speech-language therapists working with PWAs in LTCFs, they proceed to discussing the limitations of their research and future directions. We cannot detail their arguments here, but we wish to note that they deftly caution the reader against unwarranted extrapolations while also providing ways to make warranted ones. There *are* qualitative equivalents to statistical inference and generalizability, and Azios et al. provide good examples.

Evaluating Azios et al. (2018)

We have pointed out repeatedly that Azios et al.'s study is more formally structured than Hinckley's (2005); by the same token, it is fully legitimate to subject it to a more structured evaluation, using the criteria and questions in Table 14–1 in the way one would a checklist. Starting with the procedural criteria, *triangulation* is explicitly reported by the authors (using both multiple data sources and cross-analyst triangulation). *Member checking* was affected but is reported using the term *lamination*—a procedure akin to triangulation that adds an interpretive layer to existing conclusions, such as the feedback of study participants in a member check. (Of note, such terminological inconsistencies are common in the qualitative literature, underscoring once more the need for critical, reflective reading.) The authors report spending extensive amounts of *time in the field* and engaging in cross-author collaboration covering *peer debriefing* and

cross-checking, which makes the lack of an *external audition* less impactful than it would have been in single-author or noncollaborative research.

Missing from their report is an explicit *disclosure of bias* as well as any *presentation of contradictory evidence*. Their bias can, however, be deduced from their writings; it is evident both in their initial research questions and in their conclusion that they have a strong preference for person-centered care, the social model of disability (Oliver, 1990), and a focus on psychosocial well-being. It would have been helpful had they stated this at the beginning of their paper; as their bias is not hidden, however, this omission does not detract from the overall quality of their study.

More concerningly, the absence of contradictory evidence begs the question if there simply was none (in which case the authors could have stated this), or if it was not presented (which would be a problem for the validity of the study). As their own research uncovered, person-centered care is not a given in LTCFs and it may well be that some residents have "made peace" with this. A presentation of contradictory evidence (if present) would not have taken away from the weight of their findings but lent more nuance to their discussion, and if there was no contradictory evidence, mentioning this would have greatly added to the study's strength. Absent these, it is quite easy for a consumer of the study to refute its findings with anecdotal evidence of the type, "I know a PWA resident who is very happy in their traditional LTCF."

Moving on to the *interpretive criteria*, we may first note that their writing is characterized by rich, thick description despite the formal nature of their approach. Interspersed throughout their detached, clinical reporting are field notes and dialogue transcripts that vividly evoke the sense of isolation and disconnection many LTCF residents likely feel. In addition, we noted previously that triangulation, member checking, time in the field, constant comparison, and cross-checking were all present; this suggests that constant comparison was, indeed, affected. In fact, Azios et al. (2018) explicitly report procedures that imply an amount of constant comparison: "conflicting views [on the data]," they write, "were resolved through (…) scanning back through the data to justify or refute themes" (p. 1479), and their first author "kept track of classification systems [for codes and themes] and explanations (…), including those eventually discarded due to insufficient support" (p. 1478). These procedures are hardly possible absent an amount of constant comparison; the presence of the latter can therefore reasonably be inferred, adding to the trustworthiness of their findings.

In sum, then, Azios et al. (2018) is a paper of high quality based on established criteria for reviewing formal qualitative studies. It not only adheres to general guidelines for research reporting (notwithstanding our critiques outlined previously) but manages to convey a degree of evocativeness despite its structured, detached presentation.

General Summary

This chapter provided information on critically reviewing both quantitative and qualitative research articles. Information to consider within each section of the research article was discussed in detail. Example reviews of both quantitative and qualitative articles were provided for the reader. It should be clear after reading this chapter that the process of analyzing quantitative and qualitative research articles varies significantly. Specifically, the review and analysis of *quantitative* articles often follows a more prescriptive process, whereas the same is not the case for *qualitative* articles where the process is less rigid (and because of this, more open to reviewer bias or differences in interpretation).

DISCUSSION QUESTIONS

1. Describe the general purposes of the Introduction, Methods, Results, and Discussion sections of a research paper.
2. Discuss the similarities between quantitative and qualitative research articles.
3. Discuss the differences between quantitative and qualitative research articles.
4. Describe the concept of author bias in qualitative research and provide two examples.

References

Azios, J. H., Damico, J. S., & Roussel, N. (2018). Communicative accessibility in aphasia: An investigation of the interactional context of long-term care facilities. *American Journal of Speech-Language Pathology, 27*(4), 1474–1490.

Charmaz, K. (2006). *Constructing grounded theory: A practical guide through qualitative analysis.* Sage.

Creswell, J. W., & Creswell, J. D. (2023). *Research design: Qualitative, quantitative, and mixed methods approaches.* Sage.

Damico, J. S., & Simmons-Mackie, N. (2003). Qualitative research and speech-language pathology: A tutorial for the clinical realm. *American Journal of Speech-Language Pathology, 12*(2), 131–143.

Denzin, N. K., & Lincoln, Y. S. (1994). Introduction: Entering the field of qualitative research. In N. K. Denzin & Y. S. Lincoln (Eds.), *Handbook of qualitative research* (pp. 1–17). Sage.

Denzin, N. K., & Lincoln, Y. S. (2005). Introduction: The discipline and practice of qualitative research. In N. K. Denzin & Y. S. Lincoln (Eds.), *Handbook of qualitative research* (3rd ed., pp. 1–32). Sage.

Hinckley, J. (2005). The piano lesson: An autoethnography about changing clinical paradigms in aphasia practice. *Aphasiology, 19*(8), 765–777.

Holman Jones, S. (2005). Autoethnography: Making the personal political. In N. K. Denzin & Y. S. Lincoln (Eds.), *Handbook of qualitative research* (3rd ed., pp. 763–792). Sage.

Janesick, V. L. (1994). The dance of qualitative research design: Metaphor, methodolatry, and meaning. In N. K. Denzin & Y. S. Lincoln (Eds.), *Handbook of qualitative research* (pp. 209–219). Sage.

McCreery, R. W., Walker, E. A., Stiles, D. J., Spratford, M., Oleson, J. J., & Lewis, D. E. (2020). Audibility-based hearing aid fitting criteria for children with mild hearing loss. *Language, Speech, and Hearing Services in Schools, 51,* 55–67.

Oliver, M. (1990). *The politics of disablement.* Macmillan.

Patton, M. Q. (2015). *Qualitative research & evaluation methods* (4th ed.). Sage.

Pirsig, R. M. (1974). *Zen and the art of motorcycle maintenance: An inquiry into values.* William Morrow and Company.

Popper, K. R. (1959). *The logic of scientific discovery.* Hutchinson & Co.

Rehorick, D. A., & Bentz, V. M. (2008). *Transformative phenomenology. Changing ourselves, lifeworlds, and professional practice.* Lexington.

Srivastava, P., & Hopwood, N. (2009). A practical iterative framework for qualitative data analysis. *International Journal of Qualitative Methods, 8*(1), 76–84.

Winiger, A. M., Alexander, J. M., & Diefendorf, A. O. (2016). Minimal hearing loss: From a failure-based approach to evidence-based practice. *American Journal of Audiology, 25*(3), 232–245.

15

Research Grants

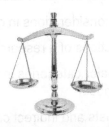

LEARNING OBJECTIVES

Upon completion of this chapter, the reader will be able to:

- Identify the three phases of the grants acquisition process
- Identify reference sources available for the seeking of grants from federal and private agencies
- List general principles of the grant-seeking process
- Discuss preliminary considerations in grant proposal writing
- Identify the major sections of a research grant proposal
- List and define the major categories in the budget section of a research grant proposal
- Differentiate direct costs and indirect costs associated with a research grant proposal
- Discuss the sources of ideas/problems for research projects
- Identify basic principles of grant proposal writing
- List suggestions for grant proposal writing
- Identify the characteristics of a fundable research grant proposal
- Describe the grant proposal review process

Introduction

There is a strong association between research activities and grants. Without grants from the government and private sector, much of the research in communication disorders (and many fields) would not be possible. In addition to any available internal funds, for those involved in research, it is essential to locate a specific external source(s) of support for their activities. For example, a university professor or hospital audiologist or school speech-language pathologist who has an interest in a specific communication disorder and wishes to pursue a research project to learn more about the disorder, may find that funds are not available within their agency to support the necessary personnel, equipment, materials, travel, and other items that are needed to conduct the research. The only feasible approach for obtaining funds for the research may be through external sources (such as the federal government or private foundations), and the only way to obtain external support is to write a grant proposal to a particular funding agency. Moreover, the importance of grants is further accentuated in academia, where support for research activities is essential for conducting research, and conducting research is essential for publications in scholarly journals, which, in turn, are essential for the awarding of tenure, which is essential for maintaining one's position in a university. Therefore, grants may be the mechanism for job stability and may play a major role in the "publish or perish" philosophy in institutions of higher education.

The Grants Acquisition Process

Acquiring grant support may appear to the uninitiated as somewhat "mystical" in nature. However, in reality, there is nothing magical about the grants acquisition process. In fact, it is a systematic process that can be considered in three phases: grant seeking, grant proposal writing, and grant management. First, the investigator seeks sources of support whose mission and interests coincide with the goals and nature of his or her project. Next, the investigator writes a grant proposal following the guidelines established by the sponsoring agency. Finally, if a grant is awarded, the investigator manages the research project, including the expenditure of awarded funds.

Grant Seeking

Grant seeking involves searching for a source of funding for a specific research project, thus matching the nature of the topic with the objectives of the support source. There are various sources of external support for research projects, the largest being the federal government. In addition, national organizations and private corporations are potential sources for competitive grants.

Foundations are another major source of support in the private sector. A foundation is a nongovernmental, nonprofit organization whose funds and programs are managed by its own trustees or directors and established to maintain or aid educational, charitable, or other activities serving the common welfare, primarily through the awarding of grants. There are different types of foundations, but the type that serves as the primary source of support for research projects is the independent foundation.

In addition to **extramural** (outside the institution) **funding** sources, colleges and universities provide support for research in the form of relatively small grants as "seed money" for starting new research projects. These **intramural** (within the institution) **funding**, although relatively small, are essential for collecting preliminary data and providing the foundation for external funding. These funds can be a very important component in the decisions for funding made by outside agencies.

Numerous references are available to locate potential funding sources in both the public and private sectors. Much of this information can be found online, most of it free and some fee-based. The following are representative samples of references available for grant-seeking purposes.

■ *Catalog of Federal Domestic Assistance* (CFDA; http://www .cfda.gov) is a valuable reference source to learn about relevant federal programs, eligibility requirements, and application deadlines. It provides access to a database of all available federal programs that can be searched in a number of ways, including key words, agency, applicant eligibility, type of assistance, and several other factors. There is a category specifically for finding grants that would be of most relevance to seekers of support for research activities. There is also a CFDA User Guide that can be downloaded.

■ *Foundation Center* (http://www .foundationcenter.org) collects, organizes, and communicates information on U.S. philanthropy; provides education and training on the grant-seeking process; and allows public access to information and services through its website, print, and electronic publications, library/learning centers, and a national network of Cooperating Collections. Included on its website are general and specialized information retrieval tools.

■ *Foundation Directory Online* (https://fconline.foundationcenter. org), developed by the Foundation Center, is part of an online subscription set of databases providing access to information on grant makers and their giving interests. Searches include text-based foundation searches, grant searches, and IRS 990 searches. (IRS 990 forms are the tax forms completed by foundations that contain information on awarded grants, including recipients and titles of projects funded, which could be very useful information to grant seekers.)

■ *infoEd Global's Sponsored Programs Information Network (SPIN)* (http://www.infoedglobal .com) is a computer database containing information on grant opportunities from federal and private sponsoring agencies. The database is targeted primarily to institutions of higher education. infoEd Global, the company that maintains the *SPIN* database, also offers an alert service called **SMARTS**, which sends email messages whenever there is a match between the grant seeker's choice of key words and the funding programs in the **SPIN** funding opportunities database. This website indicates that their database is the world's largest database of sponsored funding opportunities (over 40,000 opportunities from more than 10,000 global sponsors). A subscription is required.

- **Grants.Gov** (http://www.grants .gov), a central storehouse for information on grant programs offered by federal grant-making agencies, allows grant seekers to electronically find and apply for competitive grant opportunities from these federal agencies. Those interested in research grants can (a) register for email notification of grant opportunities; (b) access, download, complete, and submit active grant application packages; and (c) check the status of grant applications submitted via Grants.gov.

- **GrantSelect** (http://www.grant select.com) provides an extensive list of funding opportunities from state and federal government agencies (including National Institutes of Health [NIH], National Science Foundation [NSF], Centers for Disease Control and Prevention [CDC], and others), corporations, foundations, research institutes, and other nonprofit organizations. Grant seekers can subscribe to the entire research grants database or choose from customized segments, including arts and humanities, biomedical and health care, children and youth,

community development, international programs, and others.

- **Guidestar** (http://www.guidestar .org) allows grant seekers to search for information on nonprofit organizations, including foundations. It provides general information as well as specifics, including foundations' current IRS Form 990, income range, contact information, mission, programs, goals, boards of directors, grants awarded, and other relevant information.

- **Pivot** (formerly **Community of Science**; http://pivot.cos.com) is a resource for hard-to-find information critical to scientific research and other projects across all disciplines. It provides grant seekers the opportunity to search a comprehensive resource for funding opportunities. It also contains prepopulated scholar profiles worldwide to match a given institution's profiles against funding opportunities and to find potential collaborators from among the scholar profiles.

- **Society of Research Administrators (SRA) International** (http:// www.srainternational.org/sra03/ grantsweb/index.cfm) is a source for finding funds available from local, state, federal, and international governments. It also contains information to locate private funding for projects, including links to foundations, nonprofit centers, and charities.

- **GrantsNet** (http://www.hhs.gov/ grantsnet) is an internet application tool created by the Department of Health and Human Services (HHS) for finding and exchanging information about HHS and other federal grant programs. In support of its mission, HHS is the largest grant-awarding agency in the federal government.

- **Ed.Gov** (http://www.ed.gov), the website of the U.S. Department of Education (ED), contains answers to frequently asked questions about funding opportunities; information on and instructions for completing grant application packages; application packages for ED grant competitions that are currently open; announcements of grant competitions; all programs and competitions under which ED has invited or expects to invite applications for new awards; deadlines for the submission of applications; and the **Guide to ED** Programs, which describes all programs administered by ED (including the National Institute on Disability and Rehabilitation Research [NIDRR]). It also provides a search tool to find ED programs relevant to grant seekers' interests.

- **National Science Foundation** (http://www.nsf.gov/) is an independent federal agency created by Congress to promote science, health, citizen welfare, and national defense. This website includes information about research projects that NSF has funded since 1989 by searching the **Award Abstracts** database. The information includes abstracts that describe the research as well as names of principal investigators and their institutions. The database includes both completed and current research projects.

- **National Institute on Deafness and Other Communication Disorders (NIDCD)**, a member of the National Institutes of Health (NIH), is mandated to conduct and support behavioral and biomedical research and research training in the normal and disordered processes of voice, speech, language, balance, smell, and taste. The Institute also conducts and supports research and research training related to special behavioral and biomedical problems associated with people who have communication impairments or disorders as well as efforts to create devices that substitute for lost and impaired communication and sensory functions. The extramural program funds research and training opportunities at universities, medical centers, and other institutions throughout the United States and abroad through research grants, career development awards, and other mechanisms.

- **American Speech-Language-Hearing Association** (http://www.asha.org) contains information on research grants offered by the American Speech-Language-Hearing Foundation (http://www.ashafoundation.org) and federal agencies (including the National Institutes of Health, Agency for Healthcare Research and Quality, Department of Education, National Science Foundation, Centers for Disease Control and Prevention, and U.S. Department of Veterans Affairs) as well as private foundations and organizations (http://www.asha.org/research/grants-funding/Funding-for-Researchers.htm). Also included on this website is information and suggestions on the grants acquisition process, including grant seeking and grant proposal writing.

- **American Academy of Audiology** (AAA; http://www.audiology.org)

contains information on research grants offered jointly by the Academy (AAA) and the Academy of Audiology Foundation (AAF; http:// www.audiology.org/about/ foundation) to support research, education and public awareness in audiology and hearing science as well as other sources, including federal agencies, private foundations, and national organizations in hearing and balance. In support of this goal, the AAA and the AAF provide research funding through the Research Grants in Hearing & Balance Program and the New Investigator Program.

■ *American Hearing Research Foundation* (http://american-hearing.org) funds research in hearing and balance disorders. It awards an average of five to ten research projects per year, with an average grant of approximately $20,000. Priority is given to investigators early in their careers who need seed funds to generate results and data that can be used to support later applications for larger grants (e.g., NIH or NSF grants) in the future. This site has links to a research grant application as well as a list of former recipients and their research topics from 1996 through the present.

■ *Capita Foundation* (http://www .capitafoundation.org) is dedicated to the support of cutting-edge innovative auditory research worldwide. The majority of Capita Foundation grants fund early-stage research and projects by early career research scientists, allowing them to produce the preliminary results needed to secure grants from the NIH and

other major funders. Grant applications are welcomed from scientists conducting research in line with the Foundation's mission statement to "support innovative research that works toward the prevention and cure of hearing disorders."

■ *Federal Grants and Contracts* (http://www.federalgrantsand contracts.com/about.aspx) is a comprehensive biweekly review of the latest funding opportunities across all federal agencies. It covers relevant grant opportunities announced each week, provides information on upcoming grant initiatives, and offers news on standing cyclical grant competitions. It researches many online and print channels of federal information and resources, and provides specific information on scope, deadline, funds, eligibility, and contact needed to start the grant application process.

■ *The Grantsmanship Center* (http:// www.tgci.com) offers training programs that include information, resources, best approaches, tips, and insights to avoid trial-and-error learning. These training programs provide an overview of the entire proposal development process, highlighting the key elements that make proposals competitive. Also addressed is an understanding of federal application guidelines and design of a proposal development work plan.

Other reference sources on research grants include the following directories. Information on their availability can be obtained via online searches (e.g., Google) as well as at other websites (e.g., Amazon.com).

- *Annual Register of Grant Support* is a directory of grant and fellowship programs of foundations and governmental agencies as well as business, professional, and other organizations.
- *Directory of Biomedical and Health Care Grants* includes U.S. and international grant programs of governmental agencies, foundations, corporations, and professional organizations.
- *Directory of Research Grants* contains a listing of grant opportunities from federal agencies as well as U.S. and international foundations, corporations, government agencies, and other organizations. Included are grants for fellowships, basic research, equipment, building construction/renovation, and other program types.
- *Taft Foundation Reporter* provides comprehensive profiles and gives analyses of America's major private foundations in annual grants to nonprofit organizations. It contains information on corporate foundations and direct giving programs.

General Principles of Grant Seeking

The following are some general principles applicable to the grant-seeking process:

- Search databases of existing grants from relevant funding agencies
- Understand a funding agency's mission and what types of topics of research it wishes to fund
- Match an agency whose goals fit your research project topic

- Contact the contact person (program officer) to discuss your proposed project in order to determine its feasibility for support

Additional information on the grant-seeking process is provided by Bauer (2017) and Licklider (2012).

Grant Proposal Writing

Preliminary Considerations

Once the grant-seeking phase has been completed and the agency has been identified as a potential funding source for the proposed research project, the next major step is to write the grant proposal. However, before the writing begins, there are some preliminary considerations:

1. Obtain an application from the sponsoring agency's website.
2. Carefully review the agency's guidelines (located in the application material) for the relevant grants program, which should contain the following important information:
   - suggested format for the proposal;
   - any necessary appendices;
   - deadline dates;
   - any applicable cost-sharing requirements for the applicant;
   - allowable indirect cost rates;
   - criteria used to judge each proposal; and
   - relative weighting of each factor in the criteria.

The guidelines should be followed exactly as specified. If any of this information is missing from the guidelines or if there are questions about the guidelines, the sponsoring agency's contact person (whose name, email and/or postal address, and telephone number are listed in the application material) should be contacted for clarifications.

The Grant Proposal

The grant proposal usually contains the following major sections:

- Introduction
- Problem Statement (Needs Assessment)
- Objectives
- Methodology
- Budget

Writing a research grant proposal is somewhat similar to writing a manuscript for publication in a journal or a master's thesis or a doctoral dissertation because all include a review of the pertinent literature, a statement of purpose of the research, and a description of the methodology to study a proposed purpose or problem. However, since a research grant proposal is written before the proposed research is conducted, it includes a budget section requesting funds to conduct the research.

The Budget

The major categories of the budget usually include the following:

- *Personnel*—the people who will be working on the project, including the principal investigator and other personnel, as well as the amount of time they will be working on the project.
- *Fringe Benefits*—whenever grant funds are used to pay salaries and wages, associated fringe benefits must also be charged to the grant. The fringe benefit rate and percentage usually include social security, unemployment/worker's compensation, retirement, and health insurance. It is a percentage of the base salary of the persons working on the research project and will vary from institution to institution.
- *Travel*—funds to travel to professional meetings to present the findings of the research project and, depending on the nature of the research, may include funds to travel to collect data and other related research activities.
- *Equipment*—any necessary instrumentation to conduct the research. For many organizations, equipment is defined as any item with a unit acquisition cost of $5,000 or more and a lifespan of two or more years.
- *Supplies*—needed supplies and materials.
- *Contractual*—any necessary contractual agreements with other agencies or individuals as part of the research project.
- *Other*—other items not covered in the previous six categories.
- *Total Direct Costs*—the sum of the seven budget categories previously listed.
- *Indirect Costs*—expenditures not included directly in any of the budget categories previously listed, such as the cost of heating/cooling, electricity, maintenance, security

of facilities used for the research project, the processing of paperwork for purchases associated with the project, administrative costs, and other related expenses.

■ **Total Project Costs**—the total cost of the research project, including all direct and indirect costs.

It should be noted that grant proposals need not include all seven budget categories previously listed. Only budget items that can be justified because they relate directly to the methodology should be included in the proposed budget for the research project.

The Idea or Problem

A fundable proposal includes a good idea/problem that is expressed well and with an appropriate plan for implementation. The idea/problem for a research grant proposal should ask an important theoretical or applied question(s) capable of being systematically studied. A few questions to ask and answer about the idea/problem for a research study are as follows:

■ Is it important (regarding discovery, improvement, or application of knowledge)?
■ Is it timely today?
■ Is it capable of being investigated (regarding the availability of personnel, expertise, techniques, instrumentation, facilities, etc.)?

Ideas/problems for a research project come from various sources, including the following:

■ the applicant's previous experiences (e.g., teaching, research, clinical practice, administration, etc.);

■ the applicant's literature reading and familiarity with the area of investigation;
■ unresolved problems in the applicant's field of study;
■ potential applications of previous research findings; and
■ priority areas for funding established by sponsoring agencies.

Unsolicited and Solicited Proposals

An **unsolicited proposal** is one that is written without any specific guidelines provided by a sponsoring agency and is not in response to a particular need or problem expressed by a sponsoring agency. Instead, it originates from a need perceived by the applicant who tries to find a sponsor to support the proposal. Unsolicited proposals have no specific deadline dates for submission and usually are reviewed and accepted by sponsoring agencies at any time rather than at specified dates each year.

On the other hand, solicited proposals originate with a sponsoring agency that recognizes a need for something to be done or learned. Solicited proposals are usually announced by a Request for Application (RFA) or Request for Proposal (RFP), which identifies problem areas and may include specific objectives to be met.

Basic Principles of Grant Proposal Writing

■ The grant proposal should contain clear, concise writing with definitions/explanations for all appropriate terms. (Grants cannot be awarded for projects that are not understood by a sponsoring agency's reviewers.)

■ All factual statements should be documented with cited references to support them.

■ An objective and strong case for funding should be provided with sufficient empirical evidence presented to support the investigator's position.

■ The idea/problem for funding should be relevant, feasible, important, and contemporary.

■ The methodology proposed should be well-designed for accomplishing the objectives of the project.

■ The project personnel should be shown (via their curriculum vitae or resume) to be qualified to conduct the research.

■ The budget should be realistic by containing only items that are justifiable and relevant to the proposed project.

A knowledge of grant application deficiencies is helpful. Some common deficiencies are inadequate control of relevant variables, deficiency in methodology, research design problem(s), poor conceptualization of problem(s), and inappropriate statistical analyses.

Suggestions for Grant Proposal Writing

■ Read and follow the sponsoring agency's guidelines.

■ Begin writing early, well in advance of the submission deadline.

■ Set a deadline to complete each section of the grant proposal.

■ Define a specific, focused problem.

■ Develop procedures to study the problem.

■ Draft the body (narrative) of the proposal.

■ Develop a realistic budget, with valid justifications for all items in the budget.

■ Add any required additional components to the proposal (e.g., relevant assurance forms).

■ If possible, share a draft of the proposal with colleagues for their review and comments.

■ Revise the proposal based on any relevant comments and suggestions before submitting the finalized proposal.

Characteristics of a Fundable Research Grant Proposal

In summary, a fundable research grant proposal, one that should receive serious consideration for funding, should contain the following features that have been expressed by numerous investigators who have been cited earlier:

■ A clearly established need for the proposed research, preferably with supporting data, is provided.

■ Clear objectives of the project are described.

■ A detailed schedule of activities for the project, with realistic timelines, is explained.

■ If relevant, commitment of all involved agencies/consultants verified with letters of commitment in the appendix is provided.

■ Any relevant cost-sharing is included in the proposal.

■ All budget items are justifiable and consistent with the proposed purpose and procedures of the research project; all budget explanations/justifications provide an adequate basis for the dollar figures used in the budget section.

■ All major items included in the funding agency's guidelines are addressed in the proposal.

■ All appropriate assurance forms are completed, indicating that all governmental and nongovernmental agency requirements have been fulfilled.

■ All sections of the proposal contain sufficient details and address all relevant issues.

■ All directions in the funding agency's guidelines have been followed.

■ Appropriate appendices have been included to provide evidence of careful planning of the research project.

■ The writing style is clear and concise.

■ The length of the proposal does not exceed the funding agency's guidelines.

■ The qualifications of project personnel are clearly indicated (via resumes, curriculum vitae, etc.) in the proposal.

Additional information on the writing of grant proposals (some of which also include grant seeking as well as grant writing) is provided by Clarke and Fox (2007), Coley and Scheinberg (2017), Geever (2012), Gerin and Kapelewski Kinkade (2018), Gitlin and Lyons (2014), Grant Central (2018), Grayson (2005), Henson (2012), Karsh and Fox (2014), Kiritz and Floersch (2017), Miner and Miner (2013), O'Neal-McElrath (2013), Pequegnat et al. (2011), Rajan and Tomal (2015), Reif-

Lehrer (2005), Savage (2017), Smith and Works (2012), Ward (2015), Wason (2011), and Yang (2012).

The Grant Proposal Review Process

Although the specific process of reviewing research grant proposals may vary from one funding agency to another, there are some commonalities applicable to all reviews. Proposals usually are reviewed by the investigator's peers, generally colleagues at other institutions or laboratories who are knowledgeable about the topic of the proposal. Sponsoring agencies base their decisions about the awarding of grants on reviewers' comments. Usually, reviewers are required to follow specific criteria and use some type of rating scale established by the sponsoring agency to judge the merits of each proposal. Moreover, some agencies, like the National Institutes of Health (NIH), have a specific rating system for all proposals and a face-to-face meeting of a panel of peers to arrive at decisions for funding proposals. Additional information on the peer-review process can be found online at the websites of various funding agencies (e.g., https://public.csr.nih.gov).

Grant Management

Each grant usually has one principal investigator (project director) who is responsible for all activities and expenditures associated with the grant. Once a grant is awarded, there needs to be competent management of the funds because the grantee is held accountable for all expended funds. In addition, there are reporting requirements, frequently annual reports to the sponsoring agency delineating progress in research activities and fund expenditures. However, some agencies require more than an annual report. The award notification letter or an addendum to the letter should specify all reporting requirements.

Usually, funds awarded in a grant are specified and earmarked for particular budget categories (e.g., personnel, equipment, travel, etc.). However, on occasion, because of unexpected expenses or unexpected increases in approved budget items, there is a need to modify the existing approved budget. Most sponsoring agencies have an established rule of allowing the transfer of no more than a specific percentage of the entire budget from specific line items to other specific line items without the need for prior approval from the sponsoring agency. However, in cases that exceed this maximum percentage, the principal investigator must make a written request to transfer funds from one budget category to another and must receive approval in writing from the person at the sponsoring agency who is authorized to do so. In addition, the same is true for other necessary nonmonetary changes in the research project: the principal investigator must make a request in writing and must receive approval in writing from the appropriate authorized representative of the sponsoring agency.

Thus, once a grant is awarded, the grantee's responsibilities begin. In addition to conducting the proposed research, the principal investigator is responsible for the expending of funds approved by the sponsoring agency (and in the amounts approved) as well as for any fiscal and programmatic reporting requirements.

Summary

Grants are essential for conducting research. The process of grants acquisition involves three phases: grant seeking, grant proposal writing, and grant management. Grant seeking is searching for funds from internal as well as external sources, including governmental agencies, private foundations, corporations, and national organizations. Grant proposal writing involves the preparation of a proposal that makes a strong case for financial support and follows the guidelines established by the sponsoring agency. Grant management involves conducting the research project and expending funds associated with the project as delineated in the grant proposal and approved by the sponsoring agency. In addition, it involves the preparation of fiscal and programmatic reports to the sponsoring agency. Detailed information and suggestions concerning each phase of the grants acquisition process were presented in this chapter.

DISCUSSION QUESTIONS

1. What are the three phases associated with the grants acquisition process?
2. What are some available online and hard copy reference sources for locating information on research grant opportunities from federal and private agencies?
3. What are some preliminary considerations in writing a research grant proposal?
4. What are the major sections of a research grant proposal?
5. What are the major categories in the budget section of a research grant proposal?
6. What is the difference between direct costs and indirect costs associated with a research grant?
7. What are some sources of ideas/problems for research projects?
8. List some basic principles of grant proposal writing.
9. List some suggestions for research grant proposal writing.
10. What are the characteristics of a fundable research grant proposal?
11. Who reviews research grant proposals and makes recommendations for funding?
12. What are the responsibilities of the principal investigator in the management of a research grant?

References

Bauer, D. G. (2017). *The "how to" grants manual: Successful grant-seeking techniques for obtaining public and private grants* (8th ed.). Rowman & Littlefield.

Clarke, C. A., & Fox, S. P. (2007). *Grant proposal makeover: Transform your request from no to yes.* JosseyBass.

Coley, S. M., & Scheinberg, C. A. (2017). *Proposal writing: Effective grantsmanship for funding* (5th ed.). Sage.

Geever, J. C. (2012). *The Foundation Center's guide to proposal writing* (6th ed.). The Foundation Center.

Gerin, W., & Kapelewski Kinkade, C. (2018). *Writing the NIH grant proposal: A step-by-step guide* (3rd ed.). The Grantsmanship Center.

Gitlin, L. N., & Lyons, K. J. (2014). *Successful grant writing: Strategies for health and human service professionals* (4th ed.). Springer.

Grant Central. (2018). *Grant writers' seminars & workshops: Training in the art of grantsmanship. (New NIH and NSF versions of The Grant Application Writer's Workbook).* http://www.grant central.com

Grayson, H. M. (2005). *Guide to government grants writing: Tools for success.* iUniverse.

Henson, K. (2012). *Grant writing in higher education: A step-by-step guide.* Pearson Education.

Karsh, E., & Fox, A. S. (2014). *The only grant-writing book you'll ever need* (3rd ed.). Basic Books.

Kiritz, N. J., & Floersch, B. (2017). *Grantsmanship: Program planning & proposal writing* (2nd ed.). The Grantsmanship Center.

Licklider, M. M. (2012). *Grant seeking in higher education: Strategies and tools for college faculty.* Jossey-Bass.

Miner, J. T., & Miner, L. E. (2013). *Models of proposal planning and writing* (5th ed.) ABC-CLIO.

O'Neal-McElrath, T. (2013). *Winning grants, step-by-step: The complete workbook for planning, developing, and writing successful proposals* (4th ed.). Jossey-Bass.

Pequegnat, W., Stover, E., & Boyce, C. A. (Eds.). (2011). *How to write a successful research grant application: A guide for social and behavioral scientists* (2nd ed.). Springer.

Rajan, R. S., & Tomal, D. R. (2015). *Grant writing: Practical strategies for scholars and professionals*. Rowman & Littlefield.

Reif-Lehrer, L. (2005). *Grant application writer's handbook* (4th ed.). Jones & Bartlett.

Savage, C. (2017). *Grant writing: A simple, clear and concise guide.*

Smith, N. B., & Works, E. G. (2012). *The complete book of grant writing: Learn to write grants like a professional* (2nd ed.). Sourcebooks.

Ward, D. (2015). *Writing grant proposals that win* (4th ed.). Jones & Bartlett.

Wason, S. D. (2011). *Webster's new world grant writing handbook*. Wiley.

Yang, O. O. (2012). *Guide to effective grant writing: How to write an effective NIH grant application* (2nd ed.). Springer.

Glossary

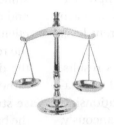

A-B design: single-case design with two phases: A represents the baseline phase and B represents the intervention phase.

A-B-A design: a single-case withdrawal design in which a second baseline phase is introduced.

Abstract: brief description of a paper, usually located at the beginning of an article.

Alternative hypothesis: opposite of null hypothesis, typically specifies significant differences between groups or conditions during statistical testing.

Analytic generalization: A view of generalization that purports that qualitative research methods study the underlying human processes of the behavior in question. Results of these analyses are applicable to a wider population because they were derived from basic, systematic human processes that are common to all humans.

Applied research: research that seeks

to answer practical questions such as those pertaining to prevention and management of communication disorders; also known as clinical research.

Artifact: any object, document, or visual representation collected (or created) during the research process that is used as data. Artifacts can include photographs, videos, texts, artworks, or physical objects. They provide researchers with tangible sources of information that offer insight into participants' experiences, behaviors, or meanings. Examples include homework portfolios in a study of students' struggling with writing, family photographs in a study of intergenerational trauma, or disused augmentative alternative communication (AAC) devices in a study of emerging technologies for communication disorders.

Assurance forms: standardized forms completed by the applicant agency to assure the funding agency that the applicant agency meets all requirements to qualify for funding.

Baseline measure: measurement of dependent variable before experimental intervention.

Basic research: research that is often theoretical; designed to seek answers that explain and/or predict phenomena.

Between-subject design: design that uses two groups of subjects, each group is assigned to a different level of the independent variable.

Bias: any influence that affects results.

Bivariate statistics: test used to analyze significance of the relationship between two variables simultaneously, for example, correlation.

Blinding: process of preventing those involved in a study (subjects, clinicians, data collectors) from having information that could bias. Same as masking.

Bricolage: a term to describe the "unsystematic" nature of the qualitative research process, which does not imply "disorganized" but rather "not stepwise." Qualitative work does not proceed in a linear fashion from step A to D via B and C (where A is, for example, a hypothesis and D an experimental result). Instead, it brings together emerging information by going from the detail to the whole and back to the detail, garnering related information along the way. Thus, rather than A $\rightarrow$ B $\rightarrow$ C $\rightarrow$ D, the process may take a form such as A $\rightarrow$ D^0 $\rightarrow$ B, A $\rightarrow$ D^1 $\rightarrow$ xyz + C $\rightarrow$ D^2 $\rightarrow$ abc $\rightarrow$ D^3, where D^3 represents the final "big picture" that may already have emerged in the second "step" (D^0) but got substantially modified by incoming information.

CADE: critically appraised topic of diagnostic evidence.

CAPE: checklist for appraising patient/practice evidence.

CAPP: checklist for appraising evidence on patient preference.

Case-control studies: when individuals are selected whether they have a particular disorder or not.

Case-to-case transfer: a type of generalization that occurs when a reader consumes a published qualitative study and decides to apply the findings to a client he/she is seeing. The reader of the research is responsible for making the decision regarding generalization rather than the researcher.

Case study research: intensive study of the background, current status, or environmental interactions of an individual, group, institution, or community.

CASM: critical appraisal of systematic review or meta-analysis.

CATE: critical appraisal of treatment evidence.

Charge master: a spreadsheet that is part of the budgetary process and includes all expenses related to the implementation of a research study.

Class I level of evidence: the highest level of evidence provided by at least one well-designed, randomized controlled clinical trial.

Class II level of evidence: evidence provided by at least one or better designed observational, clinical studies with concurrent controls, that is, single case-control or cohort-control studies.

Class III level of evidence: the lowest level of evidence; provided by expert opinion, case studies, case reports, and studies with historical controls.

Clinical practice guidelines: literature review usually a consensus by a group of experts for use in making clinical decisions. There are three types: traditional clinical practice guidelines, systematic reviews, and evidence-based clinical practice guidelines.

Clinical research: research designed to generate knowledge to guide the clinical practice in speech-language pathology and audiology; also known as applied research.

Clinical trial: study designed to investigate outcome.

Code: a verbal label or tag assigned to segments of data. Good codes explicate underlying concepts, themes, or patterns in the data and help researchers identify recurring ideas, behaviors, or phenomena within the dataset. As an example, an interviewee in a study on the first day of wearing hearing aids at school might describe their experience as follows: "All the kids were staring at me. It was embarrassing." Researchers may code this as "shame"; if they encounter a similar statement, they may then give it the same code, or a similar one such as "stigma." Related or same codes are synthesized into themes. As such, coding is the crucial first step in qualitative data analysis.

Cohort study: follows the temporal sequence of factors that may have impacted the development of a disorder.

Complementary design: the result of the dominant research method being enhanced or clarified by results from the findings of the other type of research.

Complex hypothesis: the hypothesis contains more than one independent and dependent variable.

Concept maps: require selecting important relevant concepts to add to the map and identifying salient cross-links as well as indicating relationships between concepts in different sections of the map.

Confidence interval: an inferential statistic for estimating range of values within which a population parameter is found.

Confirmability: refers to sharing findings with participants by informant checks or feedback sessions to confirm the view of the person being studied.

Conflict of commitment: conflicting demands on professionals who have obligations to their patients and to others including students and other professionals.

Conflict of interest: situations where personal and/or financial considerations compromise judgment in any professional activity.

Consent process: involves meeting with a potential subject, finding out whether he or she is capable of giving consent, and discussing the purpose, risks, and benefits of participation.

Constant comparison: the ongoing process, during qualitative data collection, of comparing new data with previously collected data to identify similarities, differences, and patterns. This iterative process helps researchers refine codes and themes, and thence promotes rigor and credibility.

Constant variable: variables that describe the population investigated by a study; variables that do not change from individual to individual (such as a diagnosis of stuttering).

Construct validity: the extent to which a test or questionnaire measures what it is supposed to measure.

Consumer of research: someone who can effectively utilize research to guide clinical decision-making based on available evidence.

Content validity: a logical examination of all behaviors that need to be measured in order to adequately answer the question.

Continuous variable: a quantitative variable that can theoretically take on values along a continuum.

Control group: a group that does not receive treatment; equivalent to the experimental group in age, sex, and so on.

Convenience sampling: using the most readily available persons as participants, sometimes called accidental sampling.

Coordinated substudies: qualitative studies that are part of a larger program project or long-term study.

Correlation: tendency for variation in one variable to be related to variation in another variable; an interrelation between two or more variables.

Correlation coefficient: a measure of the direction and strength of the relationship between variables usually ranging from +1.00 (perfect positive) through zero (no relationship) to −1.00 (perfect negative) relationships.

Correlational research: used to determine possible relationships among factors.

Cost-benefit analysis: an evaluation comparing financial costs with financial gains attributed to a program or intervention.

Cost-sharing requirements: expenses associated with a grant that are to be incurred by the applicant agency to share the expense of the research project with the funding agency.

Cover letter: typically includes the purpose, conveys appreciation to the participant, states that the survey has been approved by the appropriate committee or advisor, and offers to provide a summary of the results.

Credibility: the extent to which data are believable and trustworthy, that is, confidence in the truth of the data.

Criterion-related (predictive) validity: the measure of an attribute to predict future performance.

Critical Appraisal Topic/Paper (CAT/ CAP): a summary of a critical review of the best evidence on a specific topic; a written outcome of the evidence-based practice (EBP) process.

Cross-sectional research: involves selecting subjects from various age groups and observing differences between the behavior and characteristics of the group.

Database: information accessed by using electronic hardware.

Deception: deliberate withholding of information or misinformation.

Dependability: the qualitative equivalent to reliability of quantitative research.

Dependent variable: variable that is the effect of unknown etiology(ies) and must be described in operational terms; an outcome variable (dependent on the independent variable).

Descriptive research: designed to systemically describe situations or events as they naturally occur, in other words, the status of phenomena of interest as they currently exist.

Descriptive statistics: procedures for describing and analyzing quantitative data.

Design: the structure of a study organized for the purpose of revealing cause-and-effect relationships by controlling variables, comparing groups, or analyzing specific characteristics of individuals or groups.

Direct costs: expenses related to personnel, fringe benefits, travel, equipment, supplies, and contractual matters.

Directional hypothesis: when a researcher states there will be a change or describes a relationship in a certain direction (i.e., high or low; positive or negative; etc.).

Discrete variable: a variable that can only be measured in separate units and that cannot be measured in intervals less than 1.

Dissertation: research project/paper typically associated with a doctoral degree.

Double-blind studies: a study in which the investigator and the subject do not know group assignment.

Editing analysis: involves interpretation of the data on which categorization is used for coding, sorting, and organizing the data.

Effectiveness: in research, it is defined as the benefits and use of the procedure under "real-world" conditions.

Effect size: a statistical expression of the magnitude of difference between two treatments or the magnitude of a relationship between variables.

Efficacy: in research, it is the benefit of an intervention plan as compared to a control or standard program.

Evaluation research: the collection and analysis of information related to the effects of a program, policy, or procedure.

Evidence-based practice: such practice increases professionalism, accountability to clients and other professionals, and the social relevance of the health services delivered in an economy with increased costs and decreased resources; utilization of the best available research to make clinical decisions about patient care.

Expansion design: involves using different methods for different components for a multimethod research project.

Experimental research: examines possible cause-and-effect relationships by exposing one or more experimental groups to one or more conditions and comparing the results to one or more control groups.

Experimental treatment: utilizes the principles of experimental research investigating the use of new or novel treatment.

Exploded pie chart: emphasizes the proportion of time devoted to a topic or area that is displayed in a pie chart.

Exploratory research: examines how one event or multiple events relate to other factors.

External validity: degree results of a study can be generalized to persons or settings outside the experimental situation.

Extramural funding: funding for research projects provided by agencies outside the researcher's institution.

Extraneous variable: a variable that confounds the relationship between the independent and dependent variable.

Extrinsic variables: variables associated with the research situation or environment; related to the place and time the research was conducted and adherence (or not) to the research specification or protocols.

Fabrication: making up data or results and recording or reporting data for experiments never conducted.

Factorial designs: manipulating two or more independent variables; one group in the design accounts for each possible combination of the levels of the independent variables.

Feasibility test: a researcher reviews factors that could influence the possibility of a study being conducted.

Fidelity: maintaining integrity in use of a test or treatment.

Focus groups: a method of interviewing a group of individuals about a specific topic or issue.

Foundation: a nongovernmental, nonprofit organization whose funds and programs are managed by its own trustees or directors and established to maintain or aid educational, charitable, or other activities serving the common welfare, primarily through the awarding of grants.

Frequency polygon: a graphic display of a frequency distribution; created by drawing a straight line between the success midpoints of class intervals.

Fringe benefits: an item in the budget section of a grant proposal that usually includes social security, workers' compensation, health insurance, unemployment compensation, and a retirement plan. It is a percentage of the base salary of personnel on a funded research project and will vary from institution to institution.

Ghost authorship: failure to name as an author an individual who has made substantial contribution that merits authorship or an unnamed individual who participated in writing the manuscript; also known as honorary authorship.

Gold standard: an instrument that is considered a valid measure and that can be used as the standard for assessing validity of other instruments.

Grant seeking: the process involved in searching for a source of funding for a specific research project, thus matching the nature of the topic with the objectives of the support source.

Grants acquisition process: the process for securing a funding source that involves three phases: grant seeking, grant proposal writing, and grant management.

Group designs: design involving comparison of average or typical performance of a group to other groups or conditions; includes between-subject designs, within-subject designs, and mixed-group designs.

Health Insurance Portability and Accountability Act of 1996 (HIPAA, Title II): required the Department of Health and Human Services (HHS) to establish national standards for electronic health-care transactions and national identifiers for providers, health plans, and employers. It also addresses the security and privacy of health data.

Histogram (graph): graphic display of frequency distribution data in which scores (often in group intervals) are plotted on the x-axis and frequency (or percent of cases) is plotted on the y-axis.

Hyperclarity: suggesting that research is likely to achieve what it is unlikely to achieve.

Hypothesis: statement concerning the relationship between variables; formulated to test theories.

Immersion method: a form of qualitative data analysis that involves total immersion in the problem; considered to be an insider's perspective.

Impact evaluation: to determine whether a program should be discontinued, replaced, modified, continued, or replicated.

Independent variable: variable with known qualities that explains the dependent variable; may be manipulated to determine effect on dependent variable.

Indirect costs: costs such as heating/cooling, electricity, maintenance, security, and administrative costs.

Inferential statistics: statistics used to test hypotheses by drawing inferences or generalizations from small groups to larger groups.

Informed consent: requires obtaining the consent of the individual to participate in a study based on full prior disclosure of risks and benefits.

Institutional Review Board (IRB): a group of diverse individuals who review research proposals to protect human and animal subjects through analysis of risks and benefits.

Interaction effect: combined effect of two or more independent variables on a dependent variable.

Interexaminer reliability: implies agreement among different observers measuring the same phenomenon.

Internal validity: degree of relationship between independent and dependent variables is free from the impact of extraneous/confounding variables.

Interpretive criteria: the intangible, elusive aspects of the written product that is the endpoint of the qualitative research process. Criteria such as thickness, richness, or quality cannot be fully defined or subjected to standardized measurement; in addition, they are never fully absent from a piece of writing, nor are they present in an idealized form. It is the responsibility of the consumer to gauge a study's interpretive criteria based on what is useful to their own purposes without glossing over any flaws they may have detected.

Interquartile range: difference between the first and third quartiles in a distribution.

Interval estimation: a statistic that indicates the upper and lower limits of a range of values in which the parameter has a given probability of occurring.

Interval scale: level of measurement in which values have equal intervals, but no true zero point.

Interview: a form of data collection in which questions are asked orally and participants' responses are recorded; may be structured, semistructured, or unstructured.

Intraexaminer reliability: implies that in repeated observations of the same subject, the same examiner gets similar results.

Intramural funding: in-house funds used to support research projects.

Intrinsic variables: variables associated with subjects of an investigation such as age, gender, socioeconomic status, and marital status.

Iterative coding: related to constant comparison, iterative coding involves continuously revisiting and revising existing codes to capture emerging meanings and especially nuances of previously captured meanings.

Level of significance: significance level selected to reject the null hypothesis established before statistical analysis to reduce the risk of making a Type I or Type II error; also known as limit of confidence.

Longitudinal research: the same group of subjects is followed over time; sometimes known as cohort study, follow-up study, incidence study, or perspective study.

Main effect: separate effect of one independent variable in a multifactor design.

Mañana syndrome: procrastination; frequently results in missing deadlines.

Mean: simple arithmetic average.

Measures of central tendency: measures representing the average or typical score in a distribution (mean, median, mode).

Median: a statistic describing the central tendency of scores in an ordinal scale; the midpoint in a set of values (same number of values as above and below the median).

Meta-analysis: a technique for quantitatively combining results of several studies on a given topic.

Mixed-group design: combines within-subject and between-subject designs to investigate effects of treatment for which carryover effects would be a problem while repeatedly sampling the behavior.

Mode: the most frequently occurring value in a distribution.

Multifactor baseline designs: include more than one independent variable and require that different combinations of the independent variable be tested across the study.

Multimethod or mixed research: combines both quantitative (outcome) and qualitative (process) features in the design, data collection, and analysis.

Multivariate designs: two or more dependent variables; provides information about the effect of the independent variable on each dependent variable and on a composite dependent variable.

Multivariate statistics: statistical procedures used to study the relationships between three or more variables.

Narrative review: nonsystematic review of the literature that synthesizes particular topics of interest; also known as a "review of the literature" in most research proposals.

Nominal scale: level of measurement for classification variables; values are assigned based on mutually exclusive and exhaustive categories with no inherent rank order.

Nonequivalent groups posttest-only design: a comparison between an experimental and control group both of whom are tested after treatment and not before treatment.

Nonexperimental research: descriptive (nonstatistical) organization of data; or ex post facto research.

Nonparametric statistics: a type of inferential statistics that does not involve vigorous assumptions about the parameters of the population from which the sample was drawn; used for nominal and ordinal measures.

Normal distribution: symmetric graphic display of the numerical values.

Null hypothesis: statement that there is no relationship between variables under study; opposite of the alternative hypothesis.

One-group postdesign: a type of pre-experimental design; involves study of the presumed effect of an independent variable in one group of subjects by administering a posttest after some treatment.

One-tailed (directional) test: a test of statistical significance in which only values at one extreme (tail) of a distribution are considered in testing significance.

Online: data that are accessed by the user who interacts directly with the electronic program to retrieve desired information.

Ordinal scale: level of measurement in which scores are ranked.

Outliers: scores that are outside the range of most scores.

Parallel designs: involve qualitative methods such as case studies, focused ethnographic observation, multiple linked in-depth interviews, or some combination of time in combination with other methods.

Parameter estimation: used to estimate a single parameter such as a mean.

Parametric statistics: a type of inferential statistics that involves making assumptions about the parameters of the population from which the research sample was drawn; used for interval or ratio measures.

Participant observer: when the researcher is an active participant in the activity being studied, that is, the researcher participates as a member of the group and is not known as the researcher.

Passive participant: is detached from the group being studied and is known as the researcher.

Peer review: the process by which the quality of research is assessed; involves multiple activities.

PESICO: framework for asking a question: P = person or problem, E = environments, S = stakeholder, I = intervention, C = comparison, O = outcome.

PICO: P = patient/population, I = intervention/treatment/exposure, C = comparison, and O = outcome; a method used in evidence-based practice/research.

Pie charts: used to represent the proportion of data falling into certain categories in the form of a circle containing segments that are also called slices, sections, or wedges.

Plagiarism: use of another person's ideas, processes, results, or words without giving appropriate credit.

Point estimation: calculated by dividing the observed values from the sample by the size of the sample.

Power: the probability of a statistical test to reject the null hypothesis when in fact it is false.

Predictive value: the degree to which a test or instrument can determine an outcome.

Predictive value negative (PV–): the probability that a person does not have a problem, given that the test result is negative.

Predictive value positive (PV+): the probability that a person has a problem, given that the test result is positive.

Preexperimental designs: sometimes referred to as pseudoexperimental designs because they do not meet at least two of the three criteria for true experiments: randomization, manipulation, or control.

Primary source: firsthand data that the researcher obtains directly from the source.

Principal investigator (PI): the project director of a research grant who is responsible for all expenditures and programmatic issues associated with the grant.

Priorities: topics/areas for research support that have been established by a funding agency for a particular fiscal year.

Procedural criteria: the material, formal aspects of the qualitative research process. They may be present or absent in the authors' report and may involve quantification. Procedural criteria include, but are not limited to, triangulation, member checking, disclosure of bias, presentation of contradictory evidence, time spent in the field, peer debriefing, external audition, and cross-checking of transcripts as well as codes.

Prospective study: researcher contacts the subjects before they develop the disorder, but after exposure to risk factors.

Protected health information: related to HIPAA privacy rule about individual's past, present, and future health conditions; treatment for conditions; and financial history related to health care.

Publish or perish: academic requirement of publishing to obtain or maintain position or be promoted.

Qualitative research: research designed to investigate real-life events or situations without reference to hypothesis or theory, allowing researchers' subjective point of view; also known as field research, hermeneutic, naturalistic inquiry, phenomenological research, symbolic interactionism, descriptive research, interpretive research, and ethnographic study.

Quality: the unmeasurable but tangibly present aspects of a piece of writing. The term comes from Robert Pirsig who, as a college writing instructor, had incoming students rate previous students' essays as a class exercise. Despite their lack of instruction and their inability to verbalize their reasons for the ratings, students' assessments correlated closely with the instructor's. Pirsig concluded that "quality" of writing is discernible intuitively, in the absence of explicit knowledge and without the use of checklists or standard criteria. This conception of quality is what consumers of qualitative research use when they decide on the richness or thickness of the article in front of them.

Quantitative or statistical analysis: the organization and integration of quantitative data according to systematic mathematical rules and procedures.

Quantitative research: research that generates data capable of being organized in graphs and descriptive statistical forms; stresses numbers, measurement, deductive logic, control, and experiments.

Quasi-experimental research: like experimental research, involves manipulation of an independent variable but does not have a comparison group or randomization; also known as preexperimental and pseudoexperimental.

Quasi-statistical analysis: involves preconceived ideas about the analysis that has been specified in a code book and then using these ideas (codes) to sort the data; also known as manifest analysis.

Randomization: a method of selecting subjects that ensures that everyone in the population has an equal chance of being included in the study.

Randomized control trial (RCT): involves the experimental group receiving the variable of interest and the control group not receiving any form of treatment; also known as the "gold standard" for clinical research.

Range: distance between the lowest and highest value in a distribution.

Ratio scale: the highest level of measurement, in which there are equal intervals between score units and a true zero point.

Reliability: repeatability; consistency among repeated measures or observations.

Research hypothesis: the question being asked by an investigator; sometimes known as the working hypothesis.

Research utilization: the application of some aspect of research to clinical practice.

Retrospective study: researcher determines subjects have already been exposed to risk factors.

Rich/thick description: the detailed and comprehensive portrayal of the research context, participants, and phenomena under study. There are various ways of incorporating rich/thick description into a qualitative article: as part of the results section, interspersed throughout the paper, or through the overall tone. In all these cases, it involves vivid, nuanced, contextualized accounts that capture the complexity and depth of participants' experiences, behaviors, and perspectives. In addition, it may incorporate sensory details, cultural nuances, and first-person perspectives as well as a variety of other devices (including artistic ones such as poetry) to foster a deep, human understanding of the phenomena under study.

Risk-benefit: comparison of relative cost and benefit.

Scales of measurement: a means of assigning numbers to events or objects according to prescribed rules; nominal, ordinal, interval, or ratio.

Scatter plot: a graphic display of the relationship between two variables; also known as scatter diagram or scattergram.

Scientific approach: a systematic, empirical, controlled, and critical examination of hypothetical propositions about the association among natural phenomena.

Scientific method: a method of efficiently or methodically generating knowledge by recognizing a problem capable of objective study, collecting data by observation or experimentation, and drawing conclusions based on analysis of the data.

Secondary analysis: involves research that uses previously gathered data; examining unanalyzed variables, testing unexplored relationships, focusing on a specific subsample, or changing the unit of analysis.

Secondary sources: secondhand documentation based on what is seen or heard by someone else, or a summary of primary information.

Seed money: funds provided by colleges and universities to support research in the form of relatively small grants for starting new research projects in the

hope that this intramural support will help secure extramural funding.

Self-plagiarism: involves duplicate submission or publication; duplicate/previous submission means that the manuscript is simultaneously being considered for publication elsewhere.

Self-reports: a method of collecting data that involves a direct report of information by the person being studied.

Semilongitudinal approach: compromise designed to maximize the strengths and minimize the weaknesses of the cross-sectional and longitudinal approaches; selecting subjects at the low end of designated age spans and following them until they reach the upper limits of that age span.

Semistructured observation: a method used in qualitative research that is more concerned with some aspects of the situation for the participants than others.

Sensitivity: a measure of validity based on the probability that someone with a disease or condition will test positive.

Sequential clinical trials (SCTs): does not require a fixed sample size before the study can begin; can be used to compare two treatments such as an "old" or standard treatment to a "new" experimental treatment.

Simple hypothesis: the hypothesis includes one independent variable and one dependent variable.

Single-blind studies: a study in which only the investigator does not know the assignment of a subject to a group.

Single or one group pretest-posttest design: compares pretest and posttest data subsequent to treatment.

Single-subject discrete trial designs: individual subjects receive each treatment condition of the experiment dozens of times.

Single-subject research: focuses on the behavior of one or a few subjects; applied behavioral analysis designs or behavioral analysis; idiographic designs; single-subject experimental designs; single-case designs; intrasubject replication designs; small approach; and within-subject designs.

Snowball sampling: selection of participants by nomination or referral from earlier participants in a study.

Solicited proposals: grant proposals that originate with a sponsoring (funding) agency that recognizes a need for something to be done or learned; usually are announced by a request for application (RFA) or request for proposal (RFP), which identifies problem areas and sometimes includes specific objectives to be met.

Specificity: a measure of validity of a procedure based on the probability that a person who does not have a disease will test negative.

Standard deviation: a variability measure of the degree to which each value deviates from the mean.

Statistic: a number derived by counting or measuring sample observations drawn from a population that is used in estimating a population parameter.

Statistical Package for Social Sciences® (SPSS): statistical program used in behavioral and social sciences published by Prentice-Hall, a division of Pearson Education, Inc.; can be used for qualitative and quantitative research analyses.

Structured observation: a method used in qualitative research; what to observe is decided in advance and there is an observational schedule.

Subtheme: within themes, more specific patterns or categories may emerge during data analysis. Such subthemes highlight nuances or variations in participants' experiences, perspectives, or behaviors as pertaining to a broader theme. Subthemes provide depth and richness to the analysis, offering insight into the complexity of the phenomenon under study.

Sum of squares: a measure of variability in a set of data, equal to the sum of squared deviations for a distribution; used in analysis of variance as the basis for partitioning between groups and within-groups variance components.

Survey research: designed to provide a detailed inspection of the prevalence of conditions, practices, or attitudes in a given environment by asking people about them rather than observing them directly.

Synthesis: collecting, analyzing, and integrating information.

Systematic review: a summary of the evidence typically conducted by an expert or expert panel that uses a rigorous process for identifying, appraising, and synthesizing studies to answer a particular question or draw a conclusion.

Template analysis: involves the development of a template or analysis guide to sort the data.

Test-retest reliability: how well subjects perform on one set of measurements as compared to their performance on a second evaluation of the same measurements.

Theme: A central idea, pattern, or concept that emerges from the analysis of qualitative data. Themes are "chunks" of similar or same codes that represent broad aspects of participants' experiences, perspectives, or behaviors. They serve to highlight key insights and meanings and to organize researchers' overall interpretation of their findings.

Theoretical sampling: selection of participants based on emerging findings as the study progresses so adequate representation of important themes is ensured; also known as purposeful sampling.

Thesis: research project/paper typically associated with a master's degree.

Time series design: involves repeated measures before and after treatment using the same instruments with the same or similar subjects over an extended period of time.

Total project cost: total cost of a research project, including all direct and indirect costs.

Transferability: the extent to which findings from a qualitative study can be transferred to similar circumstances.

Treatment outcome: a broadly defined term that refers to change, or the lack of it, that may occur as a result of time, treatment, or both.

Trend chart: illustrates frequencies or percentages of change in a dataset which is organized in a developmental or temporal order.

Triangulated designs: both quantitative and qualitative methods are used to study the same entity or concept with a focus on convergence (similarities) and increased validity.

Triangulation: refers to the use of multiple methods to improve the credibility of findings or the truth and it may involve comparison of data from different sources or analyses to reduce or eliminate bias and errors.

True experimental design: characterized by manipulation (treatment or intervention), randomizations, and use of a control group.

Trustworthiness: umbrella term for qualitative equivalents of validity and reliability. Includes concepts such as credibility, rigor, and transferability. Credibility relates to the authenticity of the data collected and the extent to which interpretations are believable. Rigor concerns the degree of reflection present in the writing, with regard to both the role researcher biases played in the research process, and the systematicity of the process where applicable. Transferability assesses the extent to which findings can be applied or generalized to other contexts or populations.

Two-tailed test: test of a hypothesis using both ends of the distribution to determine a range of improbable values.

Type I error: incorrectly rejecting the null hypothesis.

Type II error: incorrectly accepting the null hypothesis.

Unsolicited proposals: grant proposals written without any guidelines provided by a sponsoring (funding) agency and are not in response to a particular need or problem expressed by the agency; originate from a need perceived by the applicant who tries to find a sponsor to support the proposal.

Unstructured observation: a method used in qualitative research when there is no attempt to manipulate the situation or environment.

Variable: a trait capable of change or modification.

Variance: a measure of variability equal to the square of the standard deviation.

V-diagrams: used to diagram the components of knowledge and clarify their relationships.

Within-subject designs: a design in which every subject in the experiment is exposed to all the experimental conditions.

Index

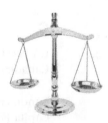

Note: Page numbers in **bold** reference non-text material.